Frontiers in Lung Cancer

(Volume 1)

Perspectives in Lung Cancer

Edited by
Keyvan Moghissi
The Yorkshire Laser Centre, Goole, UK

Jack Kastelik
Hull University Teaching Hospitals NHS Trust, Hull, UK

Philip Barber
Manchester University, NHS Foundation Trust, Manchester, UK

&

Peyman Sardari Nia
Maastricht University Medical Center, Maastricht, Netherlands

Frontiers in Lung Cancer

Volume # 1

Perspectives in Lung Cancer

Editors: Keyvan Moghissi, Jack Kastelik, Philip Barber and Peyman Sardari Nia

ISBN (Online): 978-981-14-5956-6

ISBN (Hardback/Hardcover): 978-981-14-5954-2

ISBN (Paperback/Softcover): 978-981-14-5955-9

Published by Bentham Science Publishers Pte. Ltd. Singapore. All Rights Reserved.

need for a court order if at any point you breach any terms of this License Agreement. In no event will any delay or failure by Bentham Science Publishers in enforcing your compliance with this License Agreement constitute a waiver of any of its rights.

3. You acknowledge that you have read this License Agreement, and agree to be bound by its terms and conditions. To the extent that any other terms and conditions presented on any website of Bentham Science Publishers conflict with, or are inconsistent with, the terms and conditions set out in this License Agreement, you acknowledge that the terms and conditions set out in this License Agreement shall prevail.

Bentham Science Publishers Pte. Ltd.
80 Robinson Road #02-00
Singapore 068898
Singapore
Email: subscriptions@benthamscience.net

BENTHAM SCIENCE

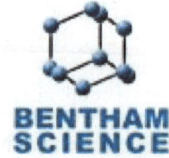

CONTENTS

PREFACE

In a career extending over six decades in Cardiothoracic Surgery, I have witnessed many innovations, advances, and changes in all aspects of lung cancer and its treatment. Some resulted from the inevitable consequences of re-organization in health care, others related to ephemeral meteors in fashion. One thing, which has not significantly altered concerns the overall outcome for lung cancer, as measured by actual - as opposed to actuarial – survival, which has remained weak.

The aims and objectives of this book are to provide an update on current understandings of lung cancer and the pathways to diagnosis and treatment for the readers, surgeons, physicians, scientists, health care professionals and others. The more general ethos has been to remind readers of some of the long-standing basics, together with contemporary and state of the art diagnostic and therapeutic methods.

I believe that, with the help of my colleagues, the authors, we have gone a long way towards the realization of this aim. I thank them for their contributions and enthusiasm.

I am greatly indebted to Kate Dixon, my colleague, and friend, for her devotion in attempting to organize both me and the book.

I acknowledge with thanks my secretary, Janet Melvin, who has spent hours in typing and formatting the manuscripts. Sirpa Pajunen-Moghissi had to re-draw many of the figures at short notice. It is a pleasure to acknowledge her effort with thanks.

Last but not the least, my sincere appreciation to Miss Mariam Mehdi, Assistant Manager (Publications) at Bentham, who has been a constant source of energy and empathy, and also Mr. Obaid Sadiq, Manager, Bentham Books, who supervised publication.

Keyvan Moghissi
The Yorkshire Laser Centre
Goole
UK

List of Contributors

Andrzej Wieczorek	Consultant Clinical Oncologist, Queens Centre for Oncology & Haematology, Castle Hill Hospital, Hull University Teaching Hospitals NHS Trust, Castle Road, Cottingham, UK
Alexandra R. Lewis	The Christie Hospital The Christie NHS Foundation Trust 550 Wilmslow Road, Manchester, M20 4BX, England
Elaine G. Boland	Consultant & Honorary Senior Lecturer in Palliative Medicine, Hull University Teaching Hospitals NHS Trust, Queen's centre for Oncology and Haematology, Castle Hill Hospital, Castle Road, Cottingham, UK
Gerard Avery	Hull & East Yorkshire NHS Trust, Hull, UK
Jack Kastelik	Castle Hill Hospital & Hull Royal Infirmary, Hull University Teaching Hospitals NHS Trust, Hull, UK
Jason W. Boland	Senior Clinical Lecturer and Honorary Consultant in Palliative Medicine, Hull York Medical School, University of Hull, Hull, UK
Keyvan Moghissi	The Yorkshire Laser Centre, Goole & District Hospital, Goole, UK
Laura Cove-Smith	The Christie Hospital The Christie NHS Foundation Trust 550 Wilmslow Road, Manchester, M20 4BX, England
Mahmoud Loubani	Hull University Teaching Hospitals NHS Trust, Hull, UK
Marcello Migliore	Thoracic Surgery, Department of Surgery and Medical Specialties, Policlinico University Hospital, University of Catania, Catania, Italy
Nilesh S. Tambe	Radiotherapy Clinical Scientist, Radiation Physics Department, Queens Centre for Oncology & Haematology, Castle Hill Hospital, Hull University Teaching Hospitals NHS Trust, Castle Road, Cottingham, UK
Peter Tcherveniakov	St James University Hospital, Leeds, UK
Philip Barber	Manchester University NHS Foundation Trust, Manchester, UK
Peyman Sardari Nia	Department of Cardiothoracic Surgery, Maastricht University Medical Center, Maastricht, the Netherlands
Scan B. Knight	Manchester Collaborative Centre for Inflammation Research, University of Manchester, Manchester, UK
Samuel Heuts	Department of Cardiothoracic Surgery, Maastricht University Medical Center, Maastricht, the Netherlands

CHAPTER 1

Surgical Anatomy of the Chest and Lung

Keyvan Moghissi[1,*] and **Peter Tcherveniakov[2]**

[1] *The Yorkshire Laser Centre, Goole & District Hospital, Goole, UK*

[2] *St James University Hospital, Leeds, UK*

Abstract: This chapter comprises of 2 sections.

Section 1 (By Keyvan Moghissi): This section gives an account of the relevant anatomy of the thorax, thoracic cavity and the bronchopulmonary segments. In addition, it also provides a brief reference to the bronchoscopic morphology.

Section 2 (By Peter Tcherveniakov): This section describes thoracoscopic anatomy as viewed on the monitor used in the Visual Assisted Thoracoscopic Surgery (VATS) system.

Keywords: Anatomy of Chest Wall and thoracic cavity, Bronchopulmonary segments, Bronchoscopic anatomy, Thoracoscopic anatomy of the thoracic cavity and applied surgery.

INTRODUCTION

THORACIC CAGE

The architectural design of the thorax consists of two vertical pillars; one is anterior, the sternum, and the other one is posterior, the vertebral column. These two are held in position by obliquely slanting ribs which are articulated to them, thus providing a firm yet flexible box referred to in many anatomy textbooks as the "thoracic cage". The anterior pillar (sternum) is shorter in length than the posterior pillar (vertebral column). Therefore, the direction of ribs from the vertebral column to the sternum is oblique and not horizontal and the lowest 5 ribs cannot directly articulate with the sternum. Three of these, namely ribs 8-10, join the 7th costal cartilage to make the costal margin. The last two ribs 11 and 12 have no attachment anteriorly and are known as floating ribs. The incomplete and fenestrated bony wall of the chest so constructed (Fig. **1**) is completed by inter-

* **Corresponding author Keyvan Moghissi:** The Yorkshire Laser Centre, Goole & District Hospital, Goole, UK; Tel: 01724 290456; E-mail: kmoghissi@yorkshirelasercentre.org

costal muscles, which thus fill in the opening between the ribs and provide a firm yet expansile closed-chest wall a necessity for inspiratory and expiratory changes in the chest volume, respectively. This basic bony and muscular structure of the chest wall is overlaid by large muscles of the chest anterior and posteriorly. These muscles which, for the most part, cover the chest also provide a firm attachment for the shoulder girdle. The thoracic cage is open at its base into the abdomen but the diaphragm closes the opening and thus separates the thoracic cavity from the abdominal cavity. The apex of the chest is the root of the neck. A membrane; Sibson's fascia, separates the thoracic cavity from the neck.

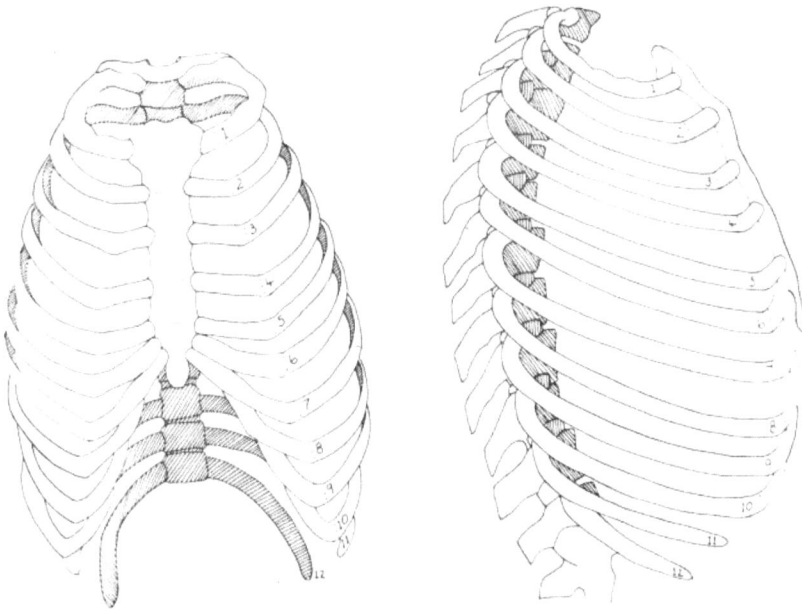

Fig. (1). Thoracic cage front and lateral view.

MUSCLES OF THE CHEST

Ribs, intercostal muscles and their neurovascular content are overlaid externally by two layers of muscles. The deeper layer consists of serratus anterior, anterolaterally, and the rhomboids (major and minor) posteriorly. These muscles are then covered by a larger superficial group which consists of pectoralis major and minor anteriorly and trapezius and latissimus dorsi posteriorly.

Knowledge of the anatomical arrangement and topography of the chest wall musculature has important practical relevance to surgical access to the thoracic cavity and to a number of other operative procedures. It is, therefore, useful to recall the anatomical characteristics of some of these muscles.

Trapezius

This large muscle covers the upper part of the posterior aspect of the neck and chest. Its fibres arise from an elongated line which extends from the occipital bone to the ligamentum nucea and spinous process of all the thoracic vertebrae including supra spinous ligament. From these origins, the muscle fibres are directed towards the posterior border of the clavicle to be attached to the lateral one-third of that bone and in continuation to the acromion and the upper border of the spine of the scapula. The lower fibres of the muscle form the upper side of a triangle known as the Triangle of Auscultation whose lower side is formed by the upper border of Latissimus Dorsi muscle. The nerve to the muscle is derived from the accessory nerve (C3, C4) which enters its deep surface together with its vessels.

Latissimus Dorsi

This muscle has also a wide origin from:

• Spine and supraspinous ligaments of the lower six thoracic vertebrae under cover of the trapezius.

• Lumbar fascia and spines of lumbar vertebrae.

• Outer lip of the posterior part of the crest of the ilium.

• Lower 4 ribs.

• Angle of scapula.

The muscle fibres converge forwards around the lateral wall of the Thorax and are inserted to the floor of the bicipital intertubercular groove of the humorous. The innervation of the muscle is from the posterior cord of the bronchial plexus (C_6, C_7, C_8 roots) which enters the anterior border of the muscle. The upper border of the muscle, on emergence from under the trapezium, forms the lower side of the Triangle of Auscultation.

Serratus Anterior

This muscle is covered partially by latissimus dorsi. It originates from the outer surfaces of the upper 8 ribs and is attached to the costal surface of the medial border of the scapula from the superior and including the inferior angle. The muscle is innervated by the long thoracic nerve.

Pectoralis Major

The anterior wall of the chest is, to a large extent, covered by the pectoralis major. This muscle arises from three distinct heads:

• Clavicular head originates from the medial half of the anterior aspect of the clavicle.

• Steno-costal head arises from the anterior surface of the sternum and adjacent six costal cartilages.

• Abdominal head takes its origin from the upper part of the aponeurosis of the external oblique muscle.

The muscle fibres from these heads are directed towards the humorous where they are inserted to the greater tubercle and the lateral lip of the bicipital (Inter Tubercular) groove.

Pectoralis Minor

The muscle takes origin from the anterior aspect of the 2nd to 4th rib near the costal cartilages. The fibres form a small triangular muscle which is inserted to the coracoid process of the scapular.

The nerve to the pectoralis muscles from the medial and lateral pectoral nerves (for pectoralis major) and medial pectoral nerve (pectoralis minor) are branches of the medial and lateral cords of the brachial plexus respectively.

SKIN AND SUBCUTANEOUS NERVES OF THE THORAX

The thoracic cage and its muscles are covered by the fascia, subcutaneous fat and skin. The skin of the thorax is thinner in front than behind. Lines of cleavage of the skin run horizontally around the chest. Incisions made along these lines heal more quickly and with a better cosmetic result than incisions made across the lines of cleavage.

The skin of the chest is supplied segmentally by the 2nd - 12th thoracic spinal nerves which also innervate the skin of the abdominal wall. A strip of skin posteriorly is supplied by the posterior primary rami of these spinal nerves. The rest of the skin anterolaterally and posterolaterally is supplied by branches of the anterior primary rami (intercostal nerves).

THORACIC CAVITY AND PLEURAL SPACE (FIG. 2 AND 3)

The external contour of the thorax is oval. The anterior bulge of the vertebral column makes the transverse section of the interior of the thoracic cavity kidney-shaped. The thoracic cavity is divided into three compartments (Fig. **2**). The two lateral compartments accommodate the lungs. The middle, the mediastinum, contains the heart and the great vessels, the trachea and its bifurcation, the oesophagus, thymus gland, lymphatics and nerves. The thoracic cavity is lined by the pleura which covers it like wallpaper. This is the parietal pleura. It then reflects to cover the lungs as the visceral pleura.

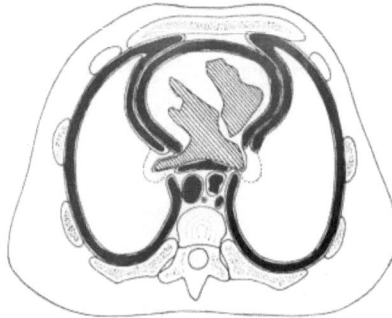

Fig. (2). Tran-section of the thorax showing the thoracic cavity and arrangement of the pleura.

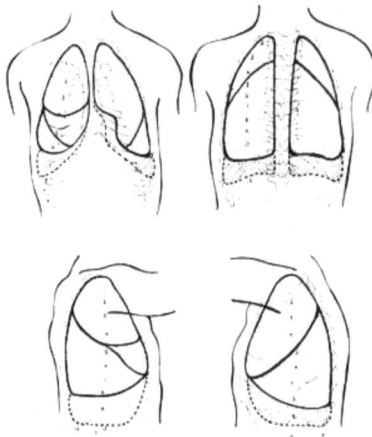

Fig. (3). Surface marking of the lung and pleura. Dotted line= parietal pleura, solid line = visceral pleura.

The pleura is a serous membrane which forms independent closed sacs on each side of the chest. Like the hemithorax itself, the pleura is in the shape of a truncated cone. The medial aspect of the pleural sac into which the lung is projected becomes inseparably attached to the lung itself. This is the visceral pleura. The parietal pleura covers the inner surface of the thoracic cavity. The original sac, now between the parietal and visceral pleura, becomes the pleural space. At the apex of the thorax, the parietal pleura strengthens Sibson's fascia. At the base it drapes the diaphragm forming the diaphragmatic pleura. Medially, the parietal pleura lines the mediastinum as the mediastinal pleura. At the root of the lung, the mediastinal pleura covers the structures of the root. It then continues as the visceral pleura to drape the lung. It is important to note that normally the parietal pleura can be stripped off the chest wall with ease and can then be seen as a glistening membrane. Such separation of visceral pleura from the lung is not possible as it is attended by damage to the pulmonary parenchyma.

The surface marking of the parietal and visceral pleura is important (Fig. **3**). The parietal pleura covers the costal surfaces of the thorax. At the apex of the chest, it projects some 2.5 cm above the medial third of the clavicle. It then turns anteromedially towards the sternoclavicular joint where it continues as the mediastinal pleura and meets its opposite number at the level of the 2nd costal cartilage. From that level to the 4th costal cartilages, the two mediastinal pleurae descend together at the back of the sternum. At the level of the 4th costal cartilage, the mediastinal pleurae diverge. The right continues vertically and the left turns laterally towards the apex of the heart, thus leaving part of the pericardium bare of pleura. Near the 6th costal cartilage, the mediastinal pleura diverges further by turning laterally to reach the mid-clavicular line and mid-axillary line at about the 8th and 10th ribs, respectively. From the mid-axillary line the pleura passes horizontally to reach the thoracic vertebrae 1-2 cm below the 12th ribs. In the process of turning laterally, the pleura covers the upper surface of the diaphragm. The lung covered by the visceral pleura closely follows the parietal pleura at the apex and on the costal walls. Inferiorly, however, it falls short of the pleura so that at the midclavicular line it is at the level of the 6th rib and at the mid-axillary line it is level with the 8th rib. It then passes posteriorly at the level of the 8th rib.

The oblique fissure of the lung is almost in line with the 6th rib. On the right side, the anterior part of the horizontal fissure is level with the 4th costal cartilage and the line of fissure passes horizontally towards the oblique fissure approximately under the 6th rib.

SURGICAL ANATOMY OF THE LUNGS AND BRONCHOPULMONARY SEGMENTS (FIGS. 4A, 4B, & 4C)

Gross anatomical description accords two lobes for the left lung (upper and lower lobes) and three lobes for the right lung (upper, middle and lower lobes) which can be identified by fissures that are visible clefts between the lobes lined by the visceral pleura.

The left lung has a single fissure, the oblique fissure, which divides the upper from the lower lobe. The right lung has an oblique fissure which, like that of the left lung, divides the lung into an upper and lower portion. In addition, a horizontal fissure divides the upper portion into upper and middle lobes. The lower portion of the right lung below the oblique fissure is the lower lobe.

Each lung has a lateral or costal surface which is convex and adapted to the configuration of the chest wall, an apex that projects behind the medial third of the clavicle into the neck, a base - which is concave - resting on the diaphragm and the medial surface which flanks the mediastinal structures, notably the pericardium. All surfaces of the lung present the impression of the intrathoracic structure against which they lie. The mediastinal surface is of particular importance as it contains the hilum, the area into which the bronchi, vessels and lymphatics pass to form the root of the lung. The hilum (or hilus) is surrounded by the pleura which covers the structure of the root forming a large cuff. Below the root, the pleura is reflected down from the hilum to form the pulmonary ligament. From the surgical point of view, the anatomical unit of the lung is the bronchopulmonary segment. It is this portion of the lung which receives a branch of the bronchus (the segmental bronchus), a branch of the pulmonary artery and one or more branches of the pulmonary vein. A bronchopulmonary segment can be dissected and resected.

Because the lobes of the lungs are lined and separated by visceral pleura covering the 'fissure', a lobectomy results in minimal air leaks from the alveoli. Segmentectomy (segmental resection) will cause a certain amount of air to leak because the boundaries of pulmonary segments are not lined, nor are they demarcated by the visceral pleura.

In both lungs, the segmental branches of the pulmonary artery to the posterior segment of the upper lobe, the middle lobe (or the lingula on the left side) and the lower lobe emerge from the main trunk after turning into the oblique fissure. This is of practical surgical importance since dissection of the fissure and division of the visceral pleural opening exposes the sheath of the artery overlaid by lymph nodes. This arrangement facilitates the dissection, ligation and division of the segmental arteries in pulmonary resection. Each lung has ten segments which are named and numbered as shown in Table **1** and Fig. (**4a**).

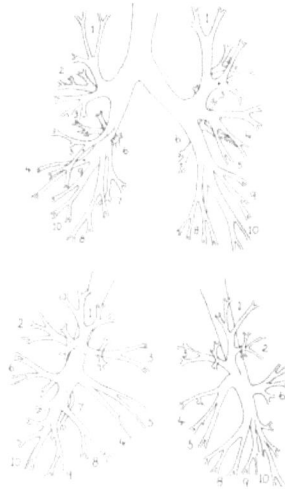

Fig. (4a). Bronchopulmonary segments.

Table 1. Bronchopulmonary Segments.

Right Lung	Left Lung
Upper lobe	*Upper lobe*
Segment 1. Apical	Segment 1. Posterior
Segment 2. Posterior	Segment 2. Posterior
Segment 3. Anterior	Segment 3. Anterior
Middle lobe	*Lingula*
Segment 4. Lateral	Segment 4. Superior
Segment 5. Medial	Segment 5. Inferior
Lower lobe	*Lower lobe*
Segment 6. Apical (dorsal)	Segment 6. Apical (dorsal)
Segment 7. Medial basal (cardiac)	Segment 7 Medial (absent)
Segment 8. Anterior basal	Segment 8. Anterior basal
Segment 9. Lateral basal	Segment 9. Lateral basal
Segment 10. Posterior basal	Segment 10. Posterior basal

Each segment of the lung receives a segmental branch of the bronchus bearing the name and the number of the pulmonary segment which it enters.

Bronchial Tree (Fig. 4b)

Two aspects of the bronchial tree are important to the surgeon:

• Anatomical.

• Endoscopic.

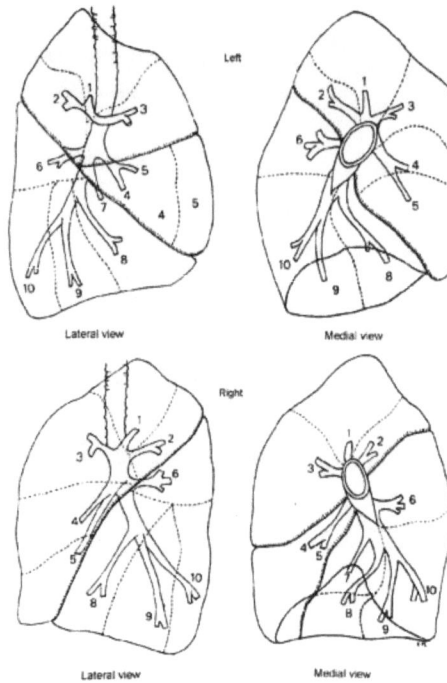

Fig. (4b). Lateral and medial view of bronchopulmonary segments.

Anatomical Aspect

This defines the main bronchi and their distribution to the lobes, segments and sub-segments of the lung. The bronchi (right and left) commence at the bifurcation of the trachea and are directed to the hilum of the right and left lung, respectively. The bifurcation is indicated in the interior of the trachea by a ridge, the carina, situated in the middle of the lower trachea in between the two bronchial openings.

• The right main bronchus gives off:

The upper lobe bronchus which subdivides into three branches, namely the apical* (1), posterior (2), and the anterior (3) segmental bronchi.

The right middle lobe bronchus which in turn subdivides into the lateral (4), and the medial (5) segmental bronchi.

The right lower lobe bronchus which subdivides into the apical (6), medial (7), anterior (8), lateral (9), and posterior (10) segmental bronchi.

• The left main bronchus gives off:

The main stem bronchus for the upper lobe and the lingula. This branch immediately divides into the left upper lobe bronchus for the upper lobe of the lung proper. This, in turn, divides into the apical (1), posterior (2), and anterior (3) segmental bronchi. The apical and posterior segmental bronchi usually emerge as one branch i.e. the apical-posterior bronchus, which then subdivides. The lingular bronchus which divides into two branches, the superior lingular (4), and inferior lingular (5) segmental bronchi.

NB. The numbers in parentheses correspond to the standard 'universal' numbering of the bronchi (Table **1**).

The left lower lobe bronchus divides, like the right lower lobe bronchus, into five segmental branches, namely: the apical (6), medial basal (7), anterior basal (8), lateral basal (9), posterior basal and (10) segmental bronchi.

The medial basal segmental bronchus on the left side is often small or non-existent. This is due to the absence of the medial basal pulmonary segment itself because of the projection of the heart into the left chest.

Endoscopic Aspect (Bronchoscopy) (Fig. 4c)

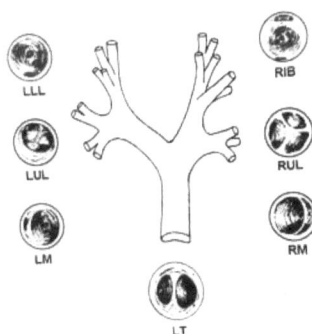

Fig. (4c). Endoscopic aspect of the bronchial tree. LT = lower trachea, RM & LM = right and left main bronchi, RUL and LUL = right and left upper lobe orifices, RIB = right intermediate bronchus (towards the lower lobe), LLL = left lower lobe bronchial orifice.

The bronchoscopic appearance of the bronchial tree is as follows.

The carina is seen as a ridge, separating the orifices of the right and left main bronchi.

At the right lateral aspect of the right main bronchus, level with the carina, is the orifice of the right upper lobe bronchus. With a rigid bronchoscope the orifice alone is usually seen without its segmental divisions. When a telescopic view is obtained using either the right-angle telescope or the flexible fibreoptic bronchoscope the orifice is seen to contain three subsidiary orifices. These are the apical, posterior and anterior segmental orifices. When the bronchoscope is introduced into the right main bronchus below the right upper lobe opening for a distance of 1.5-2 cm the following bronchial segmental orifices are seen:

• Anteriorly at about 12 o'clock there is the middle lobe orifice.

• Almost opposite posteriorly at 6 o'clock is the apical segmental orifice of the lower lobe.

• Just below these two orifices are seen the openings of the segmental bronchi for the basal segments of the lower lobe, *viz*: the anterior, posterior medial and the lateral segmental bronchial openings.

On the left of the carina, the opening of the left main bronchus is seen leading to the bronchial lumen, which is directed downwards and laterally, making an angle of about 60 degrees with the mid-line of the carina. 2-2.5 cm below the carina, on the lateral wall of the main bronchus, the common opening of the left upper lobe and that of the lingular segments is seen. The former emerges almost at a right angle, whereas the latter is directed more obliquely downwards. Normally, with a rigid bronchoscope placed within the left main bronchus, only the common orifice of the upper lobe is seen. The division of the upper lobe bronchus into two main branches (upper lobe proper, and lingula) becomes visible using a right-angle telescope or a flexible fibreoptic bronchoscope. When the latter instrument is directed within the opening of the main stem of the upper lobe bronchus the two divisions are easily seen. The opening of the left upper lobe bronchus proper is seen to divide into a further two or, at times, three segmental bronchi which are the apical-posterior segmental and the anterior segmental bronchi.

As has been noted, the apical and posterior segmental bronchi of the left upper lobe arise as a single stem dividing into two, unlike the right upper lobe where they arise individually.

The lingular segmental bronchus forms the lower division of the common left upper lobe opening. Its orifice is seen below the opening of the bronchus for the upper lobe proper. It soon divides into its two branches, the superior and inferior segmental bronchi of the lingula. Less than 0.5 cm below the stem of the left upper lobe opening, the orifice of the main lower lobe bronchus is seen. Its lumen is directed downwards and more medially than that of the upper lobe, in continuation with the left main bronchus. The openings of the segmental bronchi to the left lobe are seen with the apical segmental orifice situated posteriorly - at '6 o'clock' - or at the floor of the bronchus, when viewed with the patient in the supine position.

THORACOSCOPIC ANATOMY OF THE THORACIC CAVITY

The thoracic cavity is enclosed by the ribs, the vertebral column and the sternum. It is separated from the abdominal cavity by the diaphragm. It contains the lungs, the middle and lower airways, the heart, the pulmonary vessels, the great arteries and the major veins (superior vena cava and inferior vena cava). The thoracic cavity also contains the oesophagus.

Thoracoscopic procedures have gained rapid popularity over the last two decades. They have become routine for a variety of operations such as diagnosis of lung and pleural disease, management of recurrent pleural effusions, empyema and pneumothoraces and radical resection for NCSLC (lobectomy and segmentectomy).

Lobectomy is considered the "gold standard" treatment for patients with early-stage NSCLC [1, 2]. In the past, this was routinely performed *via* a thoracotomy. There is clear, growing evidence that using video-assisted thoracoscopic surgery (VATS) to perform anatomical lung resections has less morbidity and can be less costly [3 - 6]. With VATS lobectomy gaining popularity (albeit more slowly than expected) this chapter will look into the specifics of thoracoscopic anatomy of the thoracic cavity.

Performing any procedure by VATS has one major disadvantage. It takes away the three-dimensional view of the surgeon and replaces it with a "flat" two-dimensional representation on a screen. In order to surmount this obstacle safely, a precise knowledge of the thoracic anatomy is vital. Variations in pulmonary anatomy are relatively common. Awareness is key in performing VATS segmental or lobar pulmonary resections. Careful pre-operative review of a contrast CT scan will help identify the majority of these variations and allow for appropriate management planning.

After placing a thoracoscope in the pleural space a number of structures are clearly visible and can be readily identified. They can be categorized as shown (Fig. **5**):

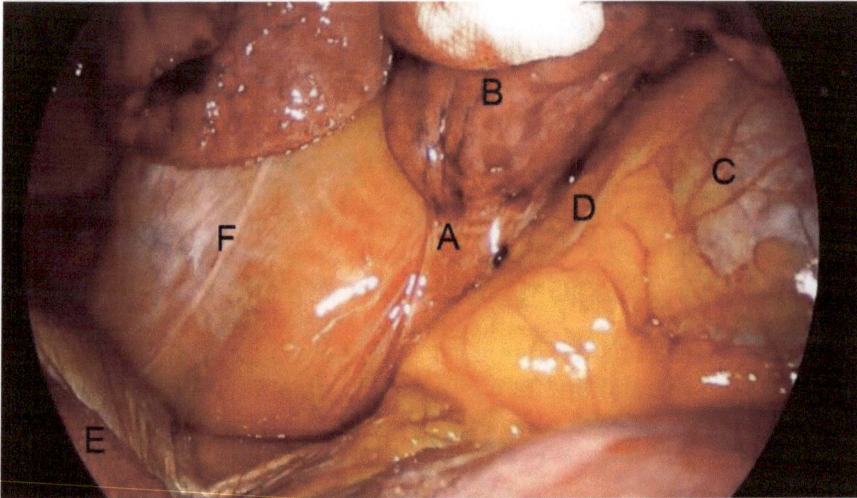

Fig. (5). A view of the right inferior pulmonary ligament (A). The lung (B) is retracted superiorly. The pericardium (C) can be seen to the right with the phrenic (D) nerve. The diaphragm (E) and sympathetic chain (F) are seen to the left.

I. Elements of the chest wall – ribs, intercostal muscles and vessels

II. Pleura – visceral and parietal

III. Lungs

IV. Pericardium

V. Major vessels – thoracic aorta, superior and inferior vena cava, internal thoracic artery and vein, azygos vein.

VI. Nerves - sympathetic chain, vagus, phrenic nerve.

Other structures such as the pulmonary artery, superior and inferior pulmonary vein, trachea, oesophagus, lymphatics and thoracic duct might not be immediately apparent and require some dissection/manipulation to visualize. This is particularly relevant for the pulmonary vessels, which are usually not clearly visible (Fig. **6**). Opening the overlying pleural reflection by sharp or blunt dissection allows for adequate exposure. When attempting an anatomical lung resection by VATS, a so-called "hilar release" should be performed prior to any dissection of the hilar structures. Mobilizing the overlying pleura not only allows for identification of the hilar structures but serves to decrease tension when further manipulation/dissection is performed, thus minimising the risk for vascular injury.

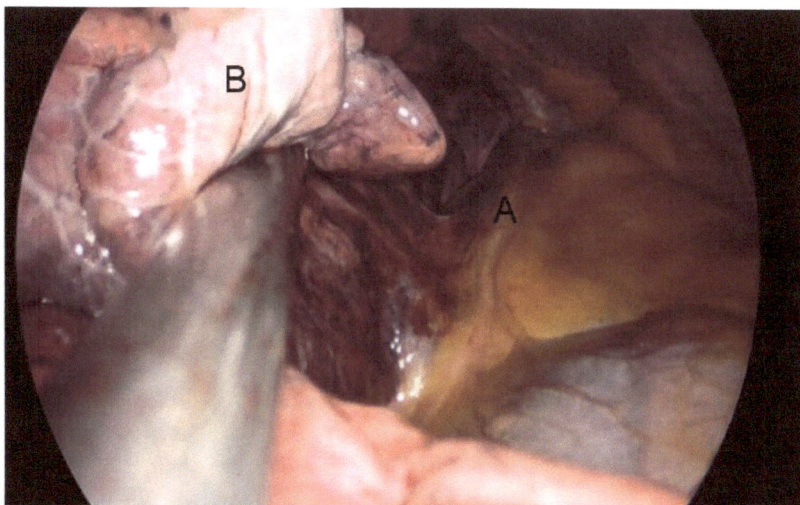

Fig. (6). View of the right pulmonary hilum. The phrenic nerve is seen running along the SVC (A) and pericardium. The lung (B) is retracted posteriorly. The hilar structures are not clearly visible.

This chapter will focus on thoracoscopic anatomy, which relates to performing VATS anatomical lung resections. The anatomical features of the chest wall, pleura, lungs and pericardium are enhanced by the thoracoscopic magnification and are usually straightforward to identify. The parietal pleura is transparent and reflects over the chest wall, great vessels, oesophagus and major airways. The ribs can be clearly visualized if the pleura is not pathologically affected, whilst the intercostal muscles and neurovascular bundle are, usually, not obvious (Fig. 7).

APPROACH TO A VATS ANATOMICAL LUNG RESECTION

During a right-sided approach, the subclavian artery and superior vena cava can be seen towards the apex, when the lung is retracted posteriorly. The azygos vein can be seen adjoining the lateral aspect of the SVC just above the pulmonary hilum. The inferior vena cava cannot usually be visualized readily, as its intrathoracic component is largely intrapericardial. The right vagus nerve enters the thoracic cavity anterior to the right subclavian artery. It follows the tracheo-oesophageal grove and gives off the right recurrent laryngeal nerve. It leaves the thoracic cavity *via* the oesophageal hiatus. The sympathetic chain can be visualized by retracting the lung anteriorly. Towards the apex, it overlies the necks of the ribs. As it descends it moves medially to run over the vertebral bodies.

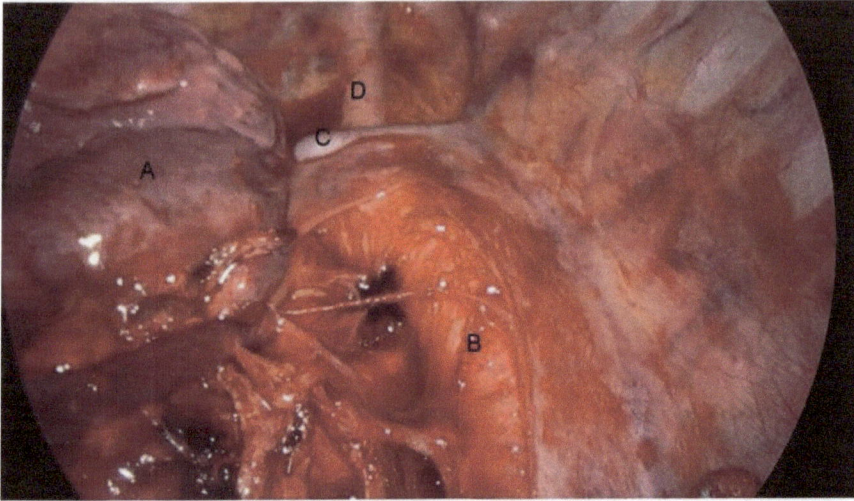

Fig. (7). View of the left posterior paravertebral area following dissection for subcarinal lymph nodes. The lung (A) is retracted anteriorly and the thoracic aorta (B) is clearly visible. The supreme intercostal vein (C) and the subclavian artery (D) are seen towards the apex.

On the left, the subclavian artery and the descending thoracic aorta can be seen towards the apex, when the lung is isolated. The origin of the internal thoracic artery from the subclavian artery can be seen and its course along the sternum can be followed.

The most common approach to a thoracoscopic lobectomy starts with hilar dissection, beginning anteriorly and continuing posteriorly. The fissure is usually not completed until all hilar structures are divided. Sometimes the pulmonary artery can be seen in a well-developed fissure (Fig. **8**).

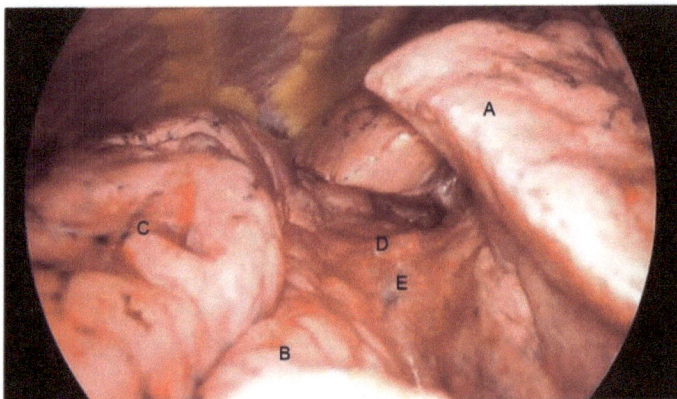

Fig. (8). Anterior view of the horizontal and oblique fissure. Aspects of the upper, middle and lower lobe can be seen. A hint of the pulmonary artery is visible posterior to a "sentinel" lymph node.

After the placement of the ports, a thoracoscopic exploration is performed, which includes confirmation of the location of the tumour, exclusion of the presence of pleural metastases and division of the inferior pulmonary ligament [7]. Hilar dissection usually starts with the mobilization of the relevant pulmonary vein. Visualization of the remaining pulmonary vein is strongly recommended. For upper lobectomy, the lung is reflected posteriorly and inferiorly to facilitate dissection. For lower lobectomy, the lung is retracted superiorly [7] (Fig. **9**).

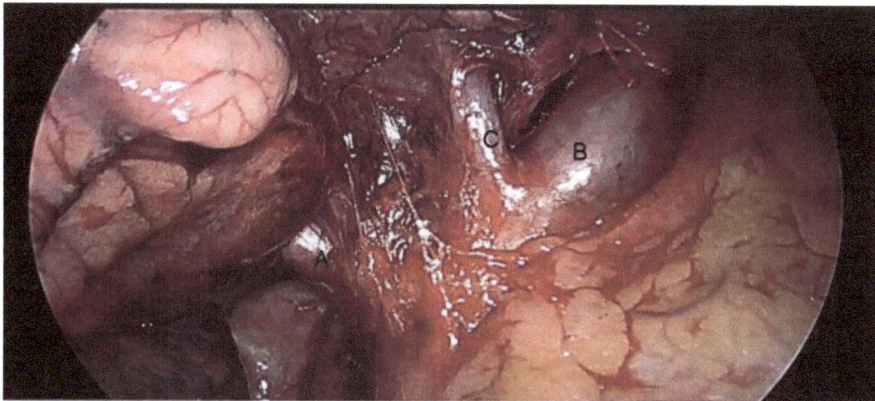

Fig. (9). Anterior view of right sided hilar dissection. The pleural reflection is mobilized. The inferior and superior pulmonary veins are seen. The middle lobe vein joins the SPV.

Left Upper Lobectomy

The lung is retracted posteriorly. The mediastinal pleura is opened and the superior pulmonary vein is identified and mobilized. The main pulmonary artery lies superior to the pulmonary vein. After stapling the vein, the apical and anterior branches of the left pulmonary artery and the upper lobe bronchus can be visualized. A careful pre-operative review of a contrast CT scan will alert the surgeon to the presence of a separate posterior pulmonary artery branch. The space between the left upper lobe bronchus and the pulmonary artery can now be developed. Alternatively, management of the bronchus may be completed first, particularly if the truncus branch of the pulmonary artery is not clearly visible. A peri-bronchial lymph node is usually encountered at the level of the secondary carina and can be used as a guide. Upon completing the bronchus the lingular branches of the pulmonary artery become clearly visible. Care must be taken to identify and preserve the pulmonary artery branch to segment 6. The fissure is completed and the specimen can be retrieved.

Left Lower Lobectomy

With the lung retracted superiorly and posteriorly, the pleura overlying the inferior pulmonary vein can be released. At this stage, the vein can be mobilized and either placed on a sling or divided. Further superior retraction of the lower lobe can demonstrate the lower lobe bronchus. The pulmonary artery can be approached in the fissure (Fig. **10**).

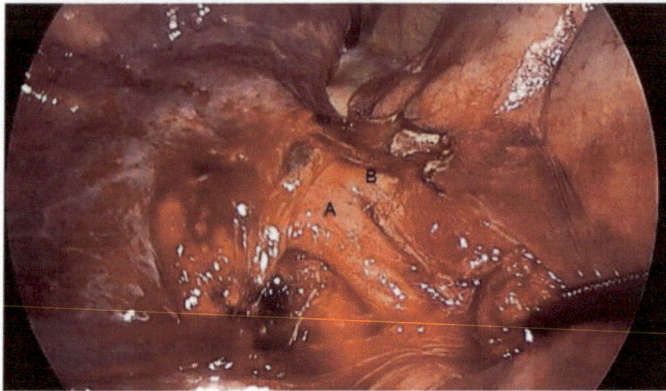

Fig. (10). Anterior view of the pulmonary artery (A) in the fissure during a left lower lobectomy. The branch to segment 6 (B) can clearly be seen.

If the pulmonary artery is difficult to identify in the fissure, dissection of the bronchus, with careful development of the space between the bronchus and artery, can be performed. This will allow the visualization of the lower- lobe pulmonary artery. The approach to right lower lobectomy is very similar. Precise identification and preservation of the lingular (left lower lobectomy) and middle lobe (right lower lobectomy) arteries are important steps of the procedure.

Right Upper Lobectomy

During a right upper lobectomy, the hilar mobilization can be initiated after releasing the inferior pulmonary ligament. The dissection can be performed posteriorly and anteriorly, with the two dissection lines coming together at the level of the azygos vein, superiorly. If the lung is retracted posteriorly, the superior pulmonary vein can be visualized. Precise identification of the middle lobe, prior to any vessel division, is an important step of the operation. It commonly joins the superior pulmonary vein (Fig. **10**). However, anatomical variations, in which it is a tributary to the inferior pulmonary vein, are not uncommon. Dissection behind the stump of the superior pulmonary vein allows the identification of the branches of the pulmonary artery to the upper lobe. A lymph node is usually encountered between the main pulmonary artery and the truncus anterior. The posterior ascending branch can be identified by opening the sheath of the pulmonary artery and exposing it to the level of the middle lobe branches. The right bronchus can be exposed as it emerges underneath the azygos vein. The right upper lobe bronchus takes off shortly afterwards.

Right Middle Lobectomy

After identifying and stapling the middle lobe vein, the middle lobe bronchus (sitting posteriorly) can be visualized. Division of the bronchus exposes pulmonary artery branches to the middle lobe artery.

Sub-lobar anatomical lung resection (segmentectomy) for malignancy, performed by VATS, is gaining popularity, particularly in patients whose fitness for undergoing lobectomy is borderline. Some studies have shown that VATS segmentectomy can be a safe and effective treatment choice for management of primary NSCLC or pulmonary metastases [8]. The term "thoracoscopic segmentectomy" refers to the resection of one or more anatomic pulmonary segments, using a completely minimally invasive approach. It involves anatomic resection, with hilar dissection, individual vessel ligation and mediastinal lymph node dissection [9]. The segmental resections that are most commonly performed are left upper trisegmentectomy, lingulectomy, superior segmentectomy and basilar segmentectomy [9].

Left Upper Lobe Trisegmentectomy

The anatomy and technique are very similar to performing a left upper lobectomy. After completing the hilar dissection, the superior vein is dissected distally until the tributaries from the trisegment are identified. Usually, the lingular vein comes in inferiorly and joins the superior pulmonary vein quite close to the hilum. The segmental bronchus sits posterior to the segmental vein and can be readily identified after its ligation. Upon dividing the bronchus, the pulmonary arteries to the trisegment can be seen.

Lingulectomy

The lingular tributary of the left superior pulmonary vein is identified in the manner described above with the segmental bronchus sitting behind it. After the bronchus is stapled and divided, the lingular segmental arterial branch can be identified.

Superior Segmentectomy

The superior segmental branch of the inferior pulmonary vein can be identified after the division of the inferior pulmonary ligament. Dissection of the posterior hilum can help with the visualization [9]. The segmental bronchus is visualized posterior to the segmental vein. After the bronchus is stapled, the pulmonary artery branches can be identified. Alternatively, if the fissure is well developed the pulmonary artery can be approached *via* that route.

Basilar Segmentectomy

The basilar segmental tributary of the inferior pulmonary vein can be identified after the division of the inferior pulmonary ligament. Anterior hilar dissection can facilitate exposure [9]. The segmental bronchus is visualized after the segmental vein is stapled. In turn, the artery can be exposed after the bronchus is stapled.

Alternatively, after the division of the basilar segmental vein, the basilar arterial trunk may be approached through the oblique fissure.

CONCLUSION

There are various ways to look at the anatomy of the thorax and its content. The most useful way, in so far as lung cancer is concerned, is to look at:

1. The architecture of the chest - that is the thoracic cage (bones) and the soft tissue which it covers. This has been described above.

2. In the current and the future perspective, one needs to consider the gross anatomy as seen through thoracoscopic instrumentation and its application to video-assisted thoracoscopic surgery (VATS).

3. Endoscopic anatomy of the airway and its arborization to the bronchial tree and the segmental anatomy of the lung are of crucial importance to understand lung cancer and the topography of lung cancer. This aspect has been referred to in some detail, describing the international code used by respiratory physicians, thoracic surgeons and oncologists.

As such, this chapter has provided the basic classically applied surgical anatomy, as well as looking at the thoracoscopic and endoscopic anatomy which is vital in lung cancer.

CONSENT FOR PUBLICATION

Not applicable.

CONFLICT OF INTEREST

The author declares that there is no conflict of interest in this chapter.

ACKNOWLEDGEMENTS

Kate Dixon & Janet Melvin are gratefully acknowledged.

REFERENCES

[1]   Ginsberg RJ, Rubinstein LV. Randomized trial of lobectomy versus limited resection for T1 N0 non-small cell lung cancer. Ann Thorac Surg 1995; 60(3): 615-22.
[http://dx.doi.org/10.1016/0003-4975(95)00537-U] [PMID: 7677489]

[2]   Ettinger DS, Akerley W, Bepler G, *et al.* Non-small cell lung cancer. J Natl Compr Canc Netw 2010; 8(7): 740-801.
[http://dx.doi.org/10.6004/jnccn.2010.0056] [PMID: 20679538]

[3]   Cattaneo SM, Park BJ, Wilton AS, *et al.* Use of video-assisted thoracic surgery for lobectomy in the elderly results in fewer complications. Ann Thorac Surg 2008; 85(1): 231-5.
[http://dx.doi.org/10.1016/j.athoracsur.2007.07.080] [PMID: 18154816]

[4]   Villamizar NR, Darrabie MD, Burfeind WR, *et al.* Thoracoscopic lobectomy is associated with lower morbidity compared with thoracotomy. J Thorac Cardiovasc Surg 2009; 138(2): 419-25.
[http://dx.doi.org/10.1016/j.jtcvs.2009.04.026] [PMID: 19619789]

[5]   Paul S, Altorki NK, Sheng S, *et al.* Thoracoscopic lobectomy is associated with lower morbidity than open lobectomy: a propensity-matched analysis from the STS database. J Thorac Cardiovasc Surg 2010; 139(2): 366-78.
[http://dx.doi.org/10.1016/j.jtcvs.2009.08.026] [PMID: 20106398]

[6]   Swanson SJ, Meyers BF, Gunnarsson CL, *et al.* Video-assisted thoracoscopic lobectomy is less costly and morbid than open lobectomy: a retrospective multiinstitutional database analysis. Ann Thorac Surg 2012; 93(4): 1027-32.
[http://dx.doi.org/10.1016/j.athoracsur.2011.06.007] [PMID: 22130269]

[7]   Burfeind WR, D'Amico TA. Thoracoscopic lobectomy. Oper Tech Thorac Cardiovasc Surg 2004; 9: 98-114.
[http://dx.doi.org/10.1053/j.optechstcvs.2004.05.002]

[8]   Atkins BZ, Harpole DH Jr, Mangum JH, *et al.* Pulmonary segmentectomy by thoracotomy or thoracoscopy: reduced hospital length of stay with a minimally-invasive approach. Ann Thorac Surg 2007; 84(4): 1107-12.
[http://dx.doi.org/10.1016/j.athoracsur.2007.05.013] [PMID: 17888955]

[9]   Pham D, Balderson S, D'Amico TA. Technique of thoracoscopic segmentectomy. Operative Techniques in Thoracic and Cardiovascular Surgery. 2008; 13(3): 188-203.

CHAPTER 2

Biology and Molecular Evolution of Lung Cancer

Sean B. Knight[*]

Manchester Collaborative Centre for Inflammation Research, University of Manchester, Manchester, UK

Abstract: Lung cancer is the worldwide leading cause of cancer-related deaths [1]. At a fundamental level, understanding the important molecular and cellular events that lead to lung cancer is critical for developing treatments to reverse this statistic. This chapter reviews the progress and limitations of our current understanding of lung cancer. It describes the initiation and progression of lung cancer from carcinogen-induced mutation of DNA to tumour formation and metastases.

Keywords: Cancer evolution, Circulating tumour cells, Driver mutation, Epithelial to mesenchymal transition, Malignant transformation, Metastases, Lung cancer, Immune evasion.

INTRODUCTION

Oncogenesis occurs largely as a consequence of deregulated cell division, which may be a consequence of inappropriate proliferation or reduced cell death. A gene-centric view posits that mutations in the DNA of genes coding for the crucial proteins involved in these processes are the cause of cancers. However, the emergence of cancer is an evolutionary path that starts with DNA mutations, followed by the acquisition of traits that involve, at their most basic level, the ability to distort local tissue architecture, allowing local invasion and evasion of the immune system. Thus, cancer is a product of the cell of origin and the unique characteristics of the local microenvironment that cancer needs to overcome to grow and metastasise.

Much is known about lung cancer in terms of epidemiological risk factors and some of the key molecular signals that initiate disease. Advances in molecular biology are now enabling us to consider the dynamics of lung cancer and how lung tumours interact with their microenvironment during progression and metast-

[*] **Corresponding author Sean B. Knight:** Manchester Collaborative Centre for Inflammation Research, University of Manchester, Manchester, UK; E-mail: sean.knight@manchester.ac.uk

Keyvan Moghissi, Jack Kastelik, Philip Barber & Peyman Sardari Nia (Eds.)

ases. This chapter will explore the origin of lung cancer and the biology of progression and metastases.

THE LUNG MICROENVIRONMENT

The mammalian lung has evolved a number of adaptations that enable its principle role in gas exchange. Passive diffusion of oxygen from inspired air is maximised by a large surface area and a diffusion barrier that is only one cell thick. Oxygen moves from the atmosphere to alveoli by convection in inspiration and carbon dioxide is expired in the opposite direction. This to and fro motion reduces the efficiency of gas exchange and is 25% less efficient than avian lungs, which have a series of parabronchi and unidirectional flow of air, but with the advantage of more flexibility in the thoracic cage [2].

The trachea-bronchial airways are lined by pseudostratified epithelium, in which each cell makes contact with the basement membrane. More distally, the epithelium becomes columnar and finally cuboidal in small airways. The major epithelial subtypes include ciliated, secretory and basal cells [3], but there are also rarer cell types, including tuft and neuroendocrine cells. Recent application of single-cell RNA sequencing to the airway epithelium has identified a new cell type, which has been named the ionocyte [4, 5].

DNA MUTATIONS AND MALIGNANT TRANSFORMATION

It is generally accepted that the process of malignant transformation begins with a mutation in a cell's DNA that leads to the acquisition of cancer-related traits. Lung cancer has one of the highest DNA mutation frequencies in comparison to other major tumour types [6]. In part, this could relate to the direct exposure of lung epithelial cells to carcinogens in cigarette smoke. A study comparing DNA mutations from different cancers showed that lung cancers in smokers are particularly associated with a mutation signature characterised by C to A substitution, which mirrors the *in-vitro* mutation profile observed after exposure to benzopyrene (a carcinogen in tobacco smoke). This phenomenon appears to be less common in cancers arising from organ systems that are not directly exposed to cigarette smoke (*e.g.*, bladder/cervical/kidney cancers) [7]. As lung cancers evolve their mutational profile alters and at later stages, other mechanisms may predominate. This has been evaluated by performing multi-regional genomic sequencing of resected tumours. Distinguishing clonal (shared between all regions) and sub-clonal (shared between a subset of regions) DNA mutations enable the construction of a timeline beginning with clonal mutations and ending with sub-clonal. Thus, the evolutionary history of cancer can be re-constructed. At later stages of lung cancer evolution, a shift in the DNA mutation signature occurs, whereby there is less C to A and more C to G/C to T substitutions [8].

This correlates with the mutational signature produced by the apolipoprotein B mRNA editing enzyme catalytic protein-like (APOBEC) family of cytosine deaminases. APOBEC was first recognised for its role in innate immunity, where it is involved in an antiviral response through deaminating cytosine in viral genomes. However, there is now much evidence that the activity of ABOPEC proteins can be up-regulated and misdirected in cancer cells leading to somatic hypermutation [9].

In general, all mechanisms of DNA mutations lead to the genetic variance of cancer cells within a tumour, which is the substrate for Darwinian natural selection to operate. Genetic variance is important for creating enough diversity to respond to selection pressures. However, evidence is growing that too much genetic instability may be detrimental through failure to faithfully transmit the essential genetic information for cellular viability to daughter cells [10].

The predominant mutational process in any given cancer will have a specific signature of DNA mutation. Studying the signatures of DNA mutation across different cancer types has revealed that most cancers (including lung cancer) have at least two different processes of DNA mutation [11]. In a sense, these are non-random, but they occur in both non-coding (the vast majority of the genome) and coding parts of the genome, meaning that most mutations would be predicted to have no consequences for cellular proliferation. Such mutations have been termed 'passenger' mutations to distinguish them from the rarer 'driver' mutations that confer a selective advantage for survival and proliferation, leading to malignant transformation [12]. Driver mutations can act dominantly, where gain-of-function occurs in a growth-promoting gene, or negatively through the loss of function of a growth-regulating (*i.e.*, tumour suppressor) gene. Next-generation DNA sequencing has provided a wealth of information about cancer genomes, but distinguishing the specific driver mutations from the much more common passenger mutations remains a challenge. Prediction algorithms can be based on frequency estimates, whereby mutations are shared by different patients to a greater extent than would be expected by random chance. Alternatively, function-based methods can be used, which entail consideration of how an individual DNA mutation will eventually lead to an alternative protein structure and hence function [13].

Several driver mutations have been identified in lung cancer. Fig. (**1a**) shows the most common gain-of-function driver mutations in lung adenocarcinomas, derived from the cancer genome atlas (TCGA) consortium [14]. These mutations tend to occur in different parts of common signalling pathways involved in survival and proliferation, as shown in Fig. (**1b**) (derived from Figure S1 [15]). Identifying driver mutations in squamous cell carcinoma of the lung have proved more difficult on account of their high rate of mutations [16]. A comprehensive analysis of tumours from 178 patients from the TCGA revealed ten genes that were significantly mutated; *TP53, CDKN2A, PTEN, PIK3CA, KEAP1, MLL2, HLA-A, NFE2L2, NOTCH1* and *RB1* [17]. Characterising the mutational landscape of small-cell lung cancer has been hampered by the paucity of surgically resected specimens given a typical diagnosis at late-stage disease [18]. Furthermore, small-cell lung cancer has an extremely high mutation rate. Whole-genome sequencing of small cell lung cancer samples from 110 patients revealed that almost all had inactivating mutations in *TP53* and *RB1*. Inactivating mutations in the *NOTCH* family genes were present in about 25% patients. Rarely, mutations in *BRAF*, *KIT* and *PIK3CA* were also present [19].

There is considerable variation in the impact of a driver mutation on the process of malignant transformation. Mutations occurring at the top of signalling cascades would be predicted to have more widespread effects than those lower down. This is illustrated by driver mutations in the epidermal growth factor receptor gene (*EGFR*). EGFR activates a number of intracellular pathways, including MAP kinase, PI3K-Akt and PLC-gamma1-PKC [30]; hence constitutive activity induced by a mutation will have numerous downstream effects on cell survival and proliferation. It is, therefore, no coincidence that mutations in *EGFR* are able to drive lung cancer in non-smokers [20], who would be predicted to have lower genomic mutation burdens than smokers.

In addition to DNA mutations that lead to an alternative protein product, genomic amplification events are common in cancer cells. These can lead to over-expression of native proteins and also contribute to oncogenesis. The role of this type of aberration in oncogenesis can be more challenging to characterise, as amplification can involve several genes making it difficult to identify which is causative. Interestingly, the same amplicon can have different genes implicated in the oncogenesis of different cell types. For example, when 8q24 amplification occurs in breast, colon and lung cancer, the proposed driver gene is *MYC*, but in acute myeloid leukaemia the same amplicon leads to *TRIB1* over-expression and oncogenesis [31]. This mechanism becomes particularly important in resistance to targeted therapies. In particular, adenocarcinomas with *EGFR* mutations escape tyrosine kinase inhibition through genomic amplification of *MET* in about 21% of cases [32].

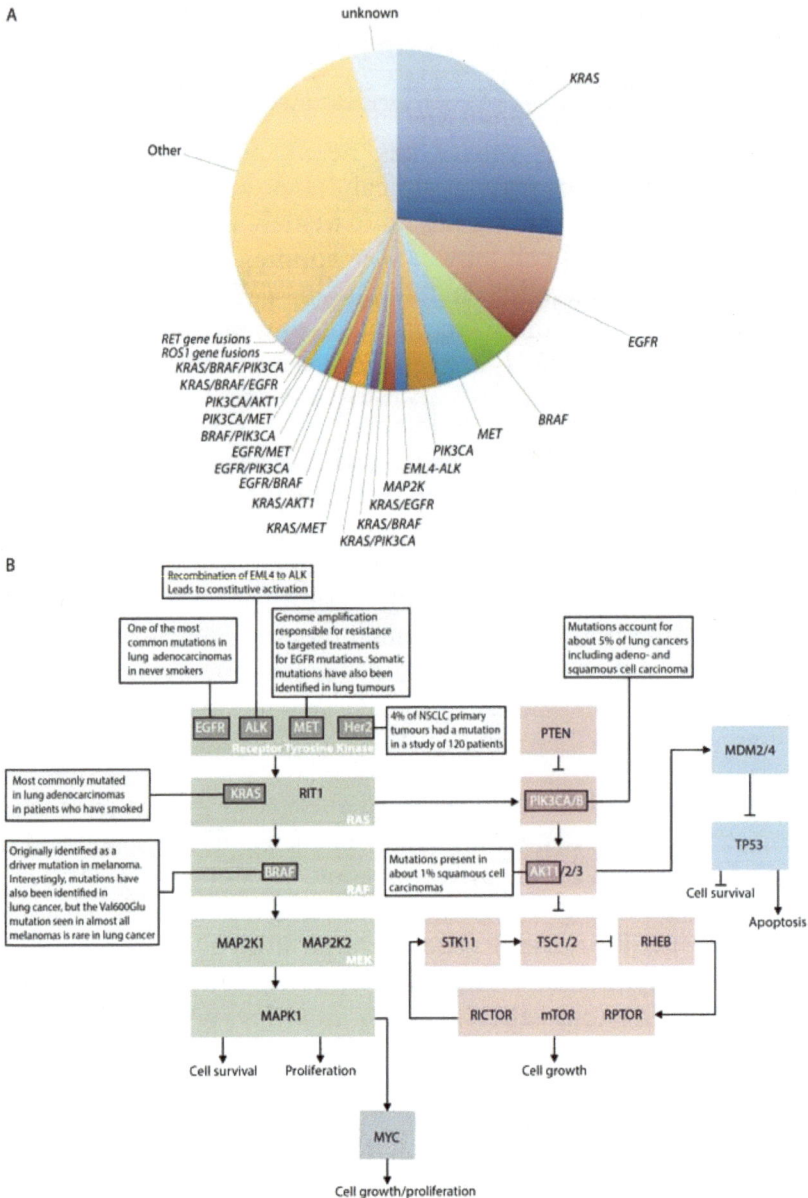

Fig. (1). A. Most common gain of function driver mutations in lung adenocarcinoma (derived from an analysis of lung adenocarcinoma driver mutations from TCGA [14]. Unknown refers to tumours where no mutations in plausible genes where found. Other refers to the many plausible mutations identified, which are not as well characterised as those specifically mentioned). B. Gain of function mutations ordered by pathway. This is a non-exhaustive diagram and several other pathways are interconnected (see Figure S1 [15]. Oncogenic signalling pathways in the cancer genome atlas for more complete representation). Mutations in EGFR [20], MET [21], ALK (EML4-ALK) [22], Her2 [23], KRAS [24, 25], BRAF [26], PIK3CA [27] and AKT1 [28, 29] are discussed.

Acquisition of a driver mutation is necessary but may not be sufficient for malignant transformation. Co-operating driver mutations/gene amplification, as well as a loss of tumour suppressor genes, may be required for full malignant transformation. This has been studied in cancers from the TCGA by comparing the ratio of non-synonymous (*i.e.*, mutations that change protein sequence) to synonymous DNA mutations (*i.e.*, mutations that do not change protein sequence) in cancers. Theoretically, synonymous mutations should not have any consequence to the cell and will not be under positive or negative selection, providing a measure of the background mutation rate. In contrast, non-synonymous mutations could be under positive/negative selection or be neutral. Applying this method to lung cancer revealed that 4 to 6 genes per tumour were under positive selection and predicted to be driver mutations for lung adenocarcinoma and squamous cell carcinoma, respectively. Interestingly when this analysis was restricted to known genes involved in cancer, only about 2 driver mutations were identified per tumour, illustrating that our list of cancer-causing genes is by no means complete [33].

LUNG CANCER CELLS OF ORIGIN

Initial hypotheses for the cells of origin for cancer were derived from superimposing the properties of cancer cells over the prevailing views of cellular differentiation. Cancer cells have an extensive capacity for proliferation and there is an inverse relationship between the degree to which they display differentiated tissue organisation and their capacity for invasion. Thus, it seems reasonable to postulate that cells already possessing some of these attributes would be most likely to be the founding population of lung cancer. To this end, there has been much focus on 'stem' cells involved in lung tissue repair and regeneration. These cells exist in a state characterised by the lack of markers of differentiated lung tissue and at steady state have a low level of turnover. However, in response to injury, they can respond robustly, proliferating and differentiating to enable tissue repair and regeneration [34].

Mouse models have provided several insights into the dynamics of lung stem cells. In particular, lineage-tracing experiments have revealed that stem cells responsible for the maintenance and regeneration of the airway epithelium represent a cell state rather than a distinct cellular population. Indeed, there is evidence that mature epithelial cell types can de-differentiate into this state after the ablation of basal stem cells [35]. This raises the possibility that any cell could give rise to cancer; however, cells that are already in a 'stem' cell state may require less steps for transformation. Furthermore, cells occupying a stem cell niche are likely to have a longer life span than differentiated cells, allowing more time for an adequate set of driver mutations to accrue [36].

The early stages of lung cancer have been best studied using mouse models, whereby specific driver mutations can be activated in different lung cell types and monitored for the onset of malignancy. The most widely used model has been the inducible *KRasG12D* model for lung adenocarcinoma, which uses the Cre/Lox system. Embryonic stem cells have been engineered such that one *KRas* allele harbours the *KRasG12D* mutation, but the expression is inhibited by an upstream stop signal flanked by loxP sites. Expression of cre-recombinase leads to the excision of this stop sequence allowing expression of *KRasG12D* at endogenous levels, therefore mimicking what is likely to happen at the onset of human lung adenocarcinomas [37]. An early study instilled adenoviral vectors containing cre-recombinase into airways of these transgenic mice to activate *KRasG12D* in a broad range of airway cell types. The first lesions to appear were atypical adenomatous hyperplasia (AAH), which stained positive for surfactant protein C (SP-C), suggesting that their origin was alveolar type II (AT2) cells, which were followed by epithelial hyperplasia (EH), adenomas and subsequently adenocarcinomas [38]. Interestingly, there was a subpopulation of cells that were positive for SP-C and CC10 (markers for AT2 and Clara cells) present in adenomas. These cells were subsequently identified at the bronchoalveolar duct junction (BADJ) in wild type mice and were thought to be bronchioalveolar stem cells (BASC). Subsequent *in vitro* and *in vivo* experiments showed that these BASCs proliferated more in response to activating *KRasG12D* mutations and were thus hypothesised to be the cell of origin for adenocarcinomas [39]. However, more recent studies have identified a much more complex origin of lung adenocarcinoma. When *KRasG12D* was exclusively expressed in CC10 positive cells, expression was limited to BASCs and Clara cells. Although hyperproliferation of cells at the BADJ occurred, all adenocarcinomas occurred in the alveoli in CC10 negative cells. Furthermore, the exclusive expression of *KRasG12D* in BASCs and AT2 cells led to the same phenotype at a higher frequency. This led the authors to propose that although several cell types can hyper-proliferate in response to *KRas* mutations, bona fide adenocarcinomas only arise when this occurs in AT2 cells [40]. These findings were replicated by using adenoviral vectors targeted to CC10 or SPC expressing cells, but interestingly, the authors came to a different conclusion, proposing that both clara cells and AT2 cells could initiate adenocarcinomas. This conclusion was drawn from two lines of evidence observed in CC10 targeted *KRasG12D* expression. Firstly, hyperproliferation at the BADJ and adenocarcinomas appeared to share the same clonal origin and secondly, adenocarcinomas had partial expression of *Sox2*, which is present in early CC10 positive hyperplasia, but not SPC positive lesions [41]. These results are interesting, as in both studies CC10 positive cells with activated *KRas* mutations were present in the airways, but only caused adenocarcinomas in the alveoli. This implies that cell type specific modulators determine whether a driver mutation initiates a tumour. To this end, inhibition of the Notch signalling pathway in CC10 positive cells at the time of *KRasG12D* activation inhibited development of adenocarcinomas, although there were hyperplastic lesions in the alveoli and BADJ. These hyperplastic lesions had up-regulated *Sox2* and had a squamous morphology. Conversely up-regulation of Notch led to airway adenocarcinomas [42].

The cell of origin for squamous cell carcinomas of the lung is more contentious and has been more difficult to study than adenocarcinomas. However, a murine model has been developed, whereby conditional deletion of the tumour suppressor genes *PTEN* and *Cdkn2a* coupled with activation of *Sox2* expression led to tumours that histologically resembled squamous cell carcinoma. Lung squamous cell carcinomas could be formed when these changes were selectively induced in basal cells, as well as CC10 and SPC positive cells. This implies that the particular mix of signalling pathway aberrations is more important in determining the cancer subtype than the cell of origin per se [43]. To this end, a recent study has demonstrated that adenocarcinomas induced by *KRasG12D* can switch to squamous cell carcinomas when the tumour suppressor gene *lkb1* is deleted [44].

The first mouse model for small cell lung cancer (SCLC) was based on the observation that *Trp53* and *Rb1* frequently carry mutations in human SCLC. Conditional deletion of both *Trp53* and *Rb1* in mouse airway epithelium led to the emergence of tumours that resembled SCLC histologically. Both deletions were necessary for this phenotype – isolated *Rb1* or *Trp53* had no malignant phenotype or only adenocarcinomas, respectively [45]. Restricting these deletions to neuroendocrine cells (Calcitonin gene-related peptide (CGRP) expressing cells) recapitulated the frequency of the SCLC phenotype observed with deletions in all airway epithelial cells. However, some SCLC tumours still emerged from AT2 and Clara cells, although at much lower frequencies [46].

EVOLUTION FROM DRIVER MUTATION TO MALIGNANCY

The landscape in which cells with driver mutations operate is likely to be dynamic. Repeated exposure to carcinogens in cigarettes is thought to create a 'field cancerisation' effect. This implies that driver mutations may occur in histologically normal tissue, leading to perhaps a survival/growth advantage, but without co-operating mutations necessary to progress to malignancy. Over time, clones with potential for cancer may grow and regress until a cell with an appropriate complement of mutations emerges and progresses to cancer. In support of this, studies have identified driver mutations in genes such as *EGFR* in histologically normal tissue adjacent to cancers [47, 48].

At all stages, from transformation to established and progressing tumours, cancers are shaped by internal and external selective pressures. Rapidly proliferating transformed cells have high metabolic needs, creating a strong demand for resources as well as a toxic microenvironment saturated with lactic acid from glycolysis and reactive oxygen species. This is compounded by external pressures that include immune surveillance and chemotherapeutic agents used in treatment. Genetic variance within tumour populations is essential for adaptation to these dynamic constraints by natural selection [49].

So far, we have considered evolution in the context of cancer initiation from non-cancerous cells through the acquisition of survival and proliferative traits. Following cancer initiation, this process becomes more complex and several models have been developed to explain how cancer progresses in different circumstances. Firstly, it is worth considering what the absence of selection would look like. This has been termed neutral evolution and predicts that over successive cell divisions, mutations will accumulate randomly, leading to a large number of mutations at low frequencies. This is predicted to occur in about 40% lung adenocarcinomas and 23% lung squamous cell carcinomas from the analysis of TCGA [50]. It is also possible for clones to be over-represented in the absence of positive selection by evolutionary drift due to stochastic events (*i.e.*, random cell death within a tumour).

Where selective pressures act on a tumour, several models have been proposed illustrated in Fig. (**2**). These include linear evolution; whereby new driver mutations provide such a strong selective advantage that they outcompete all previous clones. This model predicts that a tumour is sequentially dominated by single clones. It has been useful for conceptualising the steps involved in cancer progression, but supporting data has largely been from single gene studies, and it fails to explain the intra-tumour heterogeneity that has been unveiled by more recent studies in cancer genomics [51]. Tumours may have multiple sub-clones that dominate in their locality, but not across the tumour as a whole. This endpoint could be reached by branching evolution, whereby the best-adapted clones are selected in their locality and evolve in parallel with other geographically distinct clones. Alternatively, in some cancers, a 'big-bang' model has been suggested. This posits that at the earliest stage after malignant transformation, intra-tumoural heterogeneity is high (*i.e.*, a large number of sub-clones). Subsequently, one or a few clones accumulate a particular set of mutations giving them a positive selective advantage and proliferate rapidly to dominate the tumour. This process is formally known as punctuated evolution and is worth distinguishing from salutatory evolution, where a dramatic genomic event occurs within a single cell division leading to rapid proliferation and dominance. Given that most of these dramatic genomic changes would be expected to be deleterious salutatory evolution is thought to be a very rare event [52].

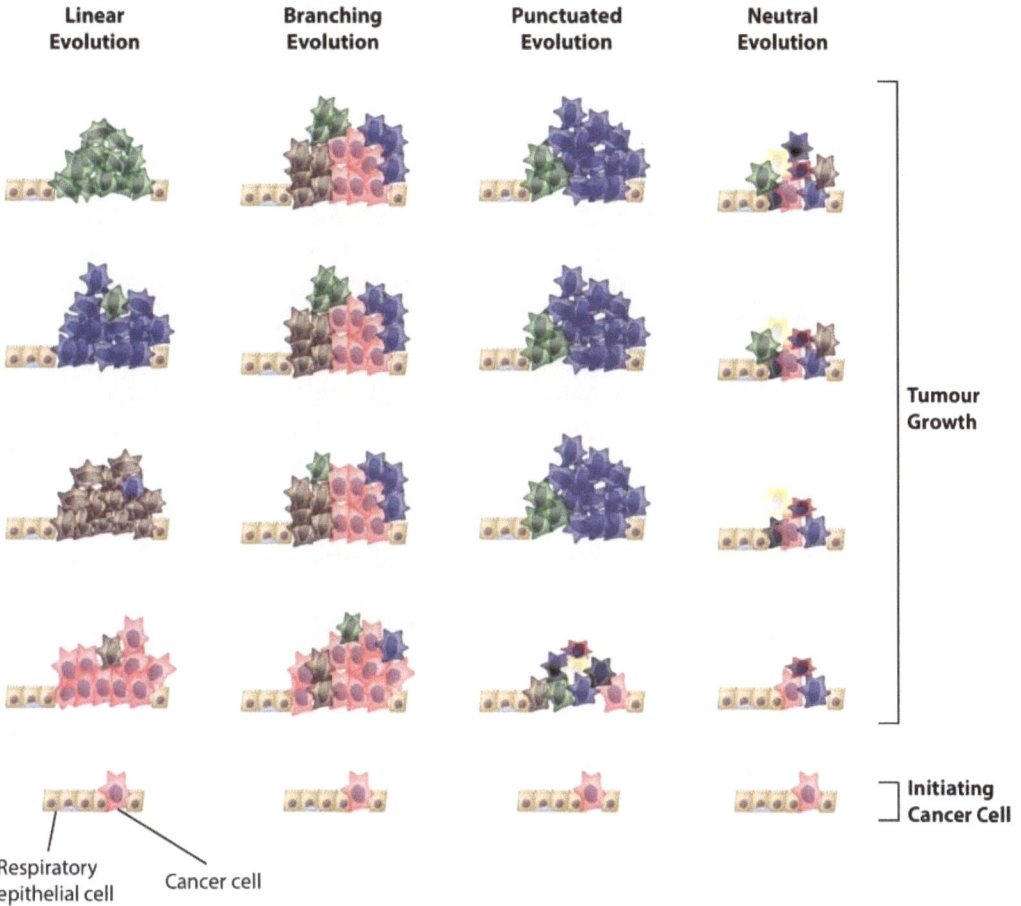

Fig. (2). Models of cancer evolution. Cells of the same colour represent clones with the same genetic profile.

Given that most of the phylogenetic studies in cancer involve analysis at a single time point, it is difficult to formally test these evolutionary models. It has been proposed that the type of mutation may influence the evolutionary path that a tumour takes. When point mutations in DNA lead to the positive selective trait, branching evolution has been proposed to dominate. In contrast, punctuated evolution appears more likely when chromosomal copy number aberrations occur [51]. It is possible that different types of evolution may dominate at different times within the lifespan of a tumour.

THE IMMUNE SYSTEM AND CANCER EVOLUTION

Mouse models have shown that T cells can directly affect the eventual genomic landscape of cancer. When sarcomas from immunodeficient mice lacking T cells were transplanted into wild type mice, escape tumours only developed if they lacked a particular immunogenic mutation that was present in the majority of the parent sarcoma population. This was in contrast to the tumours that emerged after transplantation into T cell-deficient mice, where most tumours possessed this mutation [53]. This has led to the concept that the immune system sculpts a tumour as it grows, directly affecting tumour evolution. This is thought to occur through the recognition of tumour associated antigens (TAAs). When these arise from non-synonymous mutations they have been termed neo-antigens and have the potential to activate an immune response, given that they are not present in health and therefore not recognised as 'self'. Analysis of the TCGA for lung adenocarcinomas has revealed that having a large number of clonal neo-antigens is associated with a better prognosis, presumably through providing targets for the immune system [54]. In addition to neo-antigens, the dysregulated transcriptome of cancer cells can also lead to the expression of tissue-restricted genes out of context, which can be another source of immunogenicity [55].

The first step in initiating a robust cytotoxic adaptive immune response to a tumour involves phagocytosis of TAAs by antigen-presenting cells (APCs), of which the most important are dendritic cells. APCs subsequently present TAAs via MHC-II molecules to naïve T cells in lymph nodes. Recognition of antigen within an MHC-II complex by a T cell is not in itself enough for activation. Co-stimulatory molecules on APCs are needed to fully induce activated effector T cells. One of the most important co-stimulators is CD80/86, which contacts CD28 on T cells. Activated T cells subsequently express CTLA-4, which has a greater affinity for CD80/86 than CD28, and acts as a brake preventing unregulated T cell expansion [56]. A cytolytic response is elicited when an activated CD8 T cell encounters the tumour associated antigen in association with MHC-I on cancer cells. In the periphery, cells expressing PD-L1 bind to PD-1 on CD8 T cells and inhibit signalling through the T cell receptor, thus preventing a cytotoxic reaction. In health, this acts to prevent inappropriate cytotoxicity to normal tissues [57].

Recognition and elimination of cancer cells by the immune system are challenging. Given that TAAs are derived from self, these antigens are not likely to strongly activate innate pattern recognition receptors on phagocytosis by APCs. Subsequently, the expression of co-stimulation molecules on APCs may not be optimal to activate T cells. Evidence for this has been observed in colorectal tumour samples, where infiltrating dendritic cells expressed low levels of CD80/86 [58]. Furthermore, the tumour microenvironment has been shown to suppress a range of different dendritic cell functions, including endocytosis and antigen presentation [59].

In the event that CD8 T cells are activated against TAAs, there are still barriers to a successful cytolytic response. CD8 T cells need to encounter a specific antigen in the context of an MHC-I complex for cytotoxicity. Usually, as part of protein homeostasis within a cell, intracellular protein degradation is coupled to MHC-I presentation. Proteins are marked for degradation by ubiquitination, which is carried out by the proteasome. Peptide fragments are subsequently exported into the endoplasmic reticulum by the transporter associated with antigen processing (TAP), where they are loaded into MHC-I for subsequent presentation on the cell surface. Down-regulation of TAP has been demonstrated in several tumour types [60] . In an SCLC cell line, a mutation was found that leads to non-functional TAP and impaired antigen presentation [61] .

Tumours can also express ligands that inhibit the activity of CD8 T cells. Soon after the discovery of PD-L1, a study demonstrated expression on lung, ovarian, melanoma and colorectal cancers. PD-L1 was not significantly expressed in histologically normal tissues. Inducing expression of PD-L1 in a cancer cell line that did not express PD-L1 led to increased apoptosis of co-cultured T cells, demonstrating that this had an immunosuppressive effect [62] . Antigen-presenting cells can also express PD-L1 and may also have a role in downregulating T cell anti-tumour cytotoxicity [63] . While it is logical that tumour cells expressing PD-L1 down-regulate an immune response as a means of immune evasion, the role of the immune system in facilitating this process is more difficult to dissect. Recent studies have provided some insight into the role of PD-L1 on immune cells through genetic deletion of PD-L1 from tumour cells in mouse models. In this context, treatment with antibodies that block the PD-1/P--L1 axis only affect non-tumour cells, allowing assessment of their contribution to anti-tumour immunity. When PD-L1 expression was knocked down in T3 sarcoma cell lines, they were rejected from immune-competent mice, unless they were seeded at higher densities, in which case tumours grew. Treatment with anti-PD-L1 antibodies induced tumour rejection, even in the absence of PD-L1 expression by the tumour cells, implying that non-tumour cells were compliant in immune evasion through the PD-1/PD-L1 axis [64] . These findings were extended using colorectal cancer cell lines in a mouse model. The knockdown of PD-L1 in host cells led to comparable control of tumour growth to tumour PD-L1 knockdown. The knockdown of both host and tumour PD-L1 achieved the best control of tumour growth [65] . Taken together, these and other studies support a role for host and tumour expressed PD-L1 in mediating immune evasion, emphasising the significance of expression of PD-L1 within the tumour micro-environment as a whole [66] .

The interactions between the immune system and lung cancer at the stage of cancer initiation have been less explored. Airway macrophages form the predominant innate immune cell population in the lung. These cells were previously thought to be derived from the peripheral haematopoietic system; however, more recent mouse models have provided compelling evidence that they are seeded during embryogenesis and self-repopulate throughout life [67] . This raises the prospect that these cells could be changed over time by the environmental insults that they are exposed to (including cigarette smoke) and could contribute to the process of tumour development indirectly. There is some evidence that the gene expression profiles of airway macrophages are different in smokers compared to non-smokers [68] , but further studies are needed to establish whether this has any impact on lung cancer development.

TRACKING EVOLUTION OF CANCERS

Much of what we know about cancer evolution is derived from the analysis of resected tumours. The rise of next-generation DNA sequencing has enabled sophisticated analysis and has allowed the reconstruction of the phylogenetic tree for any given cancer. However, there are caveats. Firstly, the resected tumour represents the final product of a long evolutionary path, and as detailed above, there are several factors that contribute to evolution, many of which (including the immune system) may not leave much in the way of a mutational signature. Secondly, genomic instability in cancer leads to intra-tumoral heterogeneity and thus, different regions of the tumour will have a different composition of cancer cells. Multi-regional sequencing, therefore, has several advantages over single site sampling for reconstructing tumour evolution. This technique has been exploited in the TRACERx study to provide insight into lung cancer evolution. In agreement with previous studies, mutational signatures associated with cigarette smoking were identified in early clonal mutations, in contrast to later sub-clonal mutations, which bore the signature of APOBEC somatic hypermutation. Many of the well-known driver mutations, including *EGFR/MET/BRAF* in adenocarcinoma, were primarily clonal and tended to occur before genome doubling, implying a role in tumour initiation. In contrast, mutations such as *PI3KCA* in squamous cell carcinomas occurred after genome doubling implying a role in cancer maintenance [69].

TRACERx has also combined multi-regional exome sequencing with circulating tumour DNA (ctDNA) analysis. ctDNA is thought to enter the systemic circulation passively through tumour necrosis and apoptosis, but may also be actively released by viable tumours [70]. In TRACERx, cancer evolution was monitored through ctDNA in patients who developed the recurrent disease after surgical resection. Bespoke multiplex PCR panels were synthesized for each patient, targeting clonal and sub-clonal single nucleotide variants (SNVs) to track phylogenetic branches over time. Interestingly, these PCR panels were able to detect ctDNA prior to or at clinical relapse and enabled the identification of the clonal origin of recurrent disease [71].

BIOLOGY OF TUMOUR GROWTH AND METASTASES

As cancer cells grow within a tumour, several morphological and structural changes occur within cancer and surrounding tissue that contribute to cancer progression. It is estimated that *in vivo*, tumours cannot expand beyond 100 – 500 microns - the diffusion limit of nutrients from the nearest capillary [72]. Tumours, therefore, need to establish access to the systemic circulation in order to grow beyond this size. This can occur by angiogenesis, the co-option of existing vessels, or vascular mimicry, where tumour cells take on certain characteristics of vascular endothelial cells. Tissue hypoxia is thought to be an important factor in driving new vessel formation through Hypoxia Inducible Factor (HIF). HIF consists of a stable beta subunit and an unstable alpha unit. In settings of low oxygen tension, the von-Hippel Lindau protein binds to and stabilises the alpha subunit, which enables HIF to increase the expression of several genes, including Vascular Endothelial Growth Factor (*VEGF*) [73]. HIF alpha subunit is not usually present in healthy lung tissue but is present in abundance in lung cancers [74]. To this end, high expression of *VEGF* has been observed in about 46% Stage I to stage IIIa tumours [75].

Ectopic expression of *VEGF* via adenoviral vectors has been used in mouse models to explore how new vessels form in tumours. There are some limitations in this model system, namely that *VEGF* expression is high initially and subsides over time, in contrast to tumours where long-term expression levels are expected to be maintained. However, it has proved useful to define the steps involved. The process starts with 'mother vessel' formation, where degradation of the basement membrane and pericyte detachment occurs in venules and capillaries and subsequently, there is an increase in cross-sectional area. Mother vessels then divide into daughter vessels, which can include capillaries, glomeruloid microvascular proliferations (GMP) and vascular malformations. In particular, GMPs are disorganised structures with increased permeability to plasma proteins. At any one time, a tumour is likely to be supplied by a disorganised heterogeneous collection of all these vessel types, providing a circulatory system that is friable and permeable, leading to oedema within the tumour [76].

The induction of new connections between the systemic circulation and a tumour serves both as a means to allow local growth and to start the process of metastases. Losing cell-cell cohesion and acquisition of cell motility are predicted to be critical steps in the progression of a tumour, as these enable cancer cells to leave their primary tumour and enter the circulation. In the context of epithelial-derived tumours, this involves a transition to a cell state more in keeping with mesenchymal cells. This epithelial to mesenchymal transition (EMT) occurs under physiological and pathological conditions and has a role in embryogenesis and wound healing but can be co-opted in the context of cancer progression. It appears to be driven by the tumour microenvironment [77], and probably involves an interplay between both cancer and non-cancer cells. In particular, fibroblasts have an important role. *In-vitro*, lung cancer cell lines can be induced to adopt EMT phenotypes following treatment with conditioned medium from cancer-associated-fibroblasts [78]. Other non-cancer cells within the tumour micro-environment almost certainly contribute, and to this end, tumour-associated macrophages have been shown to produce many of the cytokines thought to be important for EMT [79].

EMT is an important step in the transition from a locally advancing tumour to forming metastatic deposits. However, it does not act as a binary switch and cancer cells that have adopted some mesenchymal attributes will retain epithelial attributes as well. Thus, EMT is more of a spectrum than a specific cell state [80]. This is particularly apparent at the invading edges of cancers, where cells can maintain cell-cell cohesion but have acquired some mesenchymal attributes, such as the ability to degrade the basement membrane and migrate. This can lead to collective cell migration. The leading edge generates traction force by actomyosin mediated protrusion and contractility and cells inside the invading group are pulled forward through a network of cell-cell adhesions [81].

Vascular mimicry sits at an interesting juncture between new vessel formation and metastases. In non-small cell lung cancer, tumours that show this morphological feature tend to express other mesenchymal markers and are less likely to express epithelial markers [82].

It has long been assumed that motile cancer cells that have intravasated into the circulation seed distant metastases. In support of this hypothesis in lung cancer, circulating tumour cells (CTCs) from patients with small-cell lung cancer have been shown to form tumours in mice that show a similar treatment response pattern to the original patients [83]. However, the CTC population is heterogeneous, and not all cells entering the circulation will be capable of forming metastatic deposits [84]. The sub-set of cells with this capability has been referred to as 'tumour-initiating cells', 'cancer stem cells' or 'stem-like cells' and are thought to be rare within the CTC population [85]. The inefficiency of metastases has been illustrated by a xenograft model using CTCs from patients with breast cancer. Only blood samples with more than 1000 CTCs per 7.5ml blood sample (an unusually large number of CTCs and only present in 5/111 patients in this study) initiated metastases in mice [86].

Cancer cells may travel in the circulation as single cells or micro-emboli (CTM), which have been described as three or more CTCs in contact [87]. Non-cancer cells may also associate with CTM and may contribute to the metastatic process. In a murine model, fibroblasts associated with transplanted cancer cells, improving viability and providing an early growth advantage to metastatic deposits [88]. Platelets have also been implicated in assisting metastases through association with CTM by protecting against immune-mediated cell lysis [89]. *In vitro*, platelets reduce natural killer (NK) cell-mediated lysis of cancer cells and *in vivo* depletion of platelets reduces metastases in a murine model of metastases by a fibrosarcoma cell line [90]. Furthermore, the thrombogenicity of a tumour has been shown to correlate positively with metastatic potential [91].

The next stage in the metastatic process involves extravasating into a distant tissue site and establishing a metastatic colony. Cancer cells need to contact the vascular epithelium prior to migrating through it, which is likely mediated by adhesion molecules. This has been observed in real-time, where SCLC taken from a pleural effusion were infused into mice and intra-vital imaging captured cells rolling along the endothelium in a manner analogous to immune cells [92].

Given that most metastases have an epithelial morphology, after extravasation, it is likely that cancer cells need to undergo the reverse of EMT, *i.e.*, mesenchymal to epithelial transition (MET) [93]. It may not be necessary for a single cancer cell to possess every single attribute needed for all the steps from primary tumour dissociation to a thriving metastatic colony. Co-operation between heterogeneous cells making up CTM has been observed using a model of metastases from melanoma cell lines. When combined at a subcutaneous site, melanoma cell lines with low or high *VEGF* expression seeded metastases with both cancer cell types in most cases. However, when implanted at separate sites, almost all the pulmonary metastases occurred from the high expressing *VEGF* primary tumour [94]. The low *VEGF* expressing cancer cells were postulated to be the benefactors of co-operation with their high expressing counterparts.

In addition to seeding metastases, there is experimental evidence that CTCs can self-seed primary tumours. When breast cancer cell lines with or without fluorescent tags were transplanted at different sites in a mouse model up to 85% of the non-fluorescent tumours acquired fluorescence (*i.e.*, self-seeded CTCs) [95].

Metastasis has traditionally been assumed to be a late event in tumourigenesis. The reduction in mortality and metastatic disease following identification and resection of early-stage lung cancers in screening trials [96] can be taken as a line of evidence that supports this assumption. However, insights from recent studies have uncovered a more complex system. A mouse model of pancreatic cancer coupled a fluorescent tag to a *KRAS* mutation allowing lineage tracing of transformed cells. Interestingly, mice with localised tumours had cancer cells beyond the basement membrane in the pancreas, and at distant sites that retained normal histological appearances. These cells were usually present as single cells near blood vessels and raise the prospect that the process of metastases may start at very early stages of tumour growth [97].

There is a growing body of evidence that CTCs may reside within certain niches in distant organs that enhance survival, protecting against therapies directed at cancer. The bone marrow is of particular interest, where CTCs may occupy stem cell niches, adopting some of the characteristics of these cells that may enhance their survival and ability to seed metastases [98]. The first line of evidence came from a mouse model, where prostate cancer cells competed with haematopoietic stem cells (HSCs) for stem cell niches in mice [99]. This phenomenon has since been observed in NSCLC, where patients with localised disease (no metastases) undergoing surgical resection with curative intent had bone marrow aspirates at the time of surgery. Almost 60% patients had cancer cells (identified by cytokeratin 18) present in bone marrow aspirates, and this was associated with an increased risk of relapse [100]. Interestingly, only a small subset of these patients developed bone metastases.

CONCLUSION

As we apply an ever-increasing array of technologies to the field of lung cancer research, our knowledge is growing, and challenging some of our underlying assumptions. Major advances in DNA sequencing over the last two decades have captured a wealth of data from cancer genomes, enabling large repositories such as TCGA to be set up. The emerging field of single-cell genomics is likely to advance our understanding further. The past and present contributions of model organisms should not be forgotten. Many of the paradigms discussed in this chapter were characterised in mouse models and these have an ongoing role.

Much is known about the underlying biology of lung cancer, but there are still gaps in our knowledge. In particular, the earliest stages of lung cancer initiation remain a challenge to study. Further work in this field has the potential for dramatic clinical impacts through earlier disease recognition and treatment.

CONSENT FOR PUBLICATION

Not applicable.

CONFLICT OF INTEREST

The author confirms that this chapter's contents have no conflict of interest.

ACKNOWLEDGEMENTS

Declared none.

REFERENCES

[1]   Torre LA, Bray F, Siegel RL, *et al.* Global cancer statistics, 2012. CA Cancer J Clin 2015; 65(2): 87-108.
        [http://dx.doi.org/10.3322/caac.21262] [PMID: 25651787]

[2]   Hsia CC, Hyde DM, Weibel ER. Lung structure and the intrinsic challenges of gas exchange. Compr Physiol 2016; 6(2): 827-95.
        [http://dx.doi.org/10.1002/cphy.c150028] [PMID: 27065169]

[3]   Crystal RG, Randell SH, Engelhardt JF, Voynow J, Sunday ME. Airway epithelial cells: current concepts and challenges. Proc Am Thorac Soc 2008; 5(7): 772-7.
        [http://dx.doi.org/10.1513/pats.200805-041HR] [PMID: 18757316]

[4]   Montoro DT, Haber AL, Biton M, *et al.* A revised airway epithelial hierarchy includes CFTR-expressing ionocytes. Nature 2018; 560(7718): 319-24.
        [http://dx.doi.org/10.1038/s41586-018-0393-7] [PMID: 30069044]

[5]   Plasschaert LW, Žilionis R, Choo-Wing R, *et al.* A single-cell atlas of the airway epithelium reveals the CFTR-rich pulmonary ionocyte. Nature 2018; 560(7718): 377-81.
        [http://dx.doi.org/10.1038/s41586-018-0394-6] [PMID: 30069046]

[6]   Kandoth C, McLellan MD, Vandin F, *et al.* Mutational landscape and significance across 12 major cancer types. Nature 2013; 502(7471): 333-9.
        [http://dx.doi.org/10.1038/nature12634] [PMID: 24132290]

[7]   Alexandrov LB, Ju YS, Haase K, *et al.* Mutational signatures associated with tobacco smoking in human cancer. Science 2016; 354(6312): 618-22.
        [http://dx.doi.org/10.1126/science.aag0299] [PMID: 27811275]

[8]   de Bruin EC, McGranahan N, Mitter R, *et al.* Spatial and temporal diversity in genomic instability processes defines lung cancer evolution. Science 2014; 346(6206): 251-6.
        [http://dx.doi.org/10.1126/science.1253462] [PMID: 25301630]

[9]   Henderson S, Fenton T. APOBEC3 genes: retroviral restriction factors to cancer drivers. Trends Mol Med 2015; 21(5): 274-84.
        [http://dx.doi.org/10.1016/j.molmed.2015.02.007] [PMID: 25820175]

[10]   Swanton C, McGranahan N, Starrett GJ, Harris RS. APOBEC Enzymes: Mutagenic Fuel for Cancer Evolution and Heterogeneity. Cancer Discov 2015; 5(7): 704-12.
        [http://dx.doi.org/10.1158/2159-8290.CD-15-0344] [PMID: 26091828]

[11]   Alexandrov LB, Nik-Zainal S, Wedge DC, *et al.* Signatures of mutational processes in human cancer. Nature 2013; 500(7463): 415-21.
        [http://dx.doi.org/10.1038/nature12477] [PMID: 23945592]

[12]   Pleasance ED, Cheetham RK, Stephens PJ, *et al.* A comprehensive catalogue of somatic mutations from a human cancer genome. Nature 2010; 463(7278): 191-6.
        [http://dx.doi.org/10.1038/nature08658] [PMID: 20016485]

[13]   Pon JR, Marra MA. Driver and passenger mutations in cancer. Annu Rev Pathol 2015; 10: 25-50.
        [http://dx.doi.org/10.1146/annurev-pathol-012414-040312] [PMID: 25340638]

[14] Cancer Genome Atlas Research Network. Comprehensive molecular profiling of lung adenocarcinoma. Nature 2014; 511(7511): 543-50.
[http://dx.doi.org/10.1038/nature13385] [PMID: 25079552]

[15] Sanchez-Vega F, Mina M, Armenia J, *et al.* Oncogenic signaling pathways in the cancer genome atlas 2018; 173(2): 37-321.e10.
[http://dx.doi.org/10.1016/j.cell.2018.03.035]

[16] Friedlaender A, Banna G, Malapelle U, Pisapia P, Addeo A. Next generation sequencing and genetic alterations in squamous cell lung carcinoma: Where are we today? Front Oncol 2019; 9: 166.
[http://dx.doi.org/10.3389/fonc.2019.00166] [PMID: 30941314]

[17] Cancer Genome Atlas Research Network. Comprehensive genomic characterization of squamous cell lung cancers. Nature 2012; 489(7417): 519-25.
[http://dx.doi.org/10.1038/nature11404] [PMID: 22960745]

[18] Pietanza MC, Ladanyi M. Bringing the genomic landscape of small-cell lung cancer into focus. Nat Genet 2012; 44(10): 1074-5.
[http://dx.doi.org/10.1038/ng.2415] [PMID: 23011222]

[19] George J, Lim JS, Jang SJ, *et al.* Comprehensive genomic profiles of small cell lung cancer. Nature 2015; 524(7563): 47-53.
[http://dx.doi.org/10.1038/nature14664] [PMID: 26168399]

[20] Lynch TJ, Bell DW, Sordella R, *et al.* Activating mutations in the epidermal growth factor receptor underlying responsiveness of non-small-cell lung cancer to gefitinib. N Engl J Med 2004; 350(21): 2129-39.
[http://dx.doi.org/10.1056/NEJMoa040938] [PMID: 15118073]

[21] Kong-Beltran M, Seshagiri S, Zha J, *et al.* Somatic mutations lead to an oncogenic deletion of met in lung cancer. Cancer Res 2006; 66(1): 283-9.
[http://dx.doi.org/10.1158/0008-5472.CAN-05-2749] [PMID: 16397241]

[22] Soda M, Choi YL, Enomoto M, *et al.* Identification of the transforming EML4-ALK fusion gene in non-small-cell lung cancer. Nature 2007; 448(7153): 561-6.
[http://dx.doi.org/10.1038/nature05945] [PMID: 17625570]

[23] Stephens P, Hunter C, Bignell G, *et al.* Lung cancer: intragenic ERBB2 kinase mutations in tumours. Nature 2004; 431(7008): 525-6.
[http://dx.doi.org/10.1038/431525b] [PMID: 15457249]

[24] Santos E, Martin-Zanca D, Reddy EP, *et al.* Malignant activation of a K-ras oncogene in lung carcinoma but not in normal tissue of the same patient. Science 1984; 223(4637): 661-4.
[http://dx.doi.org/10.1126/science.6695174] [PMID: 6695174]

[25] Román M, Baraibar I, López I, *et al.* KRAS oncogene in non-small cell lung cancer: clinical perspectives on the treatment of an old target. Mol Cancer 2018; 17(1): 33.
[http://dx.doi.org/10.1186/s12943-018-0789-x] [PMID: 29455666]

[26] Pao W, Girard N. New driver mutations in non-small-cell lung cancer. Lancet Oncol 2011; 12(2): 175-80.
[http://dx.doi.org/10.1016/S1470-2045(10)70087-5] [PMID: 21277552]

[27] Okudela K, Suzuki M, Kageyama S, *et al.* PIK3CA mutation and amplification in human lung cancer. Pathol Int 2007; 57(10): 664-71.
[http://dx.doi.org/10.1111/j.1440-1827.2007.02155.x] [PMID: 17803655]

[28] Carpten JD, Faber AL, Horn C, *et al.* A transforming mutation in the pleckstrin homology domain of AKT1 in cancer. Nature 2007; 448(7152): 439-44.
[http://dx.doi.org/10.1038/nature05933] [PMID: 17611497]

[29] Malanga D, Scrima M, De Marco C, *et al.* Activating E17K mutation in the gene encoding the protein

kinase AKT1 in a subset of squamous cell carcinoma of the lung. Cell Cycle 2008; 7(5): 665-9.
[http://dx.doi.org/10.4161/cc.7.5.5485] [PMID: 18256540]

[30]   Wee P, Wang Z. Epidermal Growth Factor Receptor Cell Proliferation Signaling Pathways. Cancers (Basel) 2017; 9(5): E52.
[PMID: 28513565]

[31]   Santarius T, Shipley J, Brewer D, Stratton MR, Cooper CS. A census of amplified and overexpressed human cancer genes. Nat Rev Cancer 2010; 10(1): 59-64.
[http://dx.doi.org/10.1038/nrc2771] [PMID: 20029424]

[32]   Bean J, Brennan C, Shih JY, *et al.* MET amplification occurs with or without T790M mutations in EGFR mutant lung tumors with acquired resistance to gefitinib or erlotinib. Proc Natl Acad Sci USA 2007; 104(52): 20932-7.
[http://dx.doi.org/10.1073/pnas.0710370104] [PMID: 18093943]

[33]   Martincorena I, Raine KM, Gerstung M, *et al.* Universal patterns of selection in cancer and somatic tissues. Cell 2017; 171(5): 1029-41.e21.
[http://dx.doi.org/10.1016/j.cell.2017.09.042]

[34]   Hogan BL, Barkauskas CE, Chapman HA, *et al.* Repair and regeneration of the respiratory system: complexity, plasticity, and mechanisms of lung stem cell function. Cell Stem Cell 2014; 15(2): 123-38.
[http://dx.doi.org/10.1016/j.stem.2014.07.012] [PMID: 25105578]

[35]   Tata PR, Mou H, Pardo-Saganta A, *et al.* Dedifferentiation of committed epithelial cells into stem cells in vivo. Nature 2013; 503(7475): 218-23.
[http://dx.doi.org/10.1038/nature12777] [PMID: 24196716]

[36]   Smalley M, Ashworth A. Stem cells and breast cancer: A field in transit. Nat Rev Cancer 2003; 3(11): 832-44.
[http://dx.doi.org/10.1038/nrc1212] [PMID: 14668814]

[37]   Kwon MC, Berns A. Mouse models for lung cancer. Mol Oncol 2013; 7(2): 165-77.
[http://dx.doi.org/10.1016/j.molonc.2013.02.010] [PMID: 23481268]

[38]   Jackson EL, Willis N, Mercer K, *et al.* Analysis of lung tumor initiation and progression using conditional expression of oncogenic K-ras. Genes Dev 2001; 15(24): 3243-8.
[http://dx.doi.org/10.1101/gad.943001] [PMID: 11751630]

[39]   Kim CF, Jackson EL, Woolfenden AE, *et al.* Identification of bronchioalveolar stem cells in normal lung and lung cancer. Cell 2005; 121(6): 823-35.
[http://dx.doi.org/10.1016/j.cell.2005.03.032] [PMID: 15960971]

[40]   Xu X, Rock JR, Lu Y, *et al.* Evidence for type II cells as cells of origin of K-Ras-induced distal lung adenocarcinoma. Proc Natl Acad Sci USA 2012; 109(13): 4910-5.
[http://dx.doi.org/10.1073/pnas.1112499109] [PMID: 22411819]

[41]   Sutherland KD, Song JY, Kwon MC, Proost N, Zevenhoven J, Berns A. Multiple cells-of-origin of mutant K-Ras-induced mouse lung adenocarcinoma. Proc Natl Acad Sci USA 2014; 111(13): 4952-7.
[http://dx.doi.org/10.1073/pnas.1319963111] [PMID: 24586047]

[42]   Xu X, Huang L, Futtner C, *et al.* The cell of origin and subtype of K-Ras-induced lung tumors are modified by Notch and Sox2. Genes Dev 2014; 28(17): 1929-39.
[http://dx.doi.org/10.1101/gad.243717.114] [PMID: 25184679]

[43]   Ferone G, Song JY, Sutherland KD, *et al.* SOX2 is the determining oncogenic switch in promoting lung squamous cell carcinoma from different cells of origin. Cancer Cell 2016; 30(4): 519-32.
[http://dx.doi.org/10.1016/j.ccell.2016.09.001] [PMID: 27728803]

[44]   Zhang H, Fillmore Brainson C, Koyama S, *et al.* Lkb1 inactivation drives lung cancer lineage switching governed by Polycomb Repressive Complex 2. Nat Commun 2017; 8: 14922.
[http://dx.doi.org/10.1038/ncomms14922] [PMID: 28387316]

[45]   Meuwissen R, Linn SC, Linnoila RI, *et al*. Induction of small cell lung cancer by somatic inactivation of both Trp53 and Rb1 in a conditional mouse model. Cancer Cell 2003; 4(3): 181-9.
       [http://dx.doi.org/10.1016/S1535-6108(03)00220-4] [PMID: 14522252]

[46]   Sutherland KD, Proost N, Brouns I, *et al*. Cell of origin of small cell lung cancer: inactivation of Trp53 and Rb1 in distinct cell types of adult mouse lung. Cancer Cell 2011; 19(6): 754-64.
       [http://dx.doi.org/10.1016/j.ccr.2011.04.019] [PMID: 21665149]

[47]   Tang X, Shigematsu H, Bekele BN, *et al*. EGFR tyrosine kinase domain mutations are detected in histologically normal respiratory epithelium in lung cancer patients. Cancer Res 2005; 65(17): 7568-72.
       [http://dx.doi.org/10.1158/0008-5472.CAN-05-1705] [PMID: 16140919]

[48]   Kadara H, Wistuba II. Field cancerization in non-small cell lung cancer: implications in disease pathogenesis. Proc Am Thorac Soc 2012; 9(2): 38-42.
       [http://dx.doi.org/10.1513/pats.201201-004MS] [PMID: 22550239]

[49]   Maley CC, Aktipis A, Graham TA, *et al*. Classifying the evolutionary and ecological features of neoplasms. Nat Rev Cancer 2017; 17(10): 605-19.
       [http://dx.doi.org/10.1038/nrc.2017.69] [PMID: 28912577]

[50]   Williams MJ, Werner B, Barnes CP, Graham TA, Sottoriva A. Identification of neutral tumor evolution across cancer types. Nat Genet 2016; 48(3): 238-44.
       [http://dx.doi.org/10.1038/ng.3489] [PMID: 26780609]

[51]   Davis A, Gao R, Navin N. Tumor evolution: Linear, branching, neutral or punctuated? Biochim Biophys Acta Rev Cancer 2017; 1867(2): 151-61.
       [http://dx.doi.org/10.1016/j.bbcan.2017.01.003] [PMID: 28110020]

[52]   Graham TA, Sottoriva A. Measuring cancer evolution from the genome. J Pathol 2017; 241(2): 183-91.
       [http://dx.doi.org/10.1002/path.4821] [PMID: 27741350]

[53]   Matsushita H, Vesely MD, Koboldt DC, *et al*. Cancer exome analysis reveals a T-cell-dependent mechanism of cancer immunoediting. Nature 2012; 482(7385): 400-4.
       [http://dx.doi.org/10.1038/nature10755] [PMID: 22318521]

[54]   McGranahan N, Furness AJ, Rosenthal R, *et al*. Clonal neoantigens elicit T cell immunoreactivity and sensitivity to immune checkpoint blockade. Science 2016; 351(6280): 1463-9.
       [http://dx.doi.org/10.1126/science.aaf1490] [PMID: 26940869]

[55]   Durgeau A, Virk Y, Corgnac S, Mami-Chouaib F. Recent advances in targeting CD8 T-Cell immunity for more effective cancer immunotherapy. Front Immunol 2018; 9: 14.
       [http://dx.doi.org/10.3389/fimmu.2018.00014] [PMID: 29403496]

[56]   Kenneth Murphy CW. Janeway's Immunobiology 9. 2017; pp. 368-72.

[57]   Wei SC, Duffy CR, Allison JP. Fundamental mechanisms of immune checkpoint blockade therapy. Cancer Discov 2018; 8(9): 1069-86.
       [http://dx.doi.org/10.1158/2159-8290.CD-18-0367] [PMID: 30115704]

[58]   Chaux P, Moutet M, Faivre J, Martin F, Martin M. Inflammatory cells infiltrating human colorectal carcinomas express HLA class II but not B7-1 and B7-2 costimulatory molecules of the T-cell activation. Lab Invest 1996; 74(5): 975-83.
       [PMID: 8642792]

[59]   Ma Y, Shurin GV, Peiyuan Z, Shurin MR. Dendritic cells in the cancer microenvironment. J Cancer 2013; 4(1): 36-44.
       [http://dx.doi.org/10.7150/jca.5046] [PMID: 23386903]

[60]   Leone P, Shin EC, Perosa F, Vacca A, Dammacco F, Racanelli V. MHC class I antigen processing and presenting machinery: organization, function, and defects in tumor cells. J Natl Cancer Inst 2013;

105(16): 1172-87.
[http://dx.doi.org/10.1093/jnci/djt184] [PMID: 23852952]

[61]   Chen HL, Gabrilovich D, Tampé R, *et al.* A functionally defective allele of TAP1 results in loss of MHC class I antigen presentation in a human lung cancer. Nat Genet 1996; 13(2): 210-3.
[http://dx.doi.org/10.1038/ng0696-210] [PMID: 8640228]

[62]   Dong H, Strome SE, Salomao DR, *et al.* Tumor-associated B7-H1 promotes T-cell apoptosis: a potential mechanism of immune evasion. Nat Med 2002; 8(8): 793-800.
[http://dx.doi.org/10.1038/nm730] [PMID: 12091876]

[63]   Ostrand-Rosenberg S, Horn LA, Haile ST. The programmed death-1 immune-suppressive pathway: barrier to antitumor immunity. Journal of immunology (Baltimore, Md : 1950) 2014; 1938: 3835-41.
[http://dx.doi.org/10.4049/jimmunol.1401572]

[64]   Noguchi T, Ward JP, Gubin MM, *et al.* Temporally distinct PD-L1 expression by tumor and host cells contributes to immune escape. Cancer Immunol Res 2017; 5(2): 106-17.
[http://dx.doi.org/10.1158/2326-6066.CIR-16-0391] [PMID: 28073774]

[65]   Lau J, Cheung J, Navarro A, *et al.* Tumour and host cell PD-L1 is required to mediate suppression of anti-tumour immunity in mice. Nat Commun 2017; 8: 14572.
[http://dx.doi.org/10.1038/ncomms14572] [PMID: 28220772]

[66]   Tang F, Zheng P. Tumor cells versus host immune cells: whose PD-L1 contributes to PD-1/PD-L1 blockade mediated cancer immunotherapy? Cell Biosci 2018; 8: 34.
[http://dx.doi.org/10.1186/s13578-018-0232-4] [PMID: 29744030]

[67]   Ginhoux F, Guilliams M. Tissue-resident macrophage ontogeny and homeostasis. Immunity 2016; 44(3): 439-49.
[http://dx.doi.org/10.1016/j.immuni.2016.02.024] [PMID: 26982352]

[68]   Heguy A, O'Connor TP, Luettich K, *et al.* Gene expression profiling of human alveolar macrophages of phenotypically normal smokers and nonsmokers reveals a previously unrecognized subset of genes modulated by cigarette smoking. J Mol Med (Berl) 2006; 84(4): 318-28.
[http://dx.doi.org/10.1007/s00109-005-0008-2] [PMID: 16520944]

[69]   Jamal-Hanjani M, Wilson GA, McGranahan N, *et al.* Tracking the Evolution of Non-Small-Cell Lung Cancer. N Engl J Med 2017; 376(22): 2109-21.
[http://dx.doi.org/10.1056/NEJMoa1616288] [PMID: 28445112]

[70]   Heitzer E, Ulz P, Geigl JB. Circulating tumor DNA as a liquid biopsy for cancer. Clin Chem 2015; 61(1): 112-23.
[http://dx.doi.org/10.1373/clinchem.2014.222679] [PMID: 25388429]

[71]   Abbosh C, Birkbak NJ, Wilson GA, *et al.* Phylogenetic ctDNA analysis depicts early-stage lung cancer evolution. Nature 2017; 545(7655): 446-51.
[http://dx.doi.org/10.1038/nature22364] [PMID: 28445469]

[72]   Bielenberg DR, Zetter BR. The contribution of angiogenesis to the process of metastasis. Cancer J 2015; 21(4): 267-73.
[http://dx.doi.org/10.1097/PPO.0000000000000138] [PMID: 26222078]

[73]   Maxwell PH, Pugh CW, Ratcliffe PJ. Activation of the HIF pathway in cancer. Curr Opin Genet Dev 2001; 11(3): 293-9.
[http://dx.doi.org/10.1016/S0959-437X(00)00193-3] [PMID: 11377966]

[74]   Zhong H, De Marzo AM, Laughner E, *et al.* Overexpression of hypoxia-inducible factor 1alpha in common human cancers and their metastases. Cancer Res 1999; 59(22): 5830-5.
[PMID: 10582706]

[75]   O'Byrne KJ, Koukourakis MI, Giatromanolaki A, *et al.* Vascular endothelial growth factor, platelet-derived endothelial cell growth factor and angiogenesis in non-small-cell lung cancer. Br J Cancer 2000; 82(8): 1427-32.

[http://dx.doi.org/10.1054/bjoc.1999.1129] [PMID: 10780522]

[76]   Nagy JA, Chang SH, Shih SC, Dvorak AM, Dvorak HF. Heterogeneity of the tumor vasculature. Semin Thromb Hemost 2010; 36(3): 321-31.
[http://dx.doi.org/10.1055/s-0030-1253454] [PMID: 20490982]

[77]   Dongre A, Weinberg RA. New insights into the mechanisms of epithelial-mesenchymal transition and implications for cancer. Nat Rev Mol Cell Biol 2019; 20(2): 69-84.
[http://dx.doi.org/10.1038/s41580-018-0080-4] [PMID: 30459476]

[78]   Shintani Y, Fujiwara A, Kimura T, *et al.* IL-6 secreted from cancer-associated fibroblasts mediates chemoresistance in NSCLC by increasing epithelial-mesenchymal transition signaling. J Thorac Oncol 2016; 11(9): 1482-92.
[http://dx.doi.org/10.1016/j.jtho.2016.05.025] [PMID: 27287412]

[79]   Chen Y, Tan W, Wang C. Tumor-associated macrophage-derived cytokines enhance cancer stem-like characteristics through epithelial-mesenchymal transition. OncoTargets Ther 2018; 11: 3817-26.
[http://dx.doi.org/10.2147/OTT.S168317] [PMID: 30013362]

[80]   Lambert AW, Pattabiraman DR, Weinberg RA. Emerging biological principles of metastasis. Cell 2017; 168(4): 670-91.
[http://dx.doi.org/10.1016/j.cell.2016.11.037] [PMID: 28187288]

[81]   Friedl P, Locker J, Sahai E, Segall JE. Classifying collective cancer cell invasion. Nat Cell Biol 2012; 14(8): 777-83.
[http://dx.doi.org/10.1038/ncb2548] [PMID: 22854810]

[82]   Yao L, Zhang D, Zhao X, *et al.* Dickkopf-1-promoted vasculogenic mimicry in non-small cell lung cancer is associated with EMT and development of a cancer stem-like cell phenotype. J Cell Mol Med 2016; 20(9): 1673-85.
[http://dx.doi.org/10.1111/jcmm.12862] [PMID: 27240974]

[83]   Hodgkinson CL, Morrow CJ, Li Y, *et al.* Tumorigenicity and genetic profiling of circulating tumor cells in small-cell lung cancer. Nat Med 2014; 20(8): 897-903.
[http://dx.doi.org/10.1038/nm.3600] [PMID: 24880617]

[84]   Yang MH, Imrali A, Heeschen C. Circulating cancer stem cells: the importance to select. Chin J Cancer Res 2015; 27(5): 437-49.
[PMID: 26543330]

[85]   Krebs MG, Metcalf RL, Carter L, Brady G, Blackhall FH, Dive C. Molecular analysis of circulating tumour cells-biology and biomarkers. Nat Rev Clin Oncol 2014; 11(3): 129-44.
[http://dx.doi.org/10.1038/nrclinonc.2013.253] [PMID: 24445517]

[86]   Baccelli I, Schneeweiss A, Riethdorf S, *et al.* Identification of a population of blood circulating tumor cells from breast cancer patients that initiates metastasis in a xenograft assay. Nat Biotechnol 2013; 31(6): 539-44.
[http://dx.doi.org/10.1038/nbt.2576] [PMID: 23609047]

[87]   Hou JM, Krebs MG, Lancashire L, *et al.* Clinical significance and molecular characteristics of circulating tumor cells and circulating tumor microemboli in patients with small-cell lung cancer. J Clin Oncol 2012; 30(5): 525-32.
[http://dx.doi.org/10.1200/JCO.2010.33.3716] [PMID: 22253462]

[88]   Duda DG, Duyverman AM, Kohno M, *et al.* Malignant cells facilitate lung metastasis by bringing their own soil. Proc Natl Acad Sci USA 2010; 107(50): 21677-82.
[http://dx.doi.org/10.1073/pnas.1016234107] [PMID: 21098274]

[89]   Menter DG, Tucker SC, Kopetz S, Sood AK, Crissman JD, Honn KV. Platelets and cancer: a casual or causal relationship: revisited. Cancer Metastasis Rev 2014; 33(1): 231-69.
[http://dx.doi.org/10.1007/s10555-014-9498-0] [PMID: 24696047]

[90]   Nieswandt B, Hafner M, Echtenacher B, Männel DN. Lysis of tumor cells by natural killer cells in

mice is impeded by platelets. Cancer Res 1999; 59(6): 1295-300.
[PMID: 10096562]

[91]   Pearlstein E, Salk PL, Yogeeswaran G, Karpatkin S. Correlation between spontaneous metastatic potential, platelet-aggregating activity of cell surface extracts, and cell surface sialylation in 10 metastatic-variant derivatives of a rat renal sarcoma cell line. Proc Natl Acad Sci USA 1980; 77(7): 4336-9.
[http://dx.doi.org/10.1073/pnas.77.7.4336] [PMID: 6933486]

[92]   Heidemann F, Schildt A, Schmid K, *et al.* Selectins mediate small cell lung cancer systemic metastasis. PLoS One 2014; 9(4)e92327
[http://dx.doi.org/10.1371/journal.pone.0092327] [PMID: 24699516]

[93]   Mohan S, Chemi F, Brady G. Challenges and unanswered questions for the next decade of circulating tumour cell research in lung cancer. Transl Lung Cancer Res 2017; 6(4): 454-72.
[http://dx.doi.org/10.21037/tlcr.2017.06.04] [PMID: 28904889]

[94]   Küsters B, Kats G, Roodink I, *et al.* Micronodular transformation as a novel mechanism of VEGF--induced metastasis. Oncogene 2007; 26(39): 5808-15.
[http://dx.doi.org/10.1038/sj.onc.1210360] [PMID: 17353901]

[95]   Kim MY, Oskarsson T, Acharyya S, *et al.* Tumor self-seeding by circulating cancer cells. Cell 2009; 139(7): 1315-26.
[http://dx.doi.org/10.1016/j.cell.2009.11.025] [PMID: 20064377]

[96]   Aberle DR, Adams AM, Berg CD, *et al.* Reduced lung-cancer mortality with low-dose computed tomographic screening. N Engl J Med 2011; 365(5): 395-409.
[http://dx.doi.org/10.1056/NEJMoa1102873] [PMID: 21714641]

[97]   Rhim AD, Mirek ET, Aiello NM, *et al.* EMT and dissemination precede pancreatic tumor formation. Cell 2012; 148(1-2): 349-61.
[http://dx.doi.org/10.1016/j.cell.2011.11.025] [PMID: 22265420]

[98]   Kang Y, Pantel K. Tumor cell dissemination: emerging biological insights from animal models and cancer patients. Cancer Cell 2013; 23(5): 573-81.
[http://dx.doi.org/10.1016/j.ccr.2013.04.017] [PMID: 23680145]

[99]   Shiozawa Y, Pedersen EA, Havens AM, *et al.* Human prostate cancer metastases target the hematopoietic stem cell niche to establish footholds in mouse bone marrow. J Clin Invest 2011; 121(4): 1298-312.
[http://dx.doi.org/10.1172/JCI43414] [PMID: 21436587]

[100] Pantel K, Izbicki J, Passlick B, *et al.* Frequency and prognostic significance of isolated tumour cells in bone marrow of patients with non-small-cell lung cancer without overt metastases. Lancet 1996; 347(9002): 649-53.
[http://dx.doi.org/10.1016/S0140-6736(96)91203-9] [PMID: 8596379]

CHAPTER 3

Population Screening for Lung Cancer

Philip Barber*

Manchester University NHS Foundation Trust, Manchester, UK

Abstract: Lung Cancer is now the commonest cause of premature death in our industrial conurbations. It presents late and tends to be investigated on prolonged pathways, often with a stage shift along the way. Survival rates are closely related to stage at diagnosis, leading to a number of approaches to early diagnosis, most of which have not been validated as population screening tools. Most early screening trials used imaging, sometimes supplemented by sputum cytology, and achieved improved survival but did not reduce overall mortality, a rigorous benchmark that avoids the pitfalls of lead-time bias and overdiagnosis. The landmark National Lung Cancer Screening Study (NLST) a targeted screening study now nearly a decade old, achieved a 20% mortality improvement but this did not lead to the clinical implementation of screening programs in Europe or in the UK, where there is still an unaccountable scepticism, despite recent confirmatory evidence that the targeted screening of high-risk populations can save many lives. The Manchester implementation pilot used community-based health-checks and CT scans to access a very deprived population, detecting one lung cancer for every 23 scans, most at early stage and nearly all suitable for curative-intent treatments, with the almost complete avoidance of inappropriate interventions for non-malignant disease. Substantial numbers of non-malignant respiratory and cardiac conditions were also identified and referred for treatment. The programme is now being rolled out across the Greater Manchester conurbation and has been incorporated into the NHS Long-term Plan. It is to be hoped that the implementation of targeted screening, together with a step-change in the pace of diagnostic and treatment pathways, will start to make a real difference, assisted by a re-invigoration of evidence-based smoking cessation programmes for this uniquely preventable disease.

Keywords: Cytology, DNA biomarkers, Fluorescence bronchoscopy, Lung cancer, Mortality, NHS plan, Risk-assessment, Screening, Stage-shift, VOC's.

INTRODUCTION

It is an oft-repeated fact that lung cancer is the commonest cause of cancer death, in fact responsible for more deaths than prostate, breast and colorectal cancer

* **Corresponding authors Philip Barber:** Manchester University NHS Foundation Trust, Manchester, UK;
E-mail: phil.barber@mft.nhs.uk

Keyvan Moghissi, Jack Kastelik, Philip Barber & Peyman Sardari Nia (Eds.)

combined. What is not so widely recognised is that lung cancer has become the single commonest cause premature death in our industrial conurbations (Fig. **1**), and is very close to the commonest in the nation as a whole (Public Health England statistics). This is despite its being uniquely preventable, eminently curable and, increasingly, predictable. These prosaic but still startling facts bespeak an unacceptable neglect of the nation's biggest killer, underscored by the fact that smoking cessation, from which our Health Service has systematically disinvested, is by far the most cost-effective intervention any health economy could ever make [1 - 3]; this is in stark contrast to the financial burden of increasingly complex chemotherapy and immunotherapy used to treat advanced disease, once the stage-boat has been missed [4, 5].

Where, then, should we be directing our efforts?

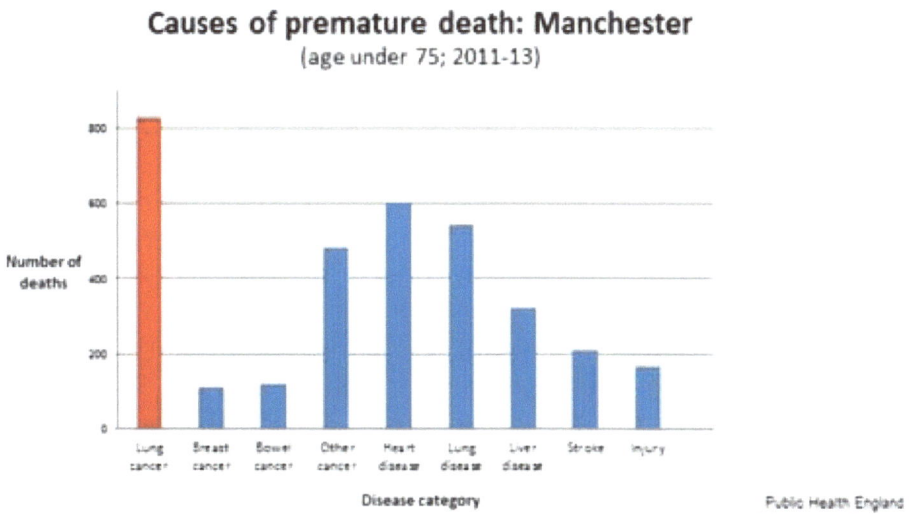

Causes of premature death: Manchester
(age under 75; 2011-13)

Fig. (1). Causes of premature death.

MOLECULAR BIOLOGY

It is possible to identify molecular and genetic abnormalities predisposing to sequential malignant change in bronchial epithelium, the so-called "genetic cascade". Thus, Kras mutations may be responsible for the activation of adenocarcinoma, and the mutation of suppressor genes such as p53 can be demonstrated in malignancy and also in the non-cancerous mucosa of cancer patients [6]. Other suppressor genes include p16, inactivated by hypermethylation [7], and the fragile histidine triad site on the short arm of chromosome 3 [8], which is subject to deletions in cancerous and pre-cancerous tissue. Deletions have also been observed on 8p, 9p, and 5q, and could predict the rate of disease progression [9]. The list is not exhaustive, and the study of gene expression in bronchial epithelial cells requires the development of gene-probe assays capable of assessing the mutational status of a large number of candidate genes. Unfortunately, the application of such techniques to population-based screening is far from practical at the present time.

The mechanism for DNA damage and repair is largely enzymic, and is thus capable of study by enzyme assay; such studies have suggested that different carcinogens may be responsible for different tumour types, but they do not, either, lend themselves to large-scale population screening, similarly with respect to the role of inflammatory cytokines responsible for a variety of effects, including invasive cell growth [10]. The identification of such biomarkers has not yet become applicable in practical and clinical terms.

EXHALED-AIR, BLOOD, AND SPUTUM ANALYSIS

A more clinical approach has been to look at volatile organic compounds (VOCs) in the exhaled air of cancer patients and controls [11]. Lung-cancer "signatures" have been identified with reportedly high sensitivity and specificity, but the technique has not yet been validated as a tool for the detection of pre-clinical disease. Sputum cytology has been extensively studied for many years and has been included in a number of screening projects, with indications that its effectiveness could be enhanced by automated sputum cytometry [12]. The current UK lungSEARCH trial is evaluating its effectiveness in the assessment of patients with obstructive lung disease [13]. Circulating tumour cells in cancer patients have also been studied, also circulating micro-RNA and DNA [14 - 19], including genetic mutations Kras, p53, and hypermethylation [20], with reportedly high levels of sensitivity and specificity, but they have never been evaluated as population screening tools. The TracerX study [20, 21] is currently looking at the post-operative circulation of specific DNA identified from resected tumours.

FLUORESCENCE BRONCHOSCOPY

Fluorescence bronchoscopy uses the autofluorescence signal differences between normal and dysplastic bronchial mucosa to enhance the detection of early micro-invasive or dysplastic disease [22 - 28]. A number of systems have used optical bronchoscopy, comparing white light with coloured light, especially blue light at 442 Nm, which stimulates green fluorescence in normal tissue, but a reddish-brown signal in dysplastic tissue. A worthwhile gain in sensitivity has been obtained, but with some loss of specificity, and mucosal inflammation and contact haemorrhage have been confounding factors. Autofluorescence, again using a blue light, is now built into some digital bronchoscopy systems, and has the advantage that contact bleeding gives a different signal. Some false positivity can still be observed however, especially in resection stumps and pre-biopsied areas. We have used it to map dysplastic areas in the course of surveillance of patients post-resection, combining it with photodynamic therapy for the treatment of recurrent/progressive early central lung cancer [29, 30]. Bronchoscopy techniques are probably too labour-intensive and patient-demanding for primary population surveillance, and decisions on the treatment of very early-stage primary central lung cancer have been compromised by a lack of evidence on its natural history and prognosis, with the potential for severe lead-time bias. Nevertheless, it is sensible, pragmatically, to treat fluorescence-detected small-volume central lung cancer with local therapy, especially if there is evidence of proliferation in morphological terms, keeping non-proliferative but histologically dysplastic areas under surveillance. Fluorescence bronchoscopy is undoubtedly a valuable adjunct to white-light bronchoscopy in the assessment and staging of central lung cancer, but probably does not lend itself to mass screening, except perhaps of very high-risk cohorts, especially survivors of treated central lung cancer, for whom we already have surveillance protocols. However, early central lung cancers, like early peripheral cancers, do mostly progress [31 - 34], but are usually radiologically occult, so a comprehensive screening programme needs arguably to take account of this somewhat different, but still lethal, form of the disease.

IMAGING

Radiological screening has been the principal basis of attempts over many years to identify lung cancer in at-risk patients and populations at a stage when it can be cured. It is well known that outcome survival in lung cancer is intimately linked to stage at diagnosis [35], five-year survival varying from over 90% for stage 1A disease, to only a few months or less for stage 4 metastatic disease, the latter accounting for up to 80% of diagnosed lung cancer in some industrial localities, and including a large number of patients diagnosed with the near-terminal disease at the time of a first (and only) emergency-room attendance.

Early detection, then, promises much, but lung cancer, like other visceral malignancies, presents late. It is, however, readily (perhaps uniquely among visceral cancers) detectable by imaging, so the radiological screening of at-risk populations looks attractive and has been the focus of interest, principally outside the UK, for many years. Within the UK, it still attracts extraordinary little attention; lung cancer is still often regarded as an irredeemable fact of life, and a consequence of smoking habits which are considered to be a lifestyle choice rather than a powerful addiction carefully nurtured by a tobacco industry which is currently busying itself with establishing Vape and low-temperature tobacco products in order to prolong addiction indefinitely into the future.

Early Studies

Radiological screening for lung cancer, carried out over the last half-century, has been on the whole disappointing but probably underrated. It has included a number of randomised controlled trials, the best known of which is the Mayo Clinic project (MLP) [36, 37], conducted between 1971 and 1983. Nearly 11,000 male smokers over the age of 45 were randomised to either 4-monthly or annual chest radiography and sputum cytology. Patients in the screened group showed improved staging and increased resectability, with a consequent improvement in five-year survival rates (33% vs 15%). However, there was no reduction of overall mortality, indeed it was slightly higher in the screened group due to an apparently higher incidence of lung cancer in that group. This phenomenon has never been fully explained, but has been encountered in more recent studies [38 - 42] and attributed to "over-diagnosis"; if this had been the case however, it would not have impacted on mortality.

Re-examinations of the project have suggested that it was underpowered, capable of detecting only a greater than 50% mortality gain. The screened group was also manifestly too broad, and the control group was 'contaminated' in that more than half the patients underwent additional chest radiography during the study period. Also, the overall rate of adherence to trial protocol was only 75% in the screened group, and a mere 50% in the control group. Finally, the assessment of cumulative mortality at 9 years is now considered sub-optimal, an assessment of 3-7 years from baseline probably more suitable. Adjusting for these potential sources of inaccuracy yields a potential mortality reduction of up to 43% [43]. This and other studies of the same era cannot therefore be regarded as definitive evidence against the benefits of screening, and the tumours identified were twice as likely to be resectable, with a consequent survival gain.

Allowance must be made, in the assessment of screening results, for a number of potential confounding factors. These include lead-time bias (advancing the time of diagnosis rather than moving back the time of death), length-time bias (the detection of less virulent tumours), and overdiagnosis (the detection of biologically insignificant tumours which would not have become clinically apparent during the patient's lifetime). There is however good evidence, from patients who have either refused or been found unfit for surgery, that untreated stage 1 lung cancer has a dismal prognosis, with five-year survivals of 0-10%. The pitfalls of lead-time bias and overdiagnosis can be overcome by the use of population mortality as a primary endpoint, rather than less rigorous parameters such as resectability or survival.

Even if one accepts the results of the Mayo Clinic and other earlier studies at face value, the findings are clearly at odds with evidence in clinical practice that diagnosis at an earlier stage improves outlook. This must mean that too few cancers have been detected by the studies, and points to a need to refine surveillance in the direction of high-risk groups. At a simple level this could simply mean older patients with a heavier smoking history. At the far end of the risk scale, it has long been possible to identify groups of patients in whom lung cancer is the commonest single cause of death; these include survivors of head and neck cancer, smokers with asbestosis, and elderly smokers with airflow limitation, especially due to emphysema. An American Lung Health study over two decades ago, looking at 6,000 smokers with airflow limitation, found that lung cancer was the commonest cause of death at the end of 5 years, exceeding heart disease and stroke. Our own locality, South Manchester, includes the single most deprived local-authority ward in England, and we became aware more than a decade ago that lung cancer accounted for an astonishing 1 in 8 deaths in that ward, a statistic of which we had great difficulty convincing our local health economy, but which has spurred us to take action on early detection and more rapid diagnostic pathways.

The Mayo Clinic project was one of three early American RCTs sponsored by the National Cancer Institute, the other two conducted by Johns Hopkins [44] and Memorial Sloan Kettering [45, 46]; these looked at the benefit of adding four-monthly sputum cytology to an annual chest x-ray, and found no improvement in mortality despite the fact that 20% of cancers in the active arm were detected by sputum cytology alone, almost all early-stage squamous cell carcinomas. The overall findings of these three studies suggest that chest x-ray screening does appear relatively ineffective in reducing lung cancer mortality, a conclusion reinforced by the findings of a large multicentred PLCO study reported in 2011, which found no benefit from an annual screening chest x-ray over 4 years, in study populations followed between November 1993 and December 2009. No stage shift was demonstrated.

Later Developments

Since that time, radiological screening for lung cancer has been transformed by two developments. The first is Risk Stratification, the second the availability of low-dose CT scanning, further refined by the development of nodule management protocols which have largely eliminated overdiagnosis, a fact that seems to have escaped the notice of many current commentators, and which distinguishes it from other organ screening programmes, many of which have failed to demonstrate convincing mortality improvements [47]. The Early Lung Cancer Action Program (ELCAP) [48] screened 3,1567 at-risk patients between 1993 and 2005, identifying 484 cancers, 85% of which were at clinical stage 1, with an 88% ten-year survival rising to 92% if resection took place within a month of diagnosis. Of note, the 8 participants with stage-1 disease who did not undergo surgery all died within 5 years of diagnosis, a telling figure for those who would overcall the issue of overdiagnosis. Operative mortality was 0.5%. The group concluded that "annual spiral CT screening can detect lung cancer that is curable" – indeed, and despite the fact that a positive result comprised any newly identified non-calcified nodule regardless of size, active management mandated only if there was enlargement of any nodule more than 3mm in diameter, or persistence of nodules of 5mm diameter or greater. The study incorporated a component of risk assessment, taking account of active/passive smoking and relevant environmental exposures, a relatively unrefined group and statistically weakened by a lower age cut-off of only 40, but the initial recruits were 60 years or older and the detection rates higher, 2.7% at baseline, 4.6% per annum at annual screening. The authors compared CT scanning followed by stage 1 surgery with later-stage treatments, and showed that the programme was highly cost-effective.

NLST and Beyond

Five years later, the hitherto elusive goal of mortality reduction was finally achieved with the landmark NLST trial [49, 50], which combined a high-risk population (55-74 years old, and a >30 pack-year smoking history) and compared low-dose CT scanning with chest radiography, obtained between August 2002 and April 2004. Data were collected until December 2009. Three screenings were performed on 53,454 patients. The study was designed for a 90% power to detect a 21% mortality reduction in the CT group in comparison with the x-ray group. 24.2% of CT scans were positive, against 6.9% chest x-rays. Across three screening rounds, when a positive screening result was obtained, around 95% of the tests in both groups were false-positive, but 1060 lung cancers were nevertheless detected in the LDCT group, 941 in the chest x-ray group. 649 cases were diagnosed after a positive LDCT screen, only 279 by chest x-ray, the remaining patients identified after a negative or missed scan, or after the screening phase had ended. There was a stage shift in favour of LDCT. There were 247 lung cancer deaths in the LDCT group, 309 in the chest x-ray group, a relative reduction of 20% (Fig. **2**). The number of scans needed to screen to detect one cancer was 320. All-cause mortality was also reduced, by 6.7%. Lung cancer accounted for 24% of all deaths in the trial. 60% of the excess deaths in the chest x-ray group were due to lung cancer and the non-lung cancer difference between the two groups was found insignificant. It has been concluded also that the results for a PLCO-eligible subset indicated that a control arm of community care (rather than annual chest x-ray) would probably have yielded a similar result.

B Death from Lung Cancer

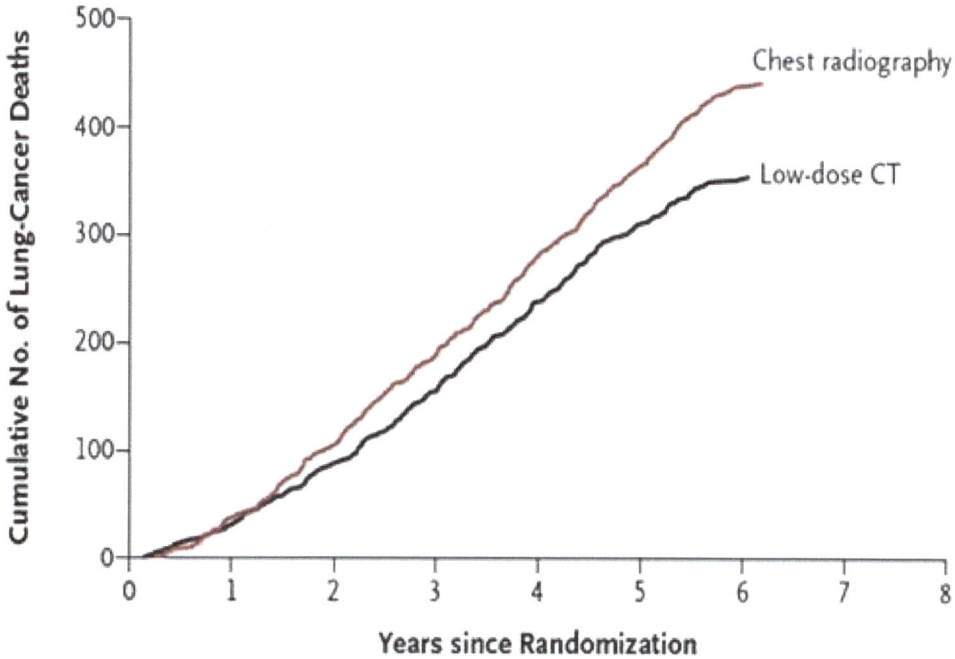

Fig. (2). NLST, NEJM, 2011.

Around that time and subsequently, a number of European studies were commencing but with less statistical power than NLST, an approach which has to be questioned; although these studies were indeed capable of providing additional information, for example on nodule management, it is arguable that NLST should have been a launch platform for practical implementation programmes incorporating, of course, additional data collection. In the UK, precisely nothing happened in practical clinical terms, but there have been attempts to refine risk stratification models, with an apparent view that the US data might be somehow inapplicable to UK populations. The UKLS study [51], a "pilot trial" looking at risk prediction identified a very high-risk group (greater than or equal to 5% over 5 years) of around 5,000 patients, 4,000 eventually randomised, with 98% participation. There were 42 screen detected cancers (2.1%), of which two thirds were at stage 1, a fifth at stage 2, a complete reversal of the normal spectrum in favour of curability, and with a greatly reduced false-positive rate of 27%, most of which underwent only further surveillance rather than inappropriate treatment. Unaccountably, a further planned study of 28,000 patients was not funded, and the UK national screening committee has remained unsupportive of population screening for lung cancer as a matter of public policy.

In the USA, the reaction was rather different. The Preventive Services Task Force recommended, in 2013 [51], low-dose CT screening for patients meeting the NLST criteria, with an extended age-range of up to 80, pointing out that "the personal and public health consequences of lung cancer are enormous, and even a small benefit from screening could save many lives". This seems an entirely reasonable response to a 20% mortality reduction demonstrated by NLST, and was strongly supported by the American Cancer Society [52 - 54]. In the same year however, a Cochrane review [55] concluded that more data were needed on cost effectiveness and potential harms before a recommendation could be made, but it was suggested that patients at risk should be offered a "discussion" on possible screening by a centre with adequate experience of nodule management and lung cancer treatment, a decidedly conservative response to a conclusive demonstration that screening saves lives.

The Refinement of Risk Prediction

Risk prediction and calculation are clearly key components of the process of maximising benefit and minimising harm. Bach and colleagues used data from 18,000 subjects enrolled in a retinoid prevention project (CARET) to derive a risk prediction model which was then used to evaluate risk in smokers enrolled in a low-dose CT scanning (LDCT) study [56]. Ten-year risk was found to vary between 0.8% and 15%, with evident and profound implications for screening enrolment. A ten-year risk table was generated from the model, but relatively few factors were included. Tammemagi and colleagues [57] modified the PLCO [58] model to ensure applicability to NLST data, using information from 80,375 persons in the control and intervention groups who had ever smoked. They used Cox models to establish whether the mortality reduction in NLST differed according to risk. The modified PLCO model (PLCO M2012) was found more sensitive than the NLST criteria for lung cancer detection. Eleven criteria were used, including no less than four smoking-related parameters; the most statistically significant factors were age, family history of lung cancer, smoking duration, and chronic airflow limitation, but BMI, socioeconomic status and ethnic group were also significant, and the addition of smoking intensity further improved the model. A spreadsheet calculator was made available, estimating lung cancer risk according to the PLCO (M2012) model. The authors concluded that the model predicted six-year risk of lung cancer with great accuracy, and it was estimated that its use in NLST would have led to 81 additional lung cancer diagnoses, saving a further 59 lives.

The Manchester Implementation Pilot [59]

In June 2014, the Macmillan Foundation launched the Macmillan Cancer

Improvement Partnership (MCIP), investigating potential improvements in diagnosis and treatment pathways for lung and breast cancer. The lung-cancer steering group looked at three areas: palliative-care interventions, a "RAPID" investigation pathway for suspected lung cancer, and prospects for early detection; this last workstream rapidly gained momentum, taking account of world chart-topping lung cancer figures in deprived sectors of the Manchester conurbation, and the stark realisation that lung cancer was the commonest cause of premature death in the city as a whole. We also considered issues of access, for what had been regarded hitherto as hard-to-reach populations, resistant to healthcare and screening initiatives. The project was ultimately enabled by direct Macmillan funding, and would never have gained traction without it - all the more rewarding for the fact that Early Detection has never been part of Macmillan core business, and has now been left to paddle its own canoe in the now-autonomous GM Health Economy and Combined Authority. We designed a community-based lung health check (LHC), using a portable CT scanner and interview facility based in local shopping centres. We used the PLCO (M2012) model at a six-year lung cancer risk threshold of 1.51, considered optimal in risk/benefit terms. Patients at or above that threshold were offered immediate LDCT, and the nodules identified were managed in accordance with BTS guidelines. Demand was high in this reportedly "resistant" population, and an incredible 56% of 1429 first attendees qualified for screening, 1384 of them scanned, the non-scanned patients being those who had already had recent scans or who were unwilling or unable to be scanned. 4.7% of scans were positive, 12.7% indeterminate. 81 individuals (5.9%) were assessed in a lung cancer clinic and 42 patients were confirmed to have lung cancer, 46 cancers diagnosed in the 42 subjects (Fig. **3**). The false-positive rate was 48%, but no single patient underwent surgical intervention for benign disease, and only four had a percutaneous biopsy, of whom 1 developed a pneumothorax, so "overdiagnosis" was not a significant issue. 63% of cancers were at stage 1, 17.4% stage 2, 8.7% stage 3, 11% stage 4 (Fig. **4**), so almost an exact mirror image of normal distribution at diagnosis, including the spectrum encountered with 399 lung cancer patients diagnosed in the same geographical locality during the previous year. The surgical resection rate was 65%, and curative-intent therapy was offered to 89% of all cases. The median deprivation rank was within the lowest English decile (Fig. **5**), markedly lower than UKLS (2873 vs 17,374), and in contrast to most screening studies, where participation tends to favour the affluent and better educated.

Lung cancer detection: prevalence round

Prevalence 3% = 1c: detected every 33s

46 Cancers Detected

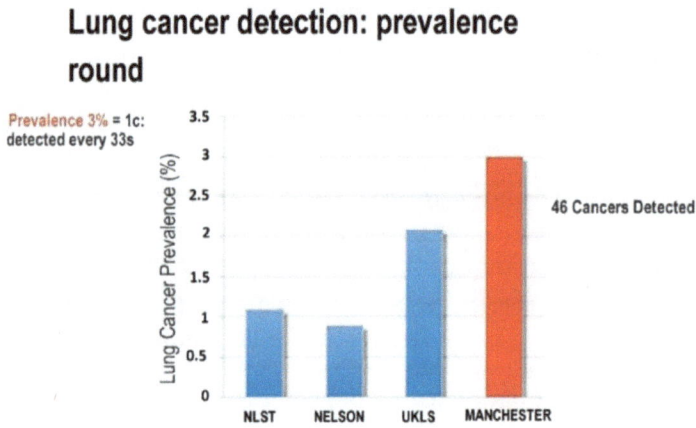

Fig. (3). Manchester Lung Health Check.

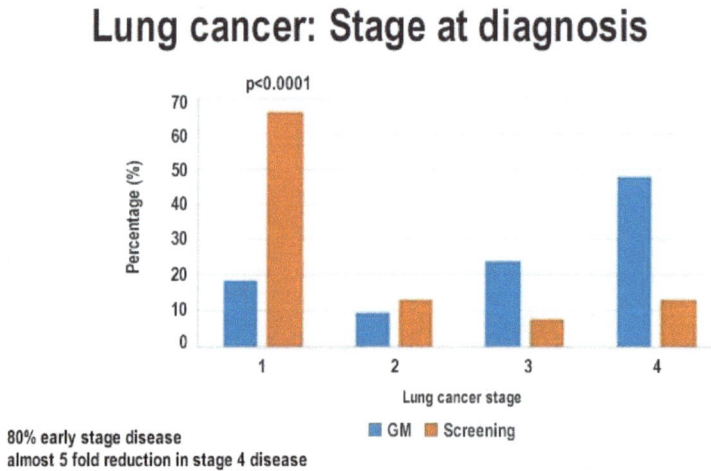

Lung cancer: Stage at diagnosis

p<0.0001

80% early stage disease
almost 5 fold reduction in stage 4 disease

Fig. (4). Manchester Lung Health Check.

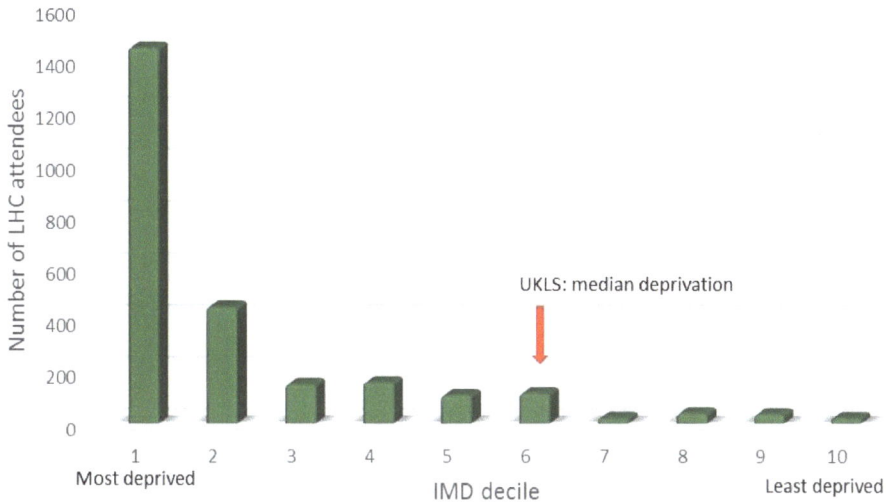

Fig. (5). Manchester Lung Health Check – reaching the hard-to-reach.

Overdiagnosis was minimised by a nodule protocol which actively investigated only those patients with PET avidity or a volume doubling time of less than 400 days, and all resected adenocarcinomas were found to have invasive (rather than lepidic) histopathology.

The second screening round yielded 2.5% positive scans, 6% indeterminate. Compliance remained high, at 90%, and of 29 patients assessed in lung cancer clinics 19 had cancers, 15 of whom were radically treated. There were no interval cancers between the two rounds. There was one resection of benign (granulomatous) disease in this second round.

Over both screening rounds, 4.4% of the cohort were diagnosed with lung cancer, equivalent to 1 cancer for every 23 persons screened. This is more than 2.5 times that seen in NLST and NELSON, and the benign surgical resection rate was ten-fold lower than in those two studies. A review of second-round cancers showed no "misses" from the first round, but retrospective scrutiny of those scans suggested that bi-annual screening could have resulted in a stage shift, with a volume doubling time estimated at only 45 days, so an evidently aggressive phenotype. The false-positive rate was much lower in the second round, probably because of the availability of a comparator baseline scan, as has been noted in other studies [58]. The service showed a baseline sensitivity of 89.4%, specificity 97%.

The Manchester project has received, on the whole, a fairly cool reception from screening experts within the UK, but is nevertheless being rolled out for a much larger population in North Manchester, with plans then to extend it to the now-autonomous Greater Manchester Combined Authority. Of note, the Manchester LHC methodology has also now been incorporated into the NHS long-term plan.

I have discussed this study in some detail because it is so far the only implementation project based on the NLST study with evaluable data. It illustrates that deprived and high-risk populations can be accessed by a targeted and community-based approach, and that a high proportion of curable early-stage cancers can be identified. "Detect, Resect" does work then, a conclusion supported by the findings of two large randomized studies. The long awaited NELSON trial [61] has shown a 26% mortality reduction in high-risk men, and an astonishing 61% reduction in high-risk women over a ten-year period, and with a stage shift comparable with other studies, identifying 65-70% of cancers at stage 1-2. An Italian study, MILD [60, 62], has shown that annual or biennial low-dose CT scanning can reduce lung cancer-specific mortality by 39%, all-cause mortality by 32%, at ten years.

The use of targeted screening provides additional health benefits: they include detection of non-malignant conditions which can benefit from early intervention, examples including coronary-artery calcification as an indicator of ischaemic heart disease, emphysema, interstitial lung disease, and a variety of other pulmonary, and some non-pulmonary, findings requiring medical attention. Lung cancer screening is also a powerful "teachable moment" for smoking cessation, as has been observed by a number of authors [63].

CONCLUSION

There have been a number of approaches to the early detection of lung cancer in the course of the last half-century. Molecular and genetic techniques looking at the biology of early lung cancer have yielded a substantial body of research evidence but have not been found applicable to population screening. Fluorescence bronchoscopy is a valuable technique in the identification and mapping of early central cancer, but does not lend itself to primary screening other than perhaps for very high-risk groups. The primary screening of high-risk populations has been attempted principally by imaging techniques, supplemented in some instances by sputum cytology. Early randomised studies using principally chest x-ray have shown highly significant increases in resectability and survival, but apparently did not improve mortality, though it now appears that this could have been to some extent due to under-powering, contamination, and limited compliance. The development of risk stratification, low-dose CT scanning, and nodule management protocols has transformed the landscape, and the NLST study of 2011 did demonstrate a convincing reduction in cancer-specific and overall mortality, but was met with complete inaction in practical and clinical terms in Europe and the UK. More recent studies, including NLST, NELSON and MILD, have confirmed that a marked stage-shift can be achieved, with substantial improvements in mortality of up to 61% over ten years, despite which no health economy has adopted lung-cancer screening, and the UK national climate remains cool. The Manchester Lung Health Check implementation project has confirmed, over a two-year period, that community-based LDCT screening in the most deprived areas of the city attracts very high compliance and has detected one lung cancer for every 23 persons screened, most at a curable stage, with acceptable levels of over-diagnosis and very few inappropriate interventions for non-malignant disease. To date, there have been no other evaluable implementations of LDCT screening, but there appears to be sufficient evidence now to proceed, and an expanded programmed is planned in the GM health economy, LHC methodology also now incorporated into the NHS plan. There are indications that the outlook for lung cancer patients can be transformed by the targeted screening of high-risk populations; in the meantime there is also a need for more rapid diagnostic pathways for patients with suspected lung cancer, a need also to greatly increase our primary prevention efforts by expanding and fully funding a comprehensive population-based smoking-cessation programme, rather than the actual disinvestment which has unaccountably taken place. A more engaged approach to at-risk smoking populations in both primary and secondary care might also be of benefit [64], perhaps with more ready access to chest x-ray, admittedly a poor substitute for CT scanning, but a marked improvement on nothing.

CONSENT FOR PUBLICATION

Not applicable.

CONFLICT OF INTEREST

The author confirms that this chapter's contents have no conflict of interest, other than his own active role in the development of the Manchester Lung Health programme.

ACKNOWLEDGEMENTS

Enza Rickers is acknowledged for preparing the text; Haval Balata, for kindly reviewing the manuscript; Janet Tonge, for her help and support in promoting the early detection of lung cancer, and Keyvan Moghissi for inviting this contribution, and for his advice and friendship over many years.

REFERENCES

[1]   Parrott S, Godfrey C, Raw M, West R, McNeill A. Guidance for commissioners on the cost effectiveness of smoking cessation interventions. Thorax 1998; 53 (Suppl. 5 Pt 2): S1-S38. [PMID: 10226676]

[2]   Orme ME, Hogue SL, Kennedy LM, Paine AC, Godfrey C. Development of the health and economic consequences of smoking interactive model. Tob Control 2001; 10(1): 55-61. [http://dx.doi.org/10.1136/tc.10.1.55] [PMID: 11226362]

[3]   Woolacott NF, Jones L, Forbes CA, *et al.* The clinical effectiveness and cost-effectiveness of bupropion and nicotine replacement therapy for smoking cessation: a systematic review and economic evaluation. Health Technol Assess 2002; 6(16): 1-245. [http://dx.doi.org/10.3310/hta6160] [PMID: 12269277]

[4]   Goodwin PJ, Shepherd FA. Economic issues in lung cancer: a review. J Clin Oncol 1998; 16(12): 3900-12. [http://dx.doi.org/10.1200/JCO.1998.16.12.3900] [PMID: 9850036]

[5]   Vera-Llonch M, Weycker D, Glass A, *et al.* Healthcare costs in patients with metastatic lung cancer receiving chemotherapy. BMC Health Serv Res 2011; 11: 305. [http://dx.doi.org/10.1186/1472-6963-11-305] [PMID: 22074001]

[6]   Lovly C. KRAS in Non-Small Cell Lung Cancer (NSCLC). My Cancer Genome 2015.https://www.mycancergenome.org/content/disease/lungcancer/kras/(Updated June 18)

[7]   Tong J, Sun X, Cheng H, *et al.* Expression of p16 in non-small cell lung cancer and its prognostic significance: a meta-analysis of published literatures. Lung Cancer 2011; 74(2): 155-63. [http://dx.doi.org/10.1016/j.lungcan.2011.04.019] [PMID: 21621871]

[8]   Mascaux B. Fragile histidine triad protein expression in non-small cell lung cancer and correlation with Ki-67 and with p53C. European Respiratory Journal 2003; 21: 753-8. [http://dx.doi.org/10.1183/09031936.03.00090202]

[9]   Sevilya. Low integrated DNA repair score and lung cancer risk. Cancer Prev Res 2013; 7(4): 398-406.

[10]   Brenner DR, Fanidi A, Grankvist K, *et al.* Inflammatory Cytokines and Lung Cancer Risk in 3 Prospective Studies. Am J Epidemiol 2017; 185(2): 86-95. [http://dx.doi.org/10.1093/aje/kww159] [PMID: 27998891]

[11]   Saalberg Y, Wolff M. VOC breath biomarkers in lung cancer. Clin Chim Acta 2016; 459(1): 5-9. [http://dx.doi.org/10.1016/j.cca.2016.05.013] [PMID: 27221203]

[12]   Kemp RA, Reinders DM, Turic B. Detection of lung cancer by automated sputum cytometry. J Thorac Oncol 2007; 2(11): 993-1000. [http://dx.doi.org/10.1097/JTO.0b013e318158d488] [PMID: 17975489]

[13]   Stephen G Spiro, Allan Hackshaw. The current UK lungSEARCH trial. Research in progress – LungSEARCH: a randomised controlled trial of surveillance for the early detection of lung cancer in a high-risk group. LungSEARCH Collaborative Group [http://dx.doi.org/10.1136/thoraxjnl-2015-207433]

[14]   Taniguchi K, Uchida J, Nishino K, *et al.* Quantitative detection of EGFR mutations in circulating tumor DNA derived from lung adenocarcinomas. Clin Cancer Res 2011; 17(24): 7808-15. [http://dx.doi.org/10.1158/1078-0432.CCR-11-1712] [PMID: 21976538]

[15]   Kimura T, Holland WS, Kawaguchi T, *et al.* Mutant DNA in plasma of lung cancer patients: potential for monitoring response to therapy. Ann N Y Acad Sci 2004; 1022: 55-60. [http://dx.doi.org/10.1196/annals.1318.010] [PMID: 15251940]

[16]   Tissot C, Toffart AC, Villar S, *et al.* Circulating free DNA concentration is an independent prognostic biomarker in lung cancer. Eur Respir J 2015; 46(6): 1773-80. [http://dx.doi.org/10.1183/13993003.00676-2015] [PMID: 26493785]

[17] Newman AM, Bratman SV, To J, *et al.* An ultrasensitive method for quantitating circulating tumor DNA with broad patient coverage. Nat Med 2014; 20(5): 548-54.
[http://dx.doi.org/10.1038/nm.3519] [PMID: 24705333]

[18] Jiang T, Ren S, Zhou C. Role of circulating-tumor DNA analysis in non-small cell lung cancer. Lung Cancer 2015; 90(2): 128-34.
[http://dx.doi.org/10.1016/j.lungcan.2015.09.013] [PMID: 26415994]

[19] Kukita Y, Uchida J, Oba S, *et al.* Quantitative identification of mutant alleles derived from lung cancer in plasma cell-free DNA via anomaly detection using deep sequencing data. PLoS One 2013; 8(11)e81468
[http://dx.doi.org/10.1371/journal.pone.0081468] [PMID: 24278442]

[20] Jamal-Hanjani M, Hackshaw A, Ngai Y, *et al.* Tracking genomic cancer evolution for precision medicine: the lung TRACERx study. PLoS Biol 2014; 12(7)e1001906
[http://dx.doi.org/10.1371/journal.pbio.1001906] [PMID: 25003521]

[21] McGranahan, Nicholas, *et al.* "Clonal status of actionable driver events and the timing of mutational processes in cancer evolution." Science translational medicine 2015; 7.283: 283ra54-4.

[22] Palcic B, Lam S, Hung J, MacAulay C. Detection and localization of early lung cancer by imaging techniques. Chest 1991; 99(3): 742-3.
[http://dx.doi.org/10.1378/chest.99.3.742] [PMID: 1995233]

[23] Hung J, Lam S, LeRiche JC, Palcic B. Autofluorescence of normal and malignant bronchial tissue. Lasers Surg Med 1991; 11(2): 99-105.
[http://dx.doi.org/10.1002/lsm.1900110203] [PMID: 2034016]

[24] Lam S, Kennedy T, Unger M, *et al.* Localization of bronchial intraepithelial neoplastic lesions by fluorescence bronchoscopy. Chest 1998; 113(3): 696-702.
[http://dx.doi.org/10.1378/chest.113.3.696] [PMID: 9515845]

[25] Kurie JM, Lee JS, Morice RC, *et al.* Autofluorescence bronchoscopy in the detection of squamous metaplasia and dysplasia in current and former smokers. J Natl Cancer Inst 1998; 90(13): 991-5.
[http://dx.doi.org/10.1093/jnci/90.13.991] [PMID: 9665147]

[26] Venmans BJ, van der Linden JC, van Boxem AJ, *et al.* Early detection of pre-invasive lesions in high risk patients. A comparison of conventional fiberoptic and fluorescence bronchoscopy. J Bronchology 1998; 5: 280-3.
[http://dx.doi.org/10.1097/00128594-199810000-00003]

[27] Kennedy TC, Hirsch FR, Miller Y, *et al.* A randomized study of fluorescence bronchoscopy versus white light bronchoscopy for early detection of lung cancer in high risk patients. Lung Cancer 2000; 29: 244a.
[http://dx.doi.org/10.1016/S0169-5002(00)80835-1]

[28] Lam S, MacAulay C, leRiche JC, Palcic B. Detection and localization of early lung cancer by fluorescence bronchoscopy. Cancer 2000; 89(11) (Suppl.): 2468-73.
[http://dx.doi.org/10.1002/1097-0142(20001201)89:11+<2468::AID-CNCR25>3.0.CO;2-V] [PMID: 11147629]

[29] Cortese DA, Edell ES. Kinsey. Photodynamic therapy of lung cancer. Semin Oncol 1994; 21: 15-9.

[30] Cortese DA, Edell ES, Kinsey JH. Photodynamic therapy for early stage squamous cell carcinoma of the lung. Mayo Clin Proc 1997; 72(7): 595-602.
[http://dx.doi.org/10.1016/S0025-6196(11)63563-5] [PMID: 9212759]

[31] Venmans BJW, van Boxem TJM, Smit EF, Postmus PE, Sutedja TG. Outcome of bronchial carcinoma in situ. Chest 2000; 117(6): 1572-6.
[http://dx.doi.org/10.1378/chest.117.6.1572] [PMID: 10858385]

[32] Breuer RH, Pasic A, Smit EF, *et al.* The natural course of preneoplastic lesions in bronchial

epithelium. Clin Cancer Res 2005; 11(2 Pt 1): 537-43.
[PMID: 15701838]

[33]   Sato M. The natural history of radiologically occult squamous cell carcinoma: a Retrospective study of overdiagnosis bias. Chest 2004; 126(1): 108-13.
[http://dx.doi.org/10.1378/chest.126.1.108] [PMID: 15249450]

[34]   Geddes DM. Natural History of Lung Cancer Review Based on Rates of Tumour Growth. British Journal of Diseases of the Chest 1979; 73: 1-17.
[http://dx.doi.org/10.1016/0007-0971(79)90002-0]

[35]   Goldstraw P, Chansky K, Crowley J, *et al.* The IASLC Lung Cancer Staging Project: Proposals for Revision of the TNM Stage Groupings in the Forthcoming (Eighth) Edition of the TNM Classification for Lung Cancer. J Thorac Oncol 2016; 11(1): 39-51.
[http://dx.doi.org/10.1016/j.jtho.2015.09.009] [PMID: 26762738]

[36]   Fontana RS, Sanderson DR, Woolner LB, Taylor WF, Miller WE, Muhm JR. Lung cancer screening: the Mayo program. J Occup Med 1986; 28(8): 746-50.
[http://dx.doi.org/10.1097/00043764-198608000-00038] [PMID: 3528436]

[37]   Marcus PM, Bergstralh EJ, Fagerstrom RM, *et al.* Lung cancer mortality in the Mayo Lung Project: impact of extended follow-up. J Natl Cancer Inst 2000; 92(16): 1308-16.
[http://dx.doi.org/10.1093/jnci/92.16.1308] [PMID: 10944552]

[38]   Danish Lung Cancer Screening Trial. Thorax 2012; 67: 296e301.
[http://dx.doi.org/10.1136/thoraxjnl-2011-200736]

[39]   Pedersen JH, Ashraf H, Dirksen A, *et al.* The Danish randomized lung cancer CT

[40]   screening trial overall design and results of the prevalence round. J Thorac Oncol 2011.

[41]   Saghir Z, Ashraf H, Dirksen A, *et al.* Contamination during 4 years of annual CT

[42]   screening in the Danish Lung Cancer Screening Trial (DLCST). Lung Cancer 2011; 71: 323e7. 2009;4:608e14.

[43]   Fontana R S. Screening for Lung Cancer – a critique of the Mayo Clinic Project. Cancer 1991 February; (Supplement): 1155-64.

[44]   Henschke CI, Yankelevitz DF. CT screening for lung cancer. Radiol Clin North Am 2000; 38(3): 487-495, viii.
[http://dx.doi.org/10.1016/S0033-8389(05)70179-2] [PMID: 10855256]

[45]   Tockman MS. Survival and mortality from lung cancer in a screened population: The Johns Hopkins Study. Chest 1986; 89: 324S-5S.
[http://dx.doi.org/10.1378/chest.89.4_Supplement.324S-a]

[46]   Melamed MR, Flehinger BJ, Zaman MB, Heelan RT, Perchick WA, Martini N. Screening for early lung cancer. Results of the Memorial Sloan-Kettering study in New York. Chest 1984; 86(1): 44-53.
[http://dx.doi.org/10.1378/chest.86.1.44] [PMID: 6734291]

[47]   Kubik A, Parkin DM, Khlat M, Erban J, Polak J, Adamec M. Lack of benefit from semi-annual screening for cancer of the lung: follow-up report of a randomized controlled trial on a population of high-risk males in Czechoslovakia. Int J Cancer 1990; 45(1): 26-33.
[http://dx.doi.org/10.1002/ijc.2910450107] [PMID: 2404878]

[48]   Henschke CI, McCauley DI, Yankelevitz DF, *et al.* Early Lung Cancer Action Project: overall design and findings from baseline screening. Lancet 1999; 354(9173): 99-105.
[http://dx.doi.org/10.1016/S0140-6736(99)06093-6] [PMID: 10408484]

[49]   Aberle DR, Adams AM, Berg CD, *et al.* Reduced lung-cancer mortality with low-dose computed tomographic screening. N Engl J Med 2011; 365(5): 395-409.
[http://dx.doi.org/10.1056/NEJMoa1102873] [PMID: 21714641]

[50] Black WC, Gareen IF, Soneji SS, *et al.* Cost-effectiveness of CT screening in the National Lung Screening Trial. N Engl J Med 2014; 371(19): 1793-802.
[http://dx.doi.org/10.1056/NEJMoa1312547] [PMID: 25372087]

[51] Field JK, Duffy SW, Baldwin DR, *et al.* UK Lung Cancer RCT Pilot Screening Trial: baseline findings from the screening arm provide evidence for the potential implementation of lung cancer screening. Thorax 2016; 71(2): 161-70.
[http://dx.doi.org/10.1136/thoraxjnl-2015-207140] [PMID: 26645413]

[52] USPSTF, updated lung cancer 2004 screening guidelines. 2004; 4.3.14.

[53] American Cancer Society lung cancer screening guidelines, first published 11113 2011.

[54] 2011.
[http://dx.doi.org/10.3322/caac.21172]

[55] Manser R, *et al.* Cochrane Database of Systematic Reviews. Screening for lung cancer published 21613 2013 Jun 21;
[http://dx.doi.org/10.1002/14651858.CD001991.pub3]

[56] Bach PB, Kattan MW, Thornquist MD, *et al.* Variations in lung cancer risk among smokers. J Natl Cancer Inst 2003; 95(6): 470-8.
[http://dx.doi.org/10.1093/jnci/95.6.470] [PMID: 12644540]

[57] Tammemägi MC, Katki HA, Hocking WG, *et al.* Selection criteria for lung-cancer screening. N Engl J Med 2013; 368(8): 728-36.
[http://dx.doi.org/10.1056/NEJMoa1211776] [PMID: 23425165]

[58] Prorok PC, *et al.* Design of the prostate, lung, colorectal and ovarian (PLCO) cancer screening trial. Controlled Clinical Trials 21;6(suppl 1): 273s-309s.

[59] Crosbie PA, *et al.* Implementing lung cancer screening: baseline and second-round results from a community-based 'Lung Health Check' pilot in deprived areas of Manchester. Thorax 2018; 0: 1-5.

[60] Lopes PA, Picozzi G, Mascalchi M, *et al.* Design, recruitment and baseline results of the ITALUNG trial for lung cancer screening with low-dose CT. Lung Cancer 2009; 64: 34e40.
[http://dx.doi.org/10.1016/j.lungcan.2008.07.003]

[61] Harry J de Koning *et al.* Reduced Lung Cancer with Volume CT Screening in a Randomized Trial. N Engl J Med 2020; 382: 503-13.

[62] Pastorino U, Silva M, Sestini S, *et al.* Prolonged lung cancer screening reduced 10-year mortality in the MILD trial: new confirmation of lung cancer screening efficacy. Annals of Oncology, mdz117 2019.
[http://dx.doi.org/10.1093/annonc/mdz117]

[63] Ostroff JS, Buckshee N, Mancuso CA, Yankelevitz DF, Henschke CI. Smoking cessation following CT screening for early detection of lung cancer. Prev Med 2001; 33(6): 613-21.
[http://dx.doi.org/10.1006/pmed.2001.0935] [PMID: 11716658]

[64] Kennedy MPT, Cheyne L, Darby M, *et al.* Lung cancer stage-shift following a symptom awareness campaign. Thorax 2018; 73(12): 1128-36.
[http://dx.doi.org/10.1136/thoraxjnl-2018-211842] [PMID: 29950525]

CHAPTER 4

Imaging for Lung Cancer

Gerard Avery[1,*] and **Keyvan Moghissi**[2]

[1] *Hull & East Yorkshire NHS Trust, Hull, UK*

[2] *The Yorkshire Laser Centre, Goole, UK*

Abstract: (Section 1) In this section, the current practice of imaging is described. Attention has been focused on the role of radiology in the staging of lung cancer and the pulmonary nodule. New methods, such as the potential use of Nano-technology in medical imaging, are briefly referred here.

(Section 2) In this short section, the physics of fluorescence is briefly described. The application of florescence imaging in clinical practice of lung cancer are presented. Autofluorescence imaging for endobronchial cancer which is now an established method and is described in some detail.

Keywords: CT Scan, Future Technology, X-Ray.

SECTION 1 CURRENT PRACTICE AND FUTURE DIRECTION OF THORACIC IMAGING DIAGNOSIS/STAGING

Chest Radiography

In the majority of situations, the chest radiograph remains the first line investigation for the evaluation of any thoracic disease. It is important that the best quality image is obtained *e.g.*: positioning (erect, posteroanterior - PA), breathing (deep inspiration), non-rotated.

Other projections that can augment the technique include: lateral, allows better visualization of the retrocardiac and posterior costophrenic areas, lordotic, angling

---

* **Corresponding author Gerard R Avery:** Hull & East Yorkshire NHS Trust, Hull, UK; Tel: +441482623205; Fax: +441482624018; E-mail: ged.avery@hey.nhs.uk

Keyvan Moghissi, Jack Kastelik, Philip Barber & Peyman Sardari Nia (Eds.)

the tube towards the head to improve the visualization of the apices, and oblique, to review pleura and ribs.

However, the sensitivity of chest radiography for detection of pulmonary nodules is low, primarily due to the image being a 2D rendering of a 3D object and CT evaluation has reduced the use of the additional views.

A "negative" chest radiograph cannot be relied upon to exclude lung cancer, but it can detect both radically treatable and metastatic lung cancer – primarily pulmonary or bone lesions.

It is estimated that up to 30% of pulmonary nodules may not be appreciated or may be misinterpreted [1, 2]. In addition, there is the potential to overcall nodules in up to 20% of the cases either due to composite opacities or lesions outside the lungs being misinterpreted [3].

There are developments in both acquisition and review which, although not currently routinely used, can improve the performance of the chest radiograph in nodule detection.

Dual-energy subtraction (DES) acquires two images; one at normal high energy, KVp, and a second at low energy, which allows better delineation of high-density structures, bone or calcification. Either image can be reviewed separately, or it is also possible to subtract the bone image to improve the detection of soft tissue abnormalities, including pulmonary nodules [4].

Digital Tomosynthesis (DTS) is an acquisition technique to acquire multiple coronal images reducing the overlap of structures, which are increasingly blurred the further they are from the in-focus plane and provides better spatial resolution than coronal reconstructions from CT [5] (Fig. **1**). This technique improves the visualization of pulmonary nodules and reduces false positive findings. A meta-analysis of 16 studies gave per-patient sensitivity and specificity for the detection of pulmonary nodules by DTS of 85% (95% CI 83-88%) and 95% (95% CI 93-96%) compared to chest radiography 47% (955 CI 44-51%) and 37% (95% CI34-40%) [6].

Computer Aided Detection (CAD) has been around as a concept since the 1960's, and commercial systems for chest radiographs are available. The development of artificial intelligence and deep learning has increased the sophistication of the systems [7]. Although its use in chest radiography has been limited, currently regarded as an adjunct to a radiologist review rather than a stand-alone assessment tool, there are recent studies using different techniques which have shown nodule detection sensitivity and specificities of 92% and 86% [8], and 62% and 96% [9].

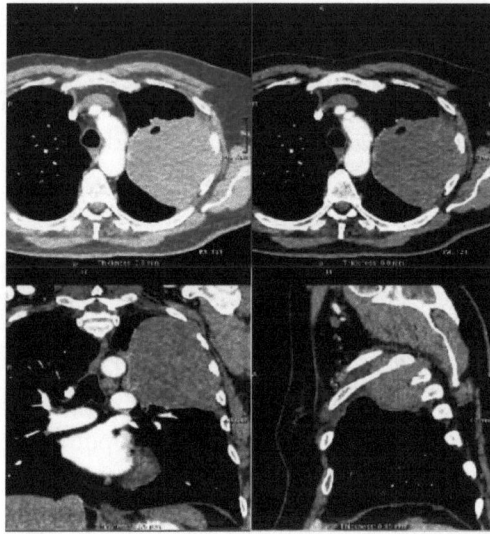

Fig. (1). Sagittal and coronal reconstructions showing to better effect chest wall/rib invasion.

Computed Tomography

The standard protocol for the assessment of suspected lung cancer is contrast enhanced CT of the chest and upper abdomen to allow assessment of the liver and adrenals. Coronal and sagittal reconstructions should be routinely performed, they have shown to provide additional information to the primary axial data set in approximately 10% of the cases (Fig. **2**) [10].

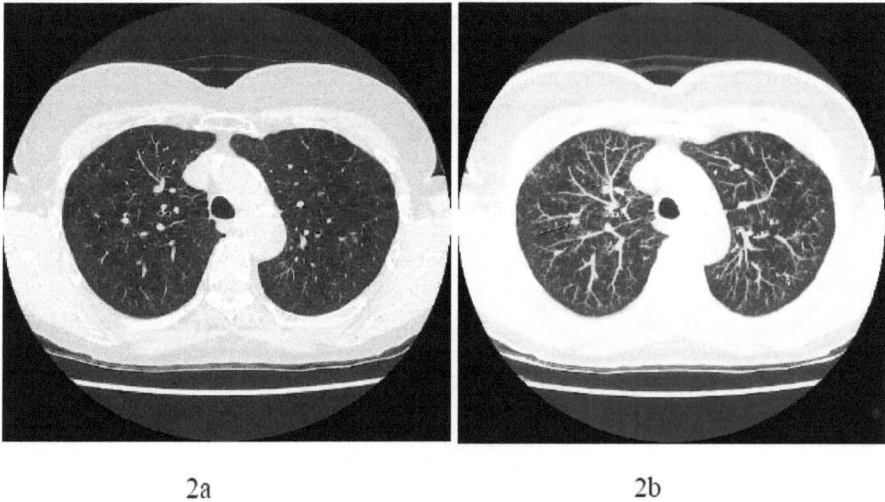

2a   2b

Fig. (2). A. Source axial image 10mm slice thickness B. Maximum intensity projection image 8mm slice thickness.

For example, they can be particularly useful for the evaluation of Pancoast tumors, mediastinal, pleural and diaphragm assessment and are essential for assessing vertebral collapse.

Maximum Intensity Projection (MIP) images are also recommended. In this reconstruction technique, only the highest attenuation voxel, along lines projected through the data set, are used to create a sliding slab of data, the thickness of which is determined at the time of reconstruction *e.g.* 5-10 mm. These images improve the detection of pulmonary nodules. Axial MIPs have been shown to perform better than coronal MIPS and one study has suggested that an 8 mm thick slab is optimal for current generation CT scanners [11].

Other reconstructions can be applied to the data *e.g.* Volume Reconstruction – this is commonly used in orthopaedic CT for bone evaluation and has been used to give 3D information on fissural integrity, vascular, and bronchial anatomy (Fig. 2c).

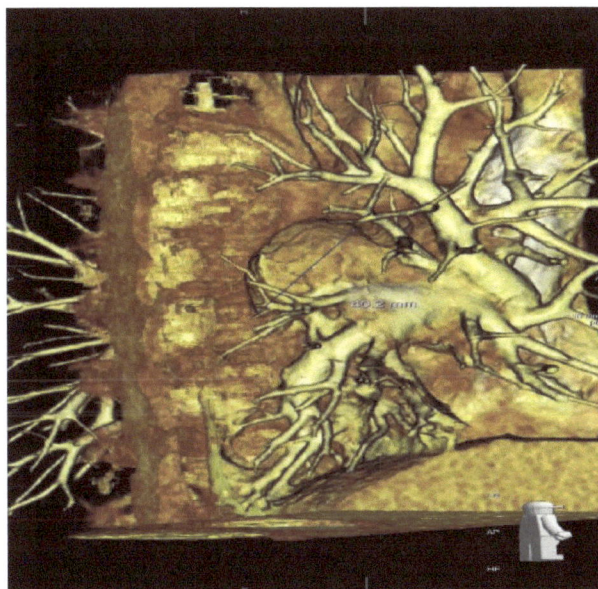

Fig. (2c). 3D rendering of right lower lobe tumor.

This can be useful in planning a surgery, including video-assisted and robotic techniques. 3D techniques also can be used to create virtual bronchoscopy allowing an endoluminal view of the major airways. The use of these depends upon the need in individual cases.

CAD of pulmonary nodules on CT is one of the most widely used applications of this technique. When used as an adjunct to a radiologist, it has shown to consistently detect nodules, which were undetected by the radiologist, of most benefit for smaller nodules, and reduces inter-observer variability [12].

The challenge is to integrate CAD into routine practice as a second read, following a primary radiologist review, this is not the current common reporting practice. However, a recent study has looked at using CAD not only in the detection of pulmonary nodules, but also in prepopulating a report template. In this small study, the additional reporting step reduced total reading times from 7-44% for the three radiologists [13].

Following the detection of a pulmonary nodule, a decision has to be made as to the significance of the finding. The prevalence of lung nodules and lung cancer varies between countries, for instance, the incidence of TB in most western European countries is <10 cases per 100,000/year whilst in Asian countries, rates are often several times higher *e.g.* China 70/100,000 and Thailand 119/100,000, which is reflected in a higher prevalence of nodules (Table **1**) [14 - 16].

Table 1. Prevalence of lung nodules and cancer by geographical area [14].

Geographical Area	Nodule Prevalence % (Mean Range)	Lung Cancer Prevalence % (Mean Range)
North America	23 (2-53)	1.7 (0-4.0)
Europe	29 (8-53)	1.2 (0.2-2.4)
East Asia	35.5 (35-36)	0.54 (0.50-0.57)

However, the prevalence of lung cancer is significantly lower than the prevalence of lung nodules and therefore, the challenge is to detect the malignant nodules, whilst minimizing the investigation/imaging of benign nodules and minimizing patient anxiety.

Pulmonary Nodule

A pulmonary nodule is defined as being between 3-30 mm in size. The size significantly affects the prevalence of malignancy (Table **2**) [17]. A nodule is also characterized by density, shape, and position, These factors influence the prevalence of malignancy and therefore, management as does the individual's clinical predictors.

Table 2. Relationship between nodule size and prevalence of malignancy [17].

Diameter mm	Prevalence of Malignancy %
<5	0-1
5-10	6-28
≥10	33-60
≥20	64-82

There are multiple pulmonary nodules management guidelines available, for example, British Thoracic Society [14], Fleischner Society [15], and Consensus Guidelines for Asia [16]. These have been developed using the data from major international lung cancer screening studies and local considerations. It is important that an appropriate guideline and standardized imaging protocols are used to allow accurate comparison between follow-up studies.

A significant challenge is to have reproducible measurement techniques to evaluate the growth of nodules on follow-up scans and the various methods include one, two, or three dimensional measurement .

One-dimensional measurement of maximal diameter is used by RECIST (Response Evaluation Criteria in Solid Tumours). Two dimensional measurements: World Health Organisation - multiply maximal longitudinal and transverse diameters on an axial image to give cross-sectional area; Fleischner Society - average diameter from maximal long and short axis on an axial image. There can be significant differences in 2D measurement between observers, most marked in subsolid nodules and asymmetrical growth may not be detected on one or two dimensional imaging.

Three dimensional measurements are considered more representative of nodule growth and are mainly automated/semi-automated programmes. However, volume estimation can be affected by technical factors *e.g.* slice thickness and reconstruction algorithm; patient factors *e.g.* cardiac/respiratory motion and nodule density; software factors *e.g.* variation between different programmes in segmentation and correction of partial volume artifact [17]. Three dimensional volume errors can be between 20-25%.

In view of these issues', guidelines use a diameter change of ≥ 2mm or a volume change of ≥ 25% as significant growth [14].

Staging

Lung cancer staging is currently undertaken using the 8th edition TNM classification, Union of International Cancer Control [18]. T staging depends upon the tumor size and involvement of structures *e.g* . pleura, mediastinum and vertebrae. N staging on CT depends upon the size of the node, measured in the short axis diameter and site. M staging depends upon the site and number of metastases.

Tumor staging is dependent upon nodule size, as mentioned above, there can be significant variation between observers therefore, guidelines for measurement have been developed for example,. window settings, and subsolid nodules are underestimated on mediastinal windows; positioning of callipers, measuring the core of a spiculated nodule not the spiculations; review of multiplanar reconstructions to obtain maximal dimensions; measurement unit, although CT scan callipers will display to 0.1 mm, measurements should be given to the nearest millimetre [21].

There are situations where CT has difficulties in determining the extent of the primary tumor. The differentiation of tumor from adjacent consolidation or atelectasis relies on different enhancement patterns between them, usually normal lung enhances to a greater extent than tumor, but this is not always the case. Similarly, the differentiation of primary tumor from adjacent node can be difficult in central tumors. Pleural involvement can be difficult to determine and the latest TNM classification reflects this with the removal of mediastinal pleural invasion as a marker of T3 disease.

CT nodal staging uses a 1cm short axis diameter to differentiate normal from enlarged nodes (1.2cm for subcarinal nodes). However, using these criteria to differentiate benign from malignant nodes gives a sensitivity of 60-83% and specificity of 77-82% [19, 20], with inflammatory nodes responsible for false positive studies and and small tumour deposits for false negative nodes. The site of the node, in respect to the primary tumor, is also important for accurate N staging. The lymph node map differentiating nodal stations is produced by the International Association for Study of Lung Cancer (IASLC) [22].

The division between right and left paratracheal nodes is the left wall of the trachea. The inferior margins of the lower paratracheal node stations, 4R and 4L, are the inferior border of the azygos vein and superior border of the left pulmonary artery, respectively. These levels form the superior boundaries of the hilar nodes, 10R and 10L, which include nodes immediately adjacent to the main bronchi.

These definitions can leave the space anterior to the tracheal bifurcation unclear and the differentiation of nodes in station 4 from station 10 is important as the staging changes from N1 to N2. Typically, nodes anterior to the bifurcation are considered to mediastinal and grouped with the lower paratracheal stations [23].

In addition, there are non-regional intrathoracic lymph nodes, including internal mammary, intercostal and diaphragmatic – *e.g.* pericardial fat or adjacent to the suprahepatic IVC. If these are considered to be involved, they are staged as distant metastases, as are axillary nodes.

CT Prognostic Information

Recent advances in CT technology may increase the ability of CT to provide prognostic information and determine the tumor type, currently dependent upon anatomical appearances. This is due to the development of dual energy CT, as with chest radiography acquiring two sets of images at different energy levels (kVp). This technique, together with the high spatial and temporal resolution of CT, allows tissue perfusion to be studied as a marker for microvascular density, angiogenesis and hypoxia, and other parameters including blood flow.

Positron Emission Tomography – Computed Tomography [PET -CT]

The routine tracer for PET-CT is [18]Flourine –fluorodeoxyglucose [FDG]. This is a marker of cellular glucose utilization. The uptake within a lesion is dependent upon blood flow, receptors status, and innate metabolic activity within the cell. It is not a marker of malignancy and its' uptake within both tumors and benign lesions, can be intense.

The evaluation compares the activity to adjacent background and usually mediastinal blood pool activity (Fig. **3**): visual assessment with abnormal activity is appreciable above adjacent background with the difference dictating the degree of concern or quantitative using a standard uptake value (SUV), this can be calculated in several ways, but most commonly using body weight to give an uptake measurement – SUV(bw).

PET –CT has roles in the evaluation of pulmonary nodules, staging of lung cancer and response assessment.

There are size limitations for the evaluation of pulmonary nodules, with the current generation of scanners nodules ≥8mm can be evaluated, although the position of the nodule within the lung can also affect the evaluation, respiratory motion artifact increases within the lung bases, potentially reducing perceived uptake although it is possible to acquire respiratory gated studies.

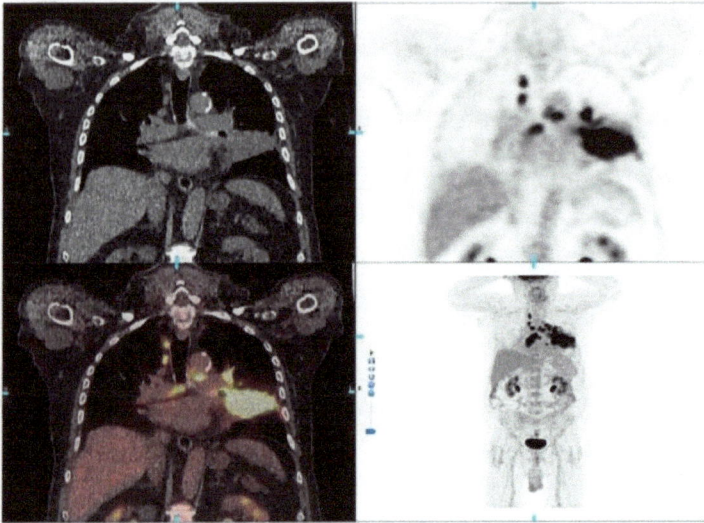

Fig. (3). ^{18}F –FDG PET CT showing increased uptake within a primary left lung tumour, ipsilateral and contralateral mediastinal lymph nodes.

PET-CT in staging is usually performed following the primary staging with CT, patients considered suitable or potentially suitable for radical treatment are evaluated [24].

PET-CT has a high sensitivity for the detection of malignancy within a solitary pulmonary nodule. A meta-analysis of 1008 nodules up to 3 cm diameter showed 95% sensitivity, the likelihood of malignancy increases above an SUV of 2.5 and in proven cancer, higher SUV values are associated with a worse prognosis. The sensitivity is reduced as some malignant tumors *e.g.* slow growing adenocarcinomas, may show low grade FDG uptake. However, the specificity was lower, 82%, reduced by the significant uptake occurring in benign lesions, such as sarcoidosis, TB or other infections including histoplasmosis [25].

There is also a reduced sensitivity in the evaluation of subsolid nodules, if malignant, these tend to be lower grade adenocarcinomas and have less intense metabolic activity. Also the heterogenous nature of the lesions with some areas of aerated tissue, together with relatively poor spatial resolution of PET, reduces the perceived uptake, the larger the solid component the less this will affect the appearance.

A recent meta- analysis on nodal staging in non-small cell lung cancer reviewed 28 studies with 3,255 patients and reported nodal sensitivity of 62% (95% CI 0.54-0.70) and specificity of 92% (95% CI 0.88-0.95) [26]. However, a Cochrane review showed higher sensitivity 0.77-0.81 and considered that the sensitivity was related to the scanner technology, NSCLC subtype and the country of origin of the study [27]. The sensitivity tends to be lower in countries with higher incidences of TB.

There are, therefore, concerns regarding the use of PET-CT as the final decider of nodal involvement. A recent study compared Endobronchial ultrasound (EBUS) in 981 patients with NSCLC who had no mediastinal involvement on PET-CT. The overall change in management, due to unexpected mediastinal upstaging, was found to be 6%. In patients staged as N0 on PET-CT, mediastinal upstaging was 0.9%, however, if staged as N1 on PET-CT 17.3% had EBUS proven mediastinal nodal disease [28].

The National Institute for Health and Care Excellence (NICE) guidance on the diagnosis and staging of lung cancer, in 2019, is based on the probability of mediastinal nodal involvement following a CT scan and the outcome of PET CT:

Low probability (nodes <10 mm): PET-CT is the preferred first test.

Intermediate probability (nodes ≥10 mm): Offer PET-CT or nodal sampling (EBUS, Endoscopic Ultrasound (EUS) or non-ultrasound guided, fine needle aspiration (FNA)) as the first test.

High probability (nodes >20 mm): Offer nodal sampling (EBUS, EUS or non-ultrasound guided FNA) as the first test.

Evaluate PET-CT-positive mediastinal nodes by mediastinal sampling (except when there is definite distant metastatic disease or a high probability that N2/N3 disease is metastatic [for example, if there is a chain of lymph nodes with high uptake] [29].

Metastatic disease is present in 18-36% of the patients with NSCLC at diagnosis and it is considered that approximately 20% of patients will relapse after radical treatment due to undetected micrometastases at the time of staging. PET-CT is a more sensitive test than CT with studies reporting up to 28% of patients having additional metastases on PET-CT and reduction in futile thoracotomies [30].

However, PET-CT has a low sensitivity for the detection of brain metastases due to the high glucose utilization of normal brain tissue and therefore, poor target to background uptake ratios and brain metastases are sometimes detected due to reduced activity in surrounding cerebral oedema rather than increased tumor uptake. In view of this, most PET-CT staging protocols do not include brain imaging and 2019 NICE guidance includes:

• Consider MRI or CT of the head in patients selected for treatment with curative

intent, especially in stage III disease.
- In patients with features suggestive of intracranial pathology, CT of the head followed by MRI, if normal, or MRI as an initial test.

PET CT can provide gross and functional tumor volume to guide radiotherapy planning. It can also evaluate response to radiotherapy and chemotherapy; activity within residual tumor, differentiation from adjacent atelectasis and post radiation fibrosis.

However, although the commonest PET tracer, FDG is non –specific targeting glucose metabolism. There are other agents which can be used to target different aspects of tumor biology for example: cellular proliferation or hypoxia; amino acid metabolism and angiogenesis. These agents are not routinely used.

^{18}F- fluorothymidine (^{18}F-FLT) is a marker for cellular proliferation, the level of uptake correlating with thymidine kinase activity and histopathological Ki-67 expression. It has a high specificity for differentiating malignant from benign lesions, but lower sensitivity than FDG for both the primary tumor and nodal disease [31].

Tumour hypoxia correlates with poorer clinical outcomes and resistance to both radiotherapy and chemotherapy [32]. The most common agent used to evaluate this is ^{18}F-fluoromisonidazole (^{18}F-FMISO),and its' potential roles include in planning dose escalation in intensity modulated radiotherapy.

Amino acid transport and metabolism is upregulated in tumors, the most frequent imaging agent used to evaluate this is ^{11}C-methionine. This agent is predominately used in imaging of brain tumors, but has been evaluated to differentiate malignant from inflammatory uptake in thoracic disease, which may be useful in countries with high incidence of non-malignant inflammatory disease *e.g.* TB [31].

Angiogenesis imaging is currently limited to small studies or pre-clinical research.

Radio-Isotope Imaging

Radio-isotope imaging of neuorendocrine tumors is routine. Somatastatin analogues labeled with either ^{18}F or ^{68}Gallium are used for PET-CT and ^{99m}Technetium and ^{111}Indium labeled agents are available for gamma camera imaging. These agents target somatastatin receptors in neuroendocrine tumor cells. The tumors are categorized into typical or atypical carcinoids. A recent meta-analysis comparing FDG PET with ^{68}Ga-DOTA peptide showed the somatostatin analog was superior to FDG for the detection of carcinoid and the SUV max ratio of DOTA peptide to FDG was an accurate predictor of histological variety with typical carcinoids, having higher peptide and lower FDG uptake [33].

Magnetic Resonance Imaging (MRI)

Currently, MRI has a limited role in the staging of the primary lung cancer and is reserved for specific issues, in particular, assessment of superior sulcus tumors and suspected extension into vertebral foramina or the spinal canal.

However, it is the best investigation for suspected brain metastases and is included in NICE guidance. MRI is a valuable technique for the evaluation of indeterminate lesions found in CT or PET-CT.

There is a potential change with the introduction of whole-body MRI (WB-MRI), the current generation scanners acquiring data from head to mid-thigh within 1 hour. A recent multicentre study compared the sensitivity and specificity of WB-MRI with standard imaging pathways of CT and PET-CT, also looking at time to complete staging and per-patient costs [34]. This found no significant difference between the sensitivity or specificity of the two pathways (Table **3**).

Table 3. Per-patient sensitivity and specificity for metastatic disease [34].

	WB-MRI	**CT/PET-CT**	**Probability**
Sensitivity	50% (95% CI 37-63)	54% (95% CI 41-67)	P=0.73
Specificity	93% (95% CI 88-96)	95% (95% CI 91-98)	P=0.45

The time to complete staging was shorter for the MRI pathway, 13(12-14) days, compared to the conventional pathway, 19(17-21) days and less costly mean per-patient costs £317 compared to £620.

It should be noted that both pathways have low sensitivity and WB-MRI performed worse for nodal assessment than the standard pathway, so that further nodal evaluation by EBUS or EUS would also have to be considered.

Ultrasound

The roles of endobronchial and endoscopic ultrasound are discussed elsewhere. However, neck and transthoracic ultrasound are important tools for staging. Involvement of supraclavicular nodes is common, and these are often accessible to ultrasound-guided biopsy or fine needle aspiration; in one study of 996 patients, 10% of them had a pathological diagnosis from this procedure [35]. In the same study, ultrasound-guided sampling of pleural effusions accounted for 5% of the pathological diagnoses.

As a dynamic technique, ultrasound allows real time assessment of tumors adjacent to the chest wall looking for signs of invasion but evaluating the relative movement. This has been evaluated by both thoracic physicians experienced in ultrasound and thoracic surgeons with sensitivities of 89%-91% and specificities of 95%-86%, compared to CT sensitivities of 42%-61% and specificities 100%-86.4% [36, 37].

Chest wall invasion is an important staging finding, upgrading tumors to T3 is associated with poorer survival and more extensive operations. In addition, it can inform the site of incision and choice of operative technique- open thoracotomy or thoracoscopic/robotic [37].

ASSESSMENT OF METASTATIC DISEASE

All the above techniques can demonstrate extra thoracic metastatic disease with variable sensitivities, and the decision as to which technique should be used will depend upon the site of suspected disease and results of earlier imaging. For instance, if a patient with known lung cancer develops hip pain then a plain radiograph is usually the first investigation. However, if the patient is being planned for radical treatment and intracranial metastatic disease is suspected or requires excluding, then MRI is the first examination.

ASSESSMENT OF TREATMENT RESPONSE

The most common imaging method of response assessment is CT and there are well defined criteria used particularly in trial situations: originally, the World Health Organisation (WHO) criteria, introduced in 1979, and later the Response Evaluation Criteria in Solid Tumours (RECIST), introduced in 2000 and revised in 2009. These use bidimensional and unidimensional measurements, respectively, to monitor target lesion size.

There have been studies looking at tumor volume for response assessment, as this is a more sensitive technique for the evaluation of growth and also potentially more reproducible.

There are concerns regarding cavitation of the tumor which can cause lesion enlargement but a reduction in viable tumor.

Pseudo progression is a recognized issue with immunomodulatory therapies and can occur in upto 5% of NSCLC patients with an initial increase in tumor size. Criteria have developed to allow assessment of response to account for this *e.g.* iRECIST, which requires follow-up scans to differentiate pseudo progression from progressive disease [38].

Other potential CT response criteria include tumor perfusion imaging, utilizing sequential post contrast imaging at different time points to evaluate contrast transfer into the extracellular space with tumor response correlating to reduction in blood flow.

FDG PET-CT is often used in the response assessment for stereotatic ablative radiotherapy (SABR). This is because the treatment can cause radiation-induced lung injury and fibrosis adjacent to the primary tumor, which can confound response assessment with CT. However, it is important to ensure that the timing of the scan is correct as the lung injury can cause transient increased uptake [39]. Imaging at 6 months minimizes this concern. There has been a study which evaluated dynamic FDG uptake and CT perfusion scanning with the acquisition taking just over 1 hour, the components showing complementary functional information [40]. This combined approach is a potential future response assessment tool for combining proliferation and hypoxia markers.

POTENTIAL FUTURE TECHNIQUES/AGENTS

PET/MRI has been evaluated in lung cancer staging and compared to PET-CT. However, two studies have not shown any overall advantage, whilst it was better at evaluation of the pulmonary veins, it was less sensitive in bronchial involvement and nodal staging [3].

MRI nano-sized contrast agents have been developed containing antibodies which can target tumour markers such as carcinoembryonic antigen and neuron-specific enolase, and have shown to increase the signal intensity in the lung cancer tissues leading to increase the accuracy and sensitivity of MRI [41].

PET tracers targeting cellular profiles are also being developed, *e.g*: Icotinib, an epidermal growth factor receptor tyrosine kinase inhibitor has been labeled with ^{18}F and shown to detect lung cancer in tumor bearing mice [42].

Daratumumab, which targets CD38, is involved in calcium transport and is also a cell surface receptor, most commonly found in haematological malignancies. It has been found in lung cancer and labeled agents have shown to detect lung cancer cells in vivo [43].

Other areas of development include PD-L1 and fibroblast-activation-protein inhibitors targeted agents. The aim of these developments is to improve diagnosis, allow biochemical biopsy in cases where it is not possible to obtain tissue, and to predict tumor therapy response.

SECTION 2

FLUORESCENCE AND FLUORESCENCE IMAGING FOR LUNG CANCER

Definition

Fluorescence refers to the re-emission of optical radiation following absorption of light energy. In a molecular system fluorescence emission is of a lower energy band (longer wavelength) than that of the excitation light.

Human tissues are made of a heterogeneous cellular mix within a matrix, each comprising of a variety of chemical compounds and their complicated optical properties.

The manner in which light interacts with a specific tissue is indicated by wavelength related absorption and scattering properties. Scattering encompasses a number of optical events and variations. Reflection is one of the events in which an incident light (Excitation light) is re-emitted with the same frequency and at a similar wave length as the excitation light. Fluorescence is another event where the re-emission is of a different wave length, usually at a higher wave length, than the excitation light.

The physics basis of fluorescence relates to the changes in electronic state(orbit) of a molecule in response to incident light energy. The lowest energy state of an electron is referred to as ground state. In response to excitation by an incident light there is enhancement of the energy level of the electrons which move to a higher energy orbit [1]. The almost immediate return to the ground state of the electron results in the release of energy (light energy/ photons) and its emission. It is during this electron energy exchange that some molecules discharge fluorescent emission in response to a specific wave length of light.

The electronic states of a molecule and their transitions from one orbit to another, with production of fluorescence emission, is usually illustrated by the Jablonsky diagram (Fig. **4**) [1, 2].

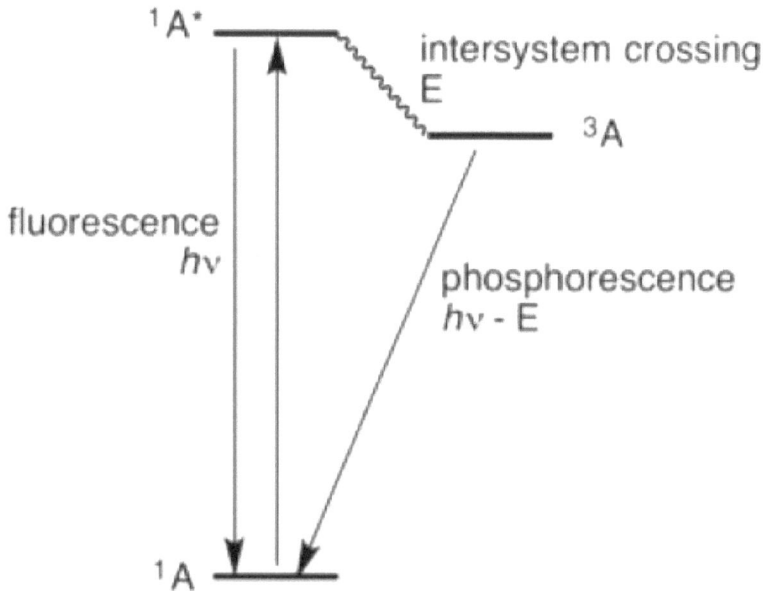

Fig. (4). A Jablonski diagram showing the excitation of molecule A to its singlet excited state ($^1A^*$) followed by intersystem crossing to the triplet state (^3A) that relaxes to the ground state by phosphorescence.

In the UV and visible part of the spectrum the optical properties of human tissues are dominated by the endogenous chromophores – atoms, which are responsible for the colour of a compound - each displaying a characteristic absorption profile. Haemoglobin, which is the principle chromophore, is non-fluorescent and demonstrates strong absorption at pre-operatively at a wave length of near 600nm. Other chromophores (such as bronchial mucosa) absorb light of bands between 250 and 500 nm but also demonstrate strong fluorescence over the range of300-700 nm. For many years now, the chemical composition of a number of these endogenous chromophores have been identified, such as collagen, elastin and flavin [3].

Fluorescence emission resulting from endogenous chromophores is referred to as auto-fluorescence (AF); it uses light in the regions of UV and blue - 400–440 nm - in the visible spectrum.

The differential fluorescence between normal and abnormal tissues forms the basis of auto fluorescence imaging and photo diagnosis.

In pulmonology medicine, auto fluorescence bronchoscopy (AFB) is one of the most important investigations for central lung cancer (CLC) [See Chapter:

Diagnosis and Therapeutic Bronchoscopy].

An incident light in the UV-blue wave length, used in AFB, will be emitted from the normal bronchial mucosa as green, whereas a neoplasm or pre-neoplastic changes usually fluoresce as red (Fig. **5**).

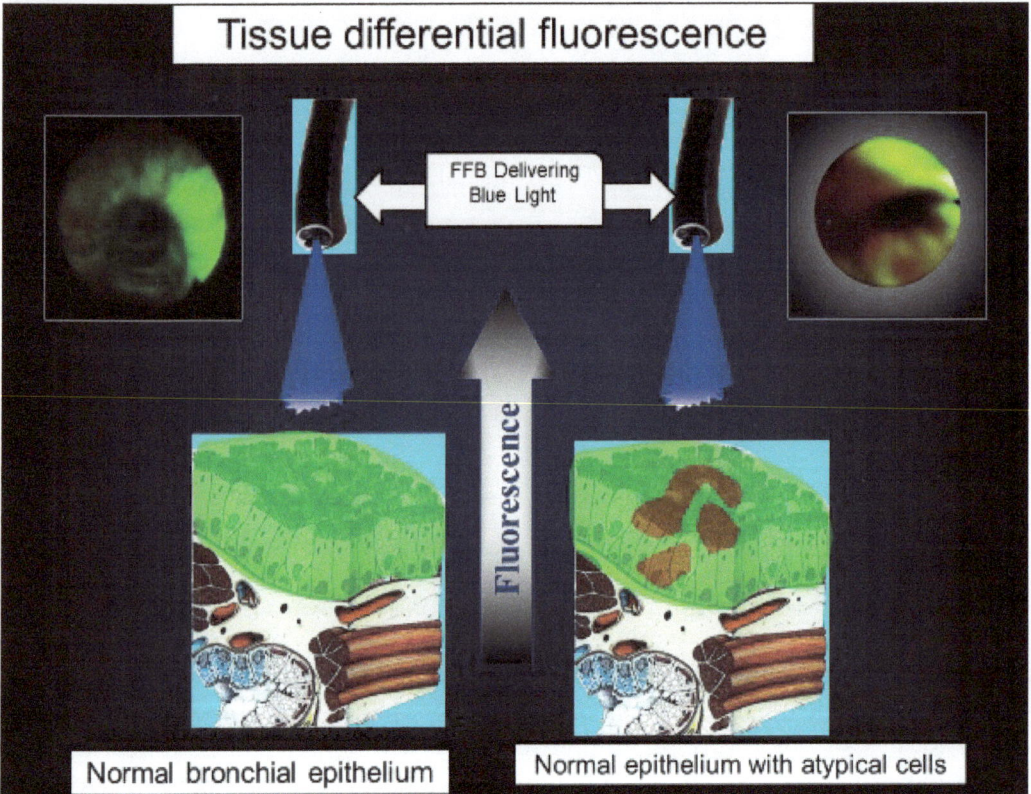

Fig. (5). Showing autofluorescence image of; the normal bronchial mucosa (left) and abnormal bronchial mucosa (right).

Auto-fluorescence can be convenient and useful in bronchology for diagnostic purposes. The sensitivity of Auto Fluorescence Bronchoscopy (AFB)is several times over and above that of standard white light bronchoscopy (WLB) [4 - 6]. An early neoplastic change of bronchial mucosa or a pre-neoplastic change at the margin of a cancer can thus be outlined by the method.

However, AFB usage for diagnostic or guided therapeutic purposes, for a lesion embedded deep in an organ, is fraught with a number of practical difficulties and erroneous results.

Firstly, the tissue penetration of the incident blue light is only 2–3 mm. Higher wavelength of light in the red or Near Infra-Red (NIR) spectrum - 700–850 nm - is needed for deeper penetration (70- 100 mm). Secondly, operative trauma and leak of blood (haemoglobin) with its strong absorption and non-fluorescent emission can falsify results.

Fluorescence emission of a tissue can be modulated by suitably designed exogenous chromophores which can be incorporated in the tissue. These will enhance the ability of the tissue to fluoresce to a light with a higher wave length band. The result will be augmentation of the differential fluorescence between normal and abnormal tissues thus increasing the diagnostic yield and increase in the discriminative power of the acquiesced fluorescent images. An exogenous chromophore is a compound which functions as a fluorescent chemical agent to generate specific fluorescence emission [7, 8]. The use of chemicals such as Aminolaevulinic acid, Methylene Blue and Indocyanine Green, which fluoresce at 630 nm, 670–700 nm and 770–800 nm respectively as chemical enhancers, are being currently evaluated and tried clinically [7 - 10].

Aminolevulinic acid guided surgery has already been successfully tried in neurosurgery [11-12] to image tumour residue at operation after resection of brain tumour, where such residues may well be indistinguishable from healthy brain tissue.

Fluorescence guided surgery (FGS) has been addressed elsewhere in this book (Chapter 15: Image-guided Surgery and Therapy for Broncho-pulmonary (Lung) Cancer). Fluorescence imaging has a number of attributes which make it, potentially, an ideal method for IGS and/or non-surgical IGT for cancer. It can identify and localize the entire tumour, including its micro-invasive components and define the boundaries of malignant and normal tissue, when coupled with appropriate devices.

More importantly, FGS can provide continuing intra-operative, real-time and updated fluorescence images, guiding the surgeon to achieve complete removal of the cancer and precancerous lesion leaving a cancer-free margin.

CONSENT FOR PUBLICATION

Not applicable.

CONFLICT OF INTEREST

The author declares that there is no conflict of interest in this chapter.

ACKNOWLEDGEMENTS

Authors would like to thank Kate Dixon and Janet Melvin.

REFERENCES (SECTION 1)

[1]   Stitik FP, Tockman MS. Radiographic screening in the early detection of lung cancer. Radiol Clin North Am 1978; 16(3): 347-66.
        [PMID: 746141]

[2]   Turkington PM, Kennan N, Greenstone MA. Misinterpretation of the chest x ray as a factor in the delayed diagnosis of lung cancer. Postgrad Med J 2002; 78(917): 158-60.
        [http://dx.doi.org/10.1136/pmj.78.917.158] [PMID: 11884698]

[3]   Erasmus JJ, Connolly JE, McAdams HP, Roggli VL. Solitary pulmonary nodules: Part I. Morphologic evaluation for differentiation of benign and malignant lesions. Radiographics 2000; 20(1): 43-58.
        [http://dx.doi.org/10.1148/radiographics.20.1.g00ja0343] [PMID: 10682770]

[4]   Li F, Engelmann R, Doi K, *et al.* Improved detection of small lung cancers with dual-energy subtraction chest radiography AJR 2008; 190: 886-891.

[5]   Chou SH, Kicska GA, Pipavath SN, Reddy GP. Digital tomosynthesis of the chest: current and emerging applications. Radiographics 2014; 34(2): 359-72.
        [http://dx.doi.org/10.1148/rg.342135057] [PMID: 24617684]

[6]   Kim JH, Lee KH, Kim K-T, *et al.* Comparison of digital tomosynthesis and chest radiography for the detection of pulmonary nodules: systematic review and meta-analysis. Br J Radiol 2016; 89(1068)20160421
        [http://dx.doi.org/10.1259/bjr.20160421] [PMID: 27759428]

[7]   Demin Yao Chunli Qin, Shi Yonghong. Computer-aided detection in chest radiography based on artificial intelligence: a survey biomedical engineering 2018. http://cs231n.stanford.edu/reports/2016/pdfs/313

[8]   Bush I. Lung nodule detection and classification 2016. http://cs231n.stanford.edu/reports/2016/pdfs/313

[9]   Wang C, Elazab A, Wu J, Hu Q. Lung nodule classification using deep feature fusion in chest radiography. Comput Med Imaging Graph 2017; 57: 10-8.
        [http://dx.doi.org/10.1016/j.compmedimag.2016.11.004] [PMID: 27986379]

[10]   Rydberg J, Sandrasegaran K, Tarver RD, *et al.* Routine isotropic computed tomography scanning of chest: value of coronal and sagittal reformations. Invest Radiol 2007; 42(1): 23-8.
        [http://dx.doi.org/10.1097/01.rli.0000248972.06586.9b] [PMID: 17213745]

[11]   Kawel N, Seifert B, Luetolf M, Boehm T. Effect of slab thickness on the CT detection of pulmonary nodules: use of sliding thin-slab maximum intensity projection and volume rendering. AJR Am J Roentgenol 2009; 192(5): 1324-9.
        [http://dx.doi.org/10.2214/AJR.08.1689] [PMID: 19380557]

[12]   Rubin GD. Lung Nodule and Cancer Detection in CT Screening. J Thorac Imaging 2015; 30(2): 130-8.
        [http://dx.doi.org/10.1097/RTI.0000000000000140] [PMID: 25658477]

[13]   Brown M, Browning P, Wahi-Anwar MW, *et al.* Integration of Chest CT CAD into the Clinical Workflow and Impact on Radiologist Efficiency Acad Radiol 2018 ; 6332(18): 8- 30373.

[14]   Callister MEJ, Baldwin DR, Akram AR, *et al.* British Thoracic Society guidelines for the investigation and management of pulmonary nodules. Thorax 2015; 70 (Suppl. 2): ii1-ii54.
        [http://dx.doi.org/10.1136/thoraxjnl-2015-207168] [PMID: 26082159]

[15]   MacMahon H, Naidich DP, Goo JM, *et al.* Guidelines for management of incidental pulmonary nodules detected on CT images: From the fleischner society 2017. Radiology 2017; 284(1): 228-43.

[http://dx.doi.org/10.1148/radiol.2017161659] [PMID: 28240562]

[16]   Bai C, Choi CM, Chu CM, *et al.* Evaluation of pulmonary nodules: Clinical practice consensus guidelines for asia. Chest 2016; 150(4): 877-93.
[http://dx.doi.org/10.1016/j.chest.2016.02.650] [PMID: 26923625]

[17]   Larici AR, Farchione A, Franchi P, *et al.* Lung nodules: size still matters. Eur Respir Rev 2017; 26(146)170025
[http://dx.doi.org/10.1183/16000617.0025-2017] [PMID: 29263171]

[18]   TNM Classification of Malignant Tumours, 8th Edition James D. Brierley (Editor), Mary K. Gospodarowicz (Editor), Christian Wittekind (Editor) ISBN: 978-1-119-26356-2 November 2016 Wiley-Blackwell.

[19]   Dales RE, Stark RM, Raman S. Computed tomography to stage lung cancer. Approaching a controversy using meta-analysis. Am Rev Respir Dis 1990; 141(5 Pt 1): 1096-101.
[http://dx.doi.org/10.1164/ajrccm/141.5_Pt_1.1096] [PMID: 2160211]

[20]   Dwamena BA, Sonnad SS, Angobaldo JO, Wahl RL. Metastases from non-small cell lung cancer: mediastinal staging in the 1990s--meta-analytic comparison of PET and CT. Radiology 1999; 213(2): 530-6.
[http://dx.doi.org/10.1148/radiology.213.2.r99nv46530] [PMID: 10551237]

[21]   Bankier AA, MacMahon H, Goo JM, *et al.* Recommendations for measuring pulmonary nodules at CT: A statement from the fleischner society. Radiology 2017; 285(2): 584-600.
[http://dx.doi.org/10.1148/radiol.2017162894] [PMID: 28650738]

[22]   Rusch VW, Asamura H, Watanabe H, *et al.* The IASLC lung cancer staging project: A proposal for a new international lymph node map in the forthcoming. 2009.

[23]   El-Sherief AH, Lau CT, Wu CC, Drake RL, Abbott GF, Rice TW. International association for the study of lung cancer (IASLC) lymph node map: radiologic review with CT illustration. Radiographics 2014; 34(6): 1680-91.
[http://dx.doi.org/10.1148/rg.346130097] [PMID: 25310423]

[24]   NICE guidance Diagnosis and staging of lung cancer. 2019. http://pathways.nice.org.uk/pathways/lung-cancer

[25]   Cronin P, Dwamena BA, Kelly AM, Carlos RC. Solitary pulmonary nodules: meta-analytic comparison of cross-sectional imaging modalities for diagnosis of malignancy. Radiology 2008; 246(3): 772-82.
[http://dx.doi.org/10.1148/radiol.2463062148] [PMID: 18235105]

[26]   K ak, S Park, GJ Cheon. Update on nodal staging in non-small cell lung cancer with integrated positron emission tomography/computed tomography: a meta-analysis Ann Nucl Med https://www.ncbi.nlm.nih.gov/pubmed/256551202015.

[27]   Schmidt-Hansen M, Baldwin DR, Hasler E, *et al.* PET-CT for assessing mediastinal lymph node involvement in patients with suspected resectable non-small cell lung cancer. Cochrane Database Syst Rev 2014; 11(11)CD009519
[http://dx.doi.org/10.1002/14651858.CD009519.pub2] [PMID: 25393718]

[28]   Naur TMH, Konge L, Clementsen PF. Endobronchial ultrasound-guided transbronchial needle aspiration for staging of patients with non-small cell lung cancer without mediastinal involvement at positron emission tomography-computed tomography. Respiration 2017; 94(3): 279-84.
[http://dx.doi.org/10.1159/000477625] [PMID: 28683462]

[29]   Diagnosis and staging of lung cancer. 2019. http://pathways.nice.org.uk/pathways/lung-cancer

[30]   Ambrosini V, Nicolini S, Caroli P. PET CT imaging in different types of lung cancer: An overview. European Journal of Radiology 2012; 81: 988-1001.

[31]   Szyszko TA, Yip C, Szlosarek P, Goh V, Cook GJ. The role of new PET tracers for lung cancer. Lung

Cancer 2016; 94: 7-14.
[http://dx.doi.org/10.1016/j.lungcan.2016.01.010] [PMID: 26973200]

[32]   Vaupel P, Mayer A. Hypoxia in cancer: significance and impact on clinical outcome. Cancer Metastasis Rev 2007; 26(2): 225-39.
[http://dx.doi.org/10.1007/s10555-007-9055-1] [PMID: 17440684]

[33]   Yuanyuan J, Guozhu H, Wuying C. The utility of 18F-FDG and 68Ga-DOTA-Peptide PET/CT in the evaluation of primary pulmonary carcinoid A systematic review and meta-analysis Medicine 2019; 98-10.

[34]   Taylor SA, Mallett S, Ball S, *et al.* Diagnostic accuracy of whole-body MRI versus standard imaging pathways for metastatic disease in newly diagnosed non-small-cell lung cancer: the prospective Streamline L trial Lancet Respir Med (published online May 9) http://dx.doi.org/10.1016/S2213-2600(19)30090-62019.

[35]   Hoosein MM, Barnes D, Khan AN, *et al.* The importance of ultrasound in staging and gaining a pathological diagnosis in patients with lung cancer - a two-year single centre experience 2011.

[36]   Bandi V, Lunn W, Ernst A, *et al.* Ultrasound vs. CT in detecting chest wall invasion by tumor: a prospective study. Chest 2008; 133(4): 881-6.
[http://dx.doi.org/10.1378/chest.07-1656] [PMID: 17951616]

[37]   Tahiri M, Khereba M, Thiffault V, *et al.* Preoperative assessment of chest wall invasion in non-small cell lung cancer using surgeon-performed ultrasound. Ann Thorac Surg 2014; 98(3): 984-9.
[http://dx.doi.org/10.1016/j.athoracsur.2014.04.111] [PMID: 25038014]

[38]   Beer L, Maximilian Hochmair H, Prosch H. Pitfalls in the radiological response assessment of immunotherapy memo 2018.

[39]   Huang K, Palma DA. Follow-up of patients after stereotactic radiation for lung cancer: a primer for the nonradiation oncologist. J Thorac Oncol 2015; 10: 412-9.
[http://dx.doi.org/10.1097/JTO.0000000000000435] [PMID: 25695219]

[40]   Yang DM, Palma D, Louie A, *et al.* Assessment of tumour response after stereotactic ablative radiation therapy for lung cancer: A prospective quantitative hybrid [18] F-fluorodeoxyglucose-positron emission tomography and CT perfusion study. J Med Imaging Radiat Oncol 2019; 63(1): 94-101.
[http://dx.doi.org/10.1111/1754-9485.12807] [PMID: 30281918]

[41]   Gao J, Li L, Liu X, Guo R, Zhao B. Contrast-enhanced magnetic resonance imaging with a novel nano-size contrast agent for the clinical diagnosis of patients with lung cancer. Exp Ther Med 2018; 15(6): 5415-21.
[http://dx.doi.org/10.3892/etm.2018.6112] [PMID: 29904421]

[42]   Lu X, Wang C, Li X, Gu P, Jia L, Zhang L. Synthesis and preliminary evaluation of ^{18}F-icotinib for EGFR-targeted PET imaging of lung cancer. Bioorg Med Chem 2019; 27(3): 545-51.
[http://dx.doi.org/10.1016/j.bmc.2018.12.034] [PMID: 30611635]

[43]   Ehlerding EB, England CG, Jiang D, *et al.* CD38 as a PET imaging target in lung cancer. Mol Pharm 2017; 14(7): 2400-6.
[http://dx.doi.org/10.1021/acs.molpharmaceut.7b00298] [PMID: 28573863]

REFERENCES (SECTION 2)

[1]   Jablonski A. Efficiency of anti-stokes fluorescence in dyes. Nature 1933; 131: 839-40.
        [http://dx.doi.org/10.1038/131839b0]

[2]   Steiner R. Fundamental of Fluorescence. 2014.

[3]   Richards-Kortum R, Sevick-Muraca E. Quantitative optical spectroscopy for tissue diagnosis. Annu
        Rev Phys Chem 1996; 47: 555-606.
        [http://dx.doi.org/10.1146/annurev.physchem.47.1.555] [PMID: 8930102]

[4]   Hung J, Lam S, LeRiche JC, Palcic B. Autofluorescence of normal and malignant bronchial tissue.
        Lasers Surg Med 1991; 11(2): 99-105.
        [http://dx.doi.org/10.1002/lsm.1900110203] [PMID: 2034016]

[5]   Lam S, Kennedy T, Unger M, *et al.* Localization of bronchial intraepithelial neoplastic lesions by
        fluorescence bronchoscopy. Chest 1998; 113(3): 696-702.
        [http://dx.doi.org/10.1378/chest.113.3.696] [PMID: 9515845]

[6]   Zeng H, McWilliam A, Lam S. Optical spectroscopy and imaging for early lung cancer detection: a
        review 2004.
        [http://dx.doi.org/10.1016/S1572-1000(04)00042-0]

[7]   Gioux S, Choi HS, Frangioni JV. Image-guided surgery using invisible near-infrared light:
        fundamentals of clinical translation. Mol Imaging 2010; 9(5): 237-55.
        [http://dx.doi.org/10.2310/7290.2010.00034] [PMID: 20868625]

[8]   Schaafsma BE, Mieog JS, Hutteman M, *et al.* The clinical use of indocyanine green as a near-infrared
        fluorescent contrast agent for image-guided oncologic surgery. J Surg Oncol 2011; 104(3): 323-32.
        [http://dx.doi.org/10.1002/jso.21943] [PMID: 21495033]

[9]   Mondal SB, Gao S, Zhu N, *et al.* Real-time fluorescence image-guided oncologic surgery. Adv Cancer
        Res 2014; 124: 171-211.
        [http://dx.doi.org/10.1016/B978-0-12-411638-2.00005-7] [PMID: 25287689]

[10]   Ujiie H, Kato T, Hu UP, *et al.* A novel minimally invasive near-infrared thoracoscopic localization
        technique of small nodules: a Phase I feasibility trial. J Thorac Cardiovasc Surg 2016; 22(6): 367-9.
        [PMID: 28495056]

[11]   Stummer W, Pichlmeier U, Meinel T, *et al.* Fluorescence-guided surgery with 5-aminolevulinic acid
        for resection of malignant glioma: a randomised controlled multicentre phase III trial. Lancet Oncol
        2006; 7(5): 392-401.
        [http://dx.doi.org/10.1016/S1470-2045(06)70665-9] [PMID: 16648043]

[12]   Eljamel S. 5-ALA fluorescence image guided resection of glioblastoma multiforme: a meta-analysis of
        the literature. Int J Mol Sci 2015; 16(5): 10443-56.
        [http://dx.doi.org/10.3390/ijms160510443] [PMID: 25961952]

CHAPTER 5

Diagnostic Approach to Lung Cancer

Jack Kastelik[*]

Castle Hill Hospital & Hull Royal Infirmary, Hull University Teaching Hospitals NHS Trust, Hull, UK

Abstract: Lung cancer is a common neoplasm. Diagnosis of lung cancer at an early stage is associated with the best prognosis. Therefore, early recognition of symptoms through increased awareness, systematic investigations and rapid diagnosis of lung cancer is of importance. Patients investigated for lung cancer would require a chest radiograph, computed tomography and Positron Emission Tomography. Imaging can provide a non-invasive approach to staging lung cancer. However, in a number of patients, more invasive methods may be required for accurate staging. Endobronchial ultrasound (EBUS) and Endoscopic ultrasound are techniques, which in conjunction with mediastinoscopy, form important techniques for mediastinal lymph node staging as well as sampling for histological diagnosis. Patients with more peripheral lesions may need biopsy using CT guidance or newer approaches such as radial EBUS or navigational bronchoscopy. Many patients with lung cancer would also require complex physiological fitness assessment, including lung function and exercise testing. A proportion of patients with lung cancer may develop pleural effusion, which would require careful assessment based on the use of systematic diagnostic protocols and understanding of the best interventional and therapeutic strategies. Therefore, investigations and management of patients with lung cancer have become complex and should be undertaken through the multidisciplinary team approach.

Keywords: Lung Cancer, Computed Tomography, Positron Emission Tomography, Endobronchial Ultrasound, Navigational Bronchoscopy, Lung Function testing, Pleural effusion, Thoracocopy.

INTRODUCTION

Each year, worldwide, approximately 1.8 million patients are diagnosed with lung cancer [1]. Unfortunately, a majority of the patients are diagnosed with advanced disease, which is not curable and has survival at 5 years in the range of 4% [1]. Only 15% to 20% of lung cancer cases are diagnosed with stage one disease, which carries a much better prognosis [2 - 5]. The Office for National Statistics in

[*] **Corresponding author Jack Kastelik:** Castle Hill Hospital & Hull Royal Infirmary, Hull University Teaching Hospitals NHS Trust, Hull, UK; Tel: +441482875875; Fax: +441482624068; E-mail: jack.kastelik@hey.nhs.uk

Keyvan Moghissi, Jack Kastelik, Philip Barber & Peyman Sardari Nia (Eds.)

England has reported 5-year survival for lung cancer in men at 12.9% and slightly higher in women at 17.7%, with other countries such as Australia reporting dissimilar 5-year survival rates of around 16%. In order to provide curative options, lung cancer requires to be diagnosed at an early stage. This can potentially be facilitated by increasing the public awareness of lung cancer and the symptoms associated with it, together with work towards improving primary care identification and early investigations of patients with suspected lung cancer. This would allow the patients to seek medical advice earlier and for the primary care physicians to rapidly initiate investigations and referrals to a specialist. In addition, there is a drive towards developing systems and programmes, including lung cancer screening, which would allow for earlier detection of lung cancer. However, before any benefits of such interventions are appreciated, clinicians are left with relying on the early recognition of symptoms, leading to rapid imaging followed by appropriate investigational protocols.

SYMPTOMS

Symptoms related to lung cancer usually occur in more advanced stages of the disease and therefore, many patients with the early stages of lung cancer may remain asymptomatic. One of the important barriers in early diagnosis is the recognition by the primary care that the symptoms that patients are presenting with may be related to lung cancer. A study from the UK revealed that the average time from the presentation and the diagnosis of lung cancer was 3 months and for patients diagnosed with the early stages of the disease, it was much longer, around 5 months [6]. Lung cancer can present with different symptoms, many of which may be non-specific. More specific symptoms of lung cancer, such as haemoptysis, may be present in only 20% of patients. The investigations are usually initiated when the symptoms become apparent typically in the form of cough, breathlessness, haemoptysis or pain. The breathlessness may occur due to the lobar collapse or mechanical compression resulting in the narrowing of the lumen of the bronchi or endo-bronchial obstruction. Voice hoarseness or breathlessness due to diaphragmatic paralysis can be a manifestation of the phrenic nerve involvement. Other presentations may be in the form of the superior vena cava obstruction syndrome or Horner's syndrome due to Pancoast's or superior sulcus tumour. The clinicians require to be aware of the modes of presentations related to so-called paraneoplastic syndromes, which may include endocrinological abnormalities such as a syndrome of inappropriate anti-diuretic hormone secretion (SIADH), hypercalcaemia or Cushing's syndrome as well as haematological abnormalities including deep vein thrombosis (DVT), superficial thrombophlebitis, disseminated intravascular coagulation (DIC) and cutaneous and musculoskeletal disorders including hypertrophic osteoarthropathy or dermatomyositis. Moreover, patients may present with neurological disorders due to the Lambert Eaton syndrome, peripheral neuropathy, cerebellar degeneration or limbic encephalitis. These syndromes may require biochemical testing to assess serum calcium, serum and urine osmolality and sodium levels or measuring serum specific anti-neuronal nuclear antibodies such as anti Hu, Yo or Ri, which may be detected in paraneoplastic neurological syndromes.

The main hurdles for early diagnosis are related to the patients' awareness of lung cancer and the reluctance to seek a medical assessment when the symptoms become apparent with studies showing a median delay of 99 days from the onset of the symptoms and the patients seeking medical opinion [7]. There is evidence that the introduction of the campaigns that increase public awareness of lung cancer and training within the primary care may result in increased referral rates for a chest radiograph and a resulting rise in the diagnosis of lung cancer. For example, a recent report of such a campaign in Leeds, a large city in the north of England, revealed an 81% rise in the community ordered chest radiographs and a shift towards diagnosing of a higher proportion of earlier stages I and II of lung cancer [8]. Another example would be the CHEST Trial, which showed an increase in consultation for new respiratory symptoms [9]. Similar findings have been reported recently from the CHEST Australia study, which showed a 40% increase in respiratory consultations within the high-risk lung cancer population [10]. Early initiation of investigations is of importance as there is evidence to suggest that the time to diagnosis for patients with lung cancer may determine the outcomes [11]. For this reason, the awareness of the symptoms of lung cancer within the population and the primary care remains an important factor for early initiation of the investigations. Once the patients are referred to a specialist centre, it is paramount that there are systems in place that would allow for systematic and timely investigational pathways, which are individualised according to each patient's requirements.

INITIAL INVESTIGATIONS

The current guideline suggests that in the UK, patients with suspected lung cancer are referred to a fast track lung cancer clinic usually as these allow for rapid investigations and diagnosis and are associated with less anxiety to the patients [12]. This is not dissimilar to the settings within the other health systems. The fast track clinics are working within the multidisciplinary team settings with a chest physician usually providing the initial assessment and the choice of investigational pathway. Cancer clinical nurse specialists form an important part of the multidisciplinary team and provide support to patients with suspected lung cancer through the investigational pathway and the diagnosis. The guidelines suggest that the investigational pathway for lung cancer should include investigations that involve the least risk to the patient and provide information on both the histological diagnosis and the staging. There is, therefore, drive towards the optimal investigational pathway that would result in rapid diagnosis and staging of the disease. There is evidence that the timely diagnosis of lung cancer can improve the outcomes. For example, a Lung-BOOST trial showed that a rapid diagnostic pathway compared to the standard care reduced time from the referral and diagnosis by 15 days and increased the median survival by 191 days [13]. In the UK, in order to improve the time interval from the referral to diagnosis and the treatment of lung cancer, the national optimal lung cancer pathway has been promoted and is being implemented [14]. Patients with suspected lung cancer should have a chest radiograph and if this is suspicious for lung cancer computed tomography (CT) of the thorax ideally on the same day (Table **1**). The staging CT scan should include imaging of the liver, the adrenals and the lower neck as this would allow to assess for any distal metastases. However, the chest wall involvement may require further imaging in the form of ultrasound or magnetic resonance imaging (MRI) [15]. Similarly, an MRI may be required to assess patients with the superior sulcus neoplasm, as this may provide more information regarding the extent of the disease. The majority of the patients with suspected lung cancer would also require a Positron Emission Tomography (PET) scan, which provides more accurate staging. PET scan compared to the CT is more accurate in assessing the mediastinal lymph nodes involvement with sensitivity and specificity of 77.4% (95% CI 65.3 to 86.1) and 90.1% (95% CI 85.3 to 93.5), respectively [16]. The PET scan may also be helpful in diagnosing distal metastases. Therefore, all patients who are considered for radical treatment should have a PET scan. However, as the PET scan is not sensitive for the brain metastatic disease detection, the current guidelines suggest that brain imaging in the form of a CT or ideally an MRI should be undertaken for patients with stage II and IIIA disease who are considered for treatment with the curative intention [12]. For the patients with stage IA disease, the CT of the brain should be considered in the presence of neurological symptoms, as the prevalence of the brain metastases is relatively low, reported at 4% [12]. In addition, any patients with neurological symptoms, including those of cord compression, which is an oncological emergency, should have brain and spine imaging in the form of an MRI.

Whilst the PET scan is sensitive for non-invasive mediastinal and hilar lymph node staging, many patients would require formal biopsy and histological assessment. Mediastinoscopy remains the gold standard for staging mediastinal lymph nodes in the context of lung cancer with a diagnostic accuracy of up to 96% and can sample mediastinoscopy can sample the American Thoracic Society (ATS) stations 1, 2, 3, 4, 7 [17, 18]. However, more often now, mediastinal and hilar lymph node staging is undertaken with Endobronchial Ultrasound (EBUS) and Endoscopic Ultrasound (EUS). An EBUS has an ultrasound probe at its tip, which is a convex probe and a 7.5 MHz transducer, which allows the real-time visualization and biopsy of the lymph nodes. Both EBUS and EUS are relatively safe procedures with reported serious complications of 0.05% to 1.43% and morbidity of 0.6% to 1.1% [19, 20]. EBUS allows for examination and sampling of the ATS stations 2, 3, 4, 7, 10, 11 and the EUS allows for examination of stations 2L, 4L, 7, 8, 9 [21]. Therefore, combined EBUS EUS allows for more complete examination, staging and sampling of the mediastinal lymph nodes [22]. The literature reports the sensitivity of EBUS of 89% to 99% and diagnostic yield of 85% to 99% [23, 24]. Um et al. reported in a prospective study that EBUS had 93% accuracy, which was higher to that of 89% for mediastinoscopy [25]. A recent meta-analysis review of 1066 patients who underwent EBUS and surgical staging of the mediastinal lymph nodes showed a sensitivity of 0.90 (CI 0.84 to 0.96) [26]. When comparing different approaches, EBUS was reported to have a diagnostic accuracy of 91%, EUS of 88% and combined EBUS and EUS of 97% [27]. In another randomized controlled study combined, EBUS and EUS had 85% sensitivity for the detection of cancer, which was similar to that of 79% for mediastinoscopy [17]. This study also showed that in cases where EBUS and EUS node sampling showed no evidence of cancer addition of mediastinoscopy increased sensitivity by 9%. Therefore, any centre that is managing patients with lung cancer should have access to EBUS, EUS, as well as surgical mediastinoscopy. When sampling mediastinal lymph nodes, it is recommended to start with the highest lymph nodes stations and then to examine the nodes in the descending station staging. This would avoid the possibility of contamination and upstaging of the nodal disease. Ideally, all lymph nodes amenable to sampling should be biopsied for staging purposes with some centres offering rapid on site examination (ROSE). Although less researched, EBUS has been used in the context of lung cancer that has already treated before curative surgery with a diagnostic accuracy of 77% for N2 nodal disease [28]. Another important consideration would be for the patients with cervical or axillary lymphadenopathy in whom ultrasound guided biopsy of those lymph nodes may provide histological diagnosis, therefore avoiding more invasive tests. Similarly, in patients with liver metastases, an ultrasound guided biopsy of these lesions may provide staging and diagnosis. Moreover, in a skill operator, EUS may be able to provide a histological diagnosis from adrenal metastases again, providing important staging and diagnostic information.

In addition to EBUS and EUS, the patients also can undergo fiberoptic bronchoscopy. This is of particular relevance in the context of central endobronchial lesions, which can be biopsied using bronchoscopy when nodal staging does not affect the treatment options such as in cases with the presence of distal metastases or. In these cases, fiberoptic bronchoscopy can provide a rapid histological diagnosis. However, in a proportion of cases, nodal staging would be required. EBUS can sample some of the peri-bronchial lung lesions. However, per-cutaneous trans-thoracic CT guided biopsy of the lung lesion may be more appropriate, especially in the early stage of the disease where there is no nodal involvement and no evidence of distal metastases. The accuracy sensitivity of per-cutaneous trans-thoracic CT guided needle lung biopsy is over 90% [29]. It is a relatively common procedure but has reported a risk of pulmonary haemorrhage between 5% and 16.9% and a recognised risk of pneumothorax with 3.3% to 15% of patients requiring intercostal chest drain insertion. Therefore, in a proportion of patients, it may not be possible to perform a CT guided biopsy [29]. In cases where CT guided biopsy may not be technically possible, there are other techniques that may be applied, such as navigational bronchoscopy or radial EBUS. The use of the investigations allows for histological diagnosis and lung cancer staging.

Table 1. Diagnostic tools for lung cancer.

Procedure	Function
Chest Radiograph	Initial imaging tool
Computed tomography	Initial staging tool
Positron Emission Tomography (PET)	Imaging staging tool, a particular advantage for mediastinal lymph node staging and distant metastases detection
Pulmonary function testing	Assessment of respiratory physiology
Cardiopulmonary Exercise testing CPex	Assessment of pulmonary physiology and fitness for surgery
Fiberoptic Bronchoscopy	Visualisation of bronchial tree, endobronchial biopsy, brushing and lavage
Endobronchial Ultrasound (EBUS)	Mediastinal lymph node staging
Endoscopic Ultrasound (EUS)	Mediastinal lymph node staging
Mediastinoscopy	Gold standard for Mediastinal Lymph node surgical staging
Thoracoscopy	Assessment of patients with pleural effusion and pleural biopsy
Thoracic ultrasound	Assessment of pleural effusion and guidance of pleural procedures
Navigational Bronchoscopy	Assessment and biopsy of lung lesions, which are beyond the reach of fiberoptic bronchoscopy
Radial EBUS	Assessment and biopsy of lung lesion, which are beyond the reach of fiberoptic bronchoscopy
CT guided biopsy	Biopsy of peripheral lung lesions

Fitness Assessment

In order to offer lung cancer therapies, patients' fitness requires to be assessed. Patients who are current smokers should be advised to stop smoking at the time of diagnosis of lung cancer as smoking increases respiratory complications following lung cancer surgery and may affect outcomes of other therapies. The presence of co-morbidities, especially respiratory, cardiac or renal disorders, may significantly affect patients' fitness for treatments. Similarly, nutritional status should be assessed through the measurements of the body mass index (BMI) and serum albumin levels, as this may have implications on the treatment options and the outcomes. All patients with lung cancer should have performance status assessed as measured using the World Health Organisation (WHO), Karnofsky or Eastern Cooperative Oncology Group (ECOG) scales. The assessment of the performance status is of importance, as this may affect patients' suitability for the therapeutic option. In fact, in the borderline cases, oncological review taking into account performance status and co-morbidities may be required to assess fitness for the systemic treatment. Similarly, in high risk group patients who may be potentially offered radical treatments, a joint assessment by a thoracic surgeon and an oncologist may be required in order to decide on the best therapeutic options with many of those decisions requiring a multidisciplinary team review.

When assessing patients with lung cancer for the radical treatment including surgery, resectability, i.e., the stage of the disease needs to be taken into consideration as well as the assessment of whether the patients are fit to undergo the treatment and if surgical resection is considered the type of surgery planned. For example, the thirty days mortality data for pneumonectomy is around 7%, which is two to three times higher than that of 2.3% for lobectomy, although both would depend on the thoracic surgeon experience and the volume of procedures performed within the units. In the context of assessing the fitness for radical treatment, including surgery, cardiovascular and respiratory factors need to be taken into consideration [30]. The cardiovascular risk assessment tools such as Thoracic Revised Cardiac Risk score ThRCRI help to estimate risks of major cardiac complications and those with high risk score should be assessed formally by a cardiologist [31, 32]. In addition, all patients would require to have a cardiovascular examination and an electrocardiogram (ECG) performed. The patients considered for surgery, especially those with underlying cardiac disease or those having pneumonectomy, may also require a pre-operative echocardiogram. Moreover, all patients who are being considered for radical treatments should have pulmonary function tests, including the lung volumes and the transfer factor. The lung function testing should be undertaken when the patients are stable and their medical treatment is maximised. Assessment of pulmonary function should include forced expiratory volume in one second (FEV$_1$), which assesses airflow and diffusing capacity for carbon monoxide (DLCO), which tests alveolar capillary transfer. The levels of FEV$_1$ and DLCO are an independent factor for predicting post-operative mortality and morbidity [33 - 35]. However, inevitably many patients will have full lung function testing, including the forced vital capacity (FVC) and the lung volumes. For the patients considered for surgery, a formal functional segment count should be undertaken to predict the post-operative lung function as the predicted post-operative FEV_1 and DLCO can be calculated and again are an independent predictive factor for estimating mortality and morbidity [33 - 35]. The formula used is as follows; estimated post operative FEV_1 = preoperative FEV_1 x (19 - number of segments to be removed)/19. Patients with estimated post operative FEV_1 of less than 40% have a high risk for planned surgical procedures. The patients with a high risk of post operative complications which may still be offered an option of surgery, providing that increased risks of complications, including breathlessness and mortality, are accepted. Perfusion scans may also be used for more accurate predictive values, especially for patients undergoing pneumonectomy. In addition, the patients should have a discussion about the alternative therapeutic options such as radical radiotherapy and radiotherapy treatments that optimise the dose to the lung cancer and minimise the risks of normal tissue damage such as stereotactic ablative radiotherapy (SABR), intensity-modulated radiotherapy (IMRT) or image-guided radiotherapy.

Current guidelines suggest that patients with FEV_1 and DLCO over 80% of predicted with the predicted post operative FEV_1 and DLCO above 60% of predicted are deemed to have low operative risk [33, 36]. Patients with post operative predicted FEV_1 and DLCO of less than 60% should undergo exercise testing such as a shuttle walk or a formal cardio pulmonary exercise testing (CPET) [33, 36]. Moreover, Brunelli et al. reported that patients with normal FEV_1 but reduced DLCO had increased peri-operative complications [37]. This is most likely through the effects that impaired alveolar capillary transfer has on the exercise capacity. There is evidence that exercise capacity inversely correlates with the post operative complications. The exercise tolerance can be objectively assessed using a six minutes walk, a shuttle walk or a stair climb test. Any de-saturation during the exercise testing of 4% or more has been accepted as an increased risk of post operative complications. There is evidence that shuttle walk of over 400 meters or stair climb test of over 22 meters, which correspond to maximal oxygen consumption (also known as maximal oxygen uptake, peak oxygen uptake or maximal aerobic capacity) abbreviated as VO_2 max of greater than 15 ml/kg/min of the CPET can be accepted as adequate for lobectomy or pneumonectomy [33, 36]. Patients who have post-operative predicted FEV_1 or DLCO of less than 30% of predicted should undergo CPET in order to determine their fitness for surgery [33, 36]. The value of VO_2 max of more than 20 ml/kg/min or more than 75% of predicted is associated with low risk even for pneumonectomy [33, 36]. Conversely, VO_2 max of 10 to 12 ml/kg/min or less is associated with higher risk and usually precludes major anatomical resection. For the intermediate group of VO_2 max of 10 to 15 ml/kg/min consideration should be given to the alternative treatments such as wedge resection, or stereotactic radiotherapy or radiofrequency ablation [33, 36]. During the CPET, the minute ventilation-to-carbon dioxide output (VE/VCO$_2$) slope, which is a measure of ventilatory efficiency, has been shown to be an independent predictor of respiratory complications after major lung resections. Thus there is evidence that patients with a VE/VCO$_2$ slope exceeding 35 had a higher incidence of respiratory complications (22% vs 7.6%, p=0.004) and mortality (7.2% vs. 0.6%, p=0.01) [38]. There are national and international guidelines on how to assess patients' fitness for radical treatment, including surgery, which provide algorithms with many common agreed protocols but also some variations. The British Thoracic Society (BTS) guidelines provide a detailed algorithm for the assessment of patients with reduced FEV$_1$ and DLCO [36]. The European Respiratory Society (ERS) and the European Society for Thoracic Surgery (ESTS) guidelines recommend CPET for everyone with FEV$_1$ or DLCO less than 80% [34]. The American College of Chest Physicians (ACCP) guidelines recommend a step approach with lung function, followed by low costs exercise testing such as shuttle walk and then CPET [39].

Staging of Lung Cancer

The precise staging of lung cancer is important from diagnostic and therapeutic aspects. The current staging is the 8th edition on Lung cancer TNM staging [40, 41]. The TNM staging describes the tumour size T, regional lymph node N and distant metastases M.

Tumour Size Staging

The tumour size less than 3 cm in the greatest dimension, surrounded by lung or visceral pleura and not positioned in the main bronchus, i.e., not more proximal than lobar bronchi is classified as T1 [40]. Furthermore, this is sub-classified as T1a if the tumour is less than 1 cm in greatest dimension, T1b if the greatest dimension of the tumour is between 1 cm but not more than 2 cm, and T1c when the greatest diameter is more than 2 cm but not more than 3 cm in greatest diameter. T2 tumour describes lesions more than 3 cm but not more than 5 cm in greatest dimension or the tumour that involves the main bronchus regardless the distance from the carina but not involving the carina, invading the visceral pleura or associated with atelectasis or obstructive pneumonitis extending to the hilar region, either involving part of the lung or the entire lung [40, 41]. This is further subdivided into T2a when the tumour is more than 3 cm but not more than 4 cm in the greatest dimension and T2b when the tumour is more than 4 cm but not more than 5 cm in the greatest dimension. The T3 describes tumour more than 5 cm but not more than 7 cm in the greatest dimension [40, 41]. T3 staging also includes any tumour that invades chest wall, phrenic nerve or parietal pericardium. The presence of a separate tumour nodule or nodules in the same lobe as the primary neoplasm also classifies T3 staging. The superior sulcus tumours are also staged as T3. T4 is defined as tumour in more than 7 cm in the greatest dimension. In addition, any tumour that invades the tracheae, recurrent laryngeal nerve, diaphragm, mediastinum, heart, great blood vessels, oesophagus or any of the vertebral bodies is classified as T4. Moreover, involvement of the carina also defines T4 staging. Any separate tumour nodules in a different ipsilateral lobe to the primary neoplasm classify the T4 stage [40, 41].

Regional Lymph Node Staging

The regional lymph nodes involvement classification describes N0 when there is no involvement, N1 metastatic ipsilateral peribronchial and or ipsilateral hilar lymph nodes and intra-pulmonary nodes, including involvement by direct extension with N1a defining a single N1 nodal station involvement and N1b multiple nodal station involvement. N2 describes metastasis in ipsilateral mediastinal and or sub carinal lymph nodes [40]. N2a1 defines the involvement of a single N2 nodal station without N1 stations involvement and N2a2 involvement of a single N2 nodal station with N1 involvement [40]. N2b is defined as the involvement of multiple N2 stations. N3 staging describes metastasis to the contralateral mediastinal or hilar, ipsilateral or contra-lateral scalene or supra-clavicular lymph nodes.

Lymph Node Stations

In order to be able to define nodal staging, the understanding of the lymph nodes anatomy is required. Station 1 lymph nodes are the low cervical, supraclavicular and sternal notch lymph nodes [40]. The presence of these lymph nodes defines an N3 disease. Superior mediastinal lymph nodes are anatomically classified as right and left upper para-tracheal 2R and 2L and lower para-tracheal 4R and 4L [40]. In addition, there are pre-vascular 3a and re-trotracheal 3p stations. The inferior mediastinal lymph nodes are classified as sub-carinal station 7, and lower zone, which include para-esophageal, which are below the carina station 8, and pulmonary ligament station 9 [40, 41]. The aortic nodes aorto pulmonary zone, which include sub aortic station 5 and para-aortic positioned around the ascending aorta and the phrenic nerve. The N1 nodes include hilar (station 10) and inter-lobar (station 11) zones as well as peri-hilar zone, which include lobar (station 12), segmental (station 13) and sub-segmental (station 14) [40].

Metastatic Disease Staging

M1 defines distant metastases, which is further sub classified as M1a and defined as separate tumour nodule(s) in a contra-lateral lobe; tumour with pleural or pericardial nodules or malignant pleural or pericardial effusion, M1b defined as a single extra thoracic metastasis in a single organ and M1c multiple extra thoracic metastases in one or several organs [40, 41]. Overall most of the pleural and pericardial effusions in the context of lung cancer are related to the neoplasm. However, in a proportion of patients, the pleural or pericardial effusion may not be related to lung neoplasm and may be considered based on clinical assessment non malignant. In these patients, sampling of the effusion would be negative for malignant cells and the fluid characteristics would be those of transudate and usually with no evidence of blood staining. These patients should have a systematic assessment of their pleural or pericardial effusion, including sampling and ideally pleural or pericardial biopsy. If all these aspects are fulfilled with no evidence for the neoplastic process, the presence of pleural or pericardial effusion can be excluded as a staging descriptor.

Visceral Pleural Invasion

Visceral pleural invasion is assessed, usually following the surgical resection although it may be possible to describe these features on some of the biopsy samples. The tumour confined within the supleural lung parenchyma or invading superficially into the pleural connective tissue is defined as PL0 [40]. If the tumour invades beyond the elastic layer it is staged as PL1. When the tumour invades into the pleura, it is staged as PL2 [40]. The PL1 and PL2 neoplasms are staged as T2. The PL3 tumours invade any component of the parietal pleura and are staged as T3 [40]. The visceral pleural invasion is usually staged on the post surgical resection samples.

Pulmonary Nodules and Early Detection of Lung Cancer

The evidence for lung cancer screening with low dose CT has been increasing and there is a European position statement, which recommends a risk stratification approach supported by quality assurance [42]. Important aspects of any proposed screening would include careful information on benefits and harms as well as smoking cessation. Moreover, newly detected solid lung nodules should be managed using semi automatically measured volume and volume doubling time. The new lung nodules greater than 200 mm^3 and non calcified lung nodules greater than 300 mm^3 should be managed using a multidisciplinary approach [43]. The evidence from the National Lung Screening Trial revealed that low dose helical CT screening, compared to the chest radiography, could reduce lung cancer mortality by 20% [44] A randomised controlled screening trial NELSON, which results were presented, showed that 270000 CT scans performed on 16,000 people aged 50 to 74 years with smoking history resulted in 0.9% lung cancer detection rate. There was over a 10 year period 26% reduction in lung cancer deaths in men and 39% for women [45, 46]. In the screening group, 50% of cancers were at an early stage and less than 10% at stage 4, compared with only 10% early stage in the control arm, where around half were diagnosed at stage 4 [45].

The screening programmes would inevitably also detect patients with pulmonary nodules [46]. There are currently guidelines on how to manage patients with pulmonary nodules detected on CT scanning [43]. There are two types of nodules detected through the screening programme [47]. The first type is the nodules that are detected at the baseline screening CT scan. The second type is the nodules that develop during the screening programme. Various reports such as the Early Lung Cancer Action Project (ELCAP) Pittsburgh Lung Screening Trial and NELSON trial, reported that between 3% to 13% would develop new nodules after baseline screening [45-49]. The European position statement on lung cancer screening recommended that the nodule risk stratification is based on nodule's lung cancer probability [42]. The high-risk nodules, usually those with more than 15% lung cancer probability, would require referral to a specialist for further assessment and investigations. In contrast, the low risk usually less than 1% lung cancer probability and intermediate risk nodules should be followed up through the additional low dose CT scanning. The volume based strategies with nodules of greater or equal 200 mm^3 being defined as high risk have been proposed. NELSON study provided evidence with regards to the new nodules detected after baseline screening [47]. Of the new solid nodules, 55% were resolving. In the patients with non-resolving new solid nodules 7% would had lung cancer in a nodule. Moreover, 5.5% of new non-resolving solid nodules that persisted as solid nodules were diagnosed as lung cancer. The volume doubling time and volume had high discriminatory power. The volume doubling time of less or equal 590 days and volume of equal or greater than 200 mm^3 were suggested to be the high risk cut off. When using applying at least one of these criteria to classify nodules as positive provided 100% sensitivity and 84% specificity for detecting lung cancer [47].

Investigations of Peripheral Lesions

It is inevitable that with earlier detection of lung cancer there will be a need for investigations of peripheral lung lesions. Currently, non bronchoscopic option of CT guided biopsy is the most commonly applied technique. There are two bronchoscopic techniques that are gaining wider use; namely radial EBUS and navigational bronchoscopy [50]. The radial EBUS is a flexible bronchoscope with an ultrasound probe that gives 360° ultrasound visualisation of solid lesions [50]. Once the lesions are located, the probe is removed, allowing for biopsy instruments to be introduced with the most commonly trans-bronchial biopsy technique being used. A meta-analysis that included 16 studies showed a diagnostic yield of 78% for lesion greater than 20mm and that of 56% for lesion less than 2 cm [51, 52]. The most serious complications of the radial EBUS included pneumothorax reported to occur in 1% of cases, with 0.4% of cases requiring a chest drain insertion. Navigational bronchoscopy is a relatively new technology that allows for the sampling of peripheral lung lesions. There are two main types of navigational bronchoscopy, namely virtual bronchoscopy and electromagnetic navigational bronchoscopy [53]. Virtual bronchoscopy is a computed guided simulation bronchoscopy, which allows to re-construct detailed bronchial tree using spatial data from the CT images of collimated thin slices of 0.5 to 1mm [50, 53]. Virtual bronchoscopy can be combined with fluoroscopy and radial endobronchial ultrasound, having shown with the later to have 94.4% diagnostic yield [53-55]. Electromagnetic navigational bronchoscopy uses electromagnetic emitter and tracking board, which creates a magnetic field around the patients allowing for tracking the position of a sensor, which is attached to a flexible wire called locatable guide, which can be passed through the working channel of the bronchoscope [53, 55]. The thin sliced CT images allow for the virtual bronchoscopy images to be created using designated computer based software and to locate the target lesion. Once this is established, a flexible bronchoscope is inserted into the patient's bronchial tree allowing for the introduction of a sensor probe thought its working channel. The sensor probe than is navigated using the magnetic field and multiple views on the screen allow to locate the target lesion. Once the target lesion is located the sensor probe is removed, leaving a sheath through which instruments such as needle, brush and biopsy forceps can be introduced to allow sampling [55]. The NAVIGATE study prospectively reported a diagnostic yield of the electromagnetic navigational bronchoscopy at 73% in 1053 procedures, with complications such as pneumothorax occurring in 4.3% procedures, of which 2.9% required chest drain insertion [56]. Therefore, electromagnetic navigational bronchoscopy is becoming an important technique for the investigation of peripheral lung lesions.

Potentially Resectable N2 Disease

In the context of stage III N2 disease, which is defined as the metastatic spread of lung cancer to the ipsilateral mediastinal lymph nodes and represents disease at one end with bulky invasive N2 nodes, which accepted treatment involves concurrent chemo-radiotherapy and at the other extreme incidental finding of N2 disease during surgical resection as well as patients with less prominent but histologically proven N2 involvement where the optimal management currently is under debate [57]. Therefore, in this group of patients, a systematic investigational protocol would be required as accurate diagnosis and staging may have prognostic as well as possible therapeutic implications. The data from the database of the International Association for the Study of Lung Cancer (IASLC) revealed that patients with a single-station N2 disease have 5-year survival of around 35%, which is similar to that of patients with multi-station N1 diseases [3, 57]. Conversely, patients with multiple-station N2 disease have a much lower 5-year survival of 20%. However, the management option for the resectable N2 disease group of patients with non-small cell lung cancer (NSCLC) remains a matter of discussion. For example, the BTS guidelines do not recommend induction chemotherapy prior to surgery, but adjuvant chemotherapy was recommended for stage IB i.e. greater than 4 cm, stage II and III [2]. The National Institute for Care and Care Excellence (NICE) guidelines accepted the limitation of the evidence currently available, but it was felt that the evidence for induction chemotherapy was less robust compared to that for adjuvant chemotherapy [1]. Although the BTS and the NICE guidelines did not specifically addressed the single node station N2 NSCLC [2, 12]. The ACCP guidelines do not recommend adjuvant chemotherapy in resectable N2 NSCLC, however, the evidence assessed here mainly concentrated on a comparison of preoperative chemotherapy and surgery against surgery alone [3]. The European Society for Medical Oncology (ESMO) guidelines on the management of early and locally advanced non-small cell lung cancer recommend in the context of a single station N2 disease, surgery and multimodality treatment, which may take form of induction chemotherapy followed by surgery, chemo-radiotherapy followed by surgery or surgery followed by adjuvant chemotherapy acknowledging that evidence is not sufficient at present [5, 58]. The suggested investigational pathway for the patient with suspected single station N2 disease is more complex. Those patients who are deemed fit for radical therapy and surgery should have an assessment of the N2 lymph mode stations, which would require sampling of at least 3 nodal stations either endoscopically (EBUS, EUS) or surgically. Moreover, the patients would need imaging in the form of PET scanning as well as the MRI imaging of the brain. The precise definition of which group of patients could be considered for surgery is not clear at this stage, but it is suggested that the at least primary neoplasm should be resectable with clear margins and that the N2 disease should be defined and that it should be free from the major mediastinal structures and with no individual nodes being greater than 3 cm. However, at present, the investigations and management of this group of patients remain challenging and further research would be required before any firm recommendations can be provided.

Pleural Effusion in Lung Cancer

Lung cancer is the commonest cause of malignant pleural effusion occurring in 30 to 40% of cases [59, 60]. Malignant pleural effusions in the context of lung cancer are usually exudates in type, but rarely, for example, in cases of carcinomateous lymphangitis it could be a transudate [61]. The presence of malignant pleural effusion in lung cancer defines advanced stage IV disease with reported 1-year survival in M1b disease with malignant pleural effusion of 12.6% compared to that of 24.8% in patients without malignant pleural effusion [62]. The risk of developing malignant pleural effusion seems higher in the presence of histological confirmation of adenocarcinoma or large cell lung cancer, the larger size of tumour and the lymph node involvement. The prognostication for patients with lung cancer and malignant pleural effusion, although still remains a challenge, has improved in recent years. The proposed prognostic malignant pleural effusion tool LENT score, which assesses pleural fluid lactate dehydrogenase, Eastern Cooperative Oncology Group performance score, neutrophil to lymphocytes ratio and the tumour type has been assessed with promising results [63]. Similarly, the PROMISE score which includes eight clinical and biological parameters such as haemoglobin, C-reactive protein, white blood cell count, Eastern Cooperative Oncology Group performance status, cancer type, pleural fluid tissue inhibitor of metalloproteinases 1 (TIMP 1) concentrations and previous chemotherapy or radiotherapy was reported to accurately estimate 3 months mortality in patients with malignant pleural effusion [64]. However, in order to develop more precise prognostication models, our understanding would require to improve the pathophysiology and the complex interactions between different biomarkers involved in malignant pleural effusion formation in lung cancer. In the broad sense, malignant pleural effusion occurs when the production of pleural fluid exceeds that of clearance. This may be due to plasma leakage as most malignant pleural effusions have high protein content, lymphatic blockage and invasion, although not in all cases, of the pleura by cancer. It is likely that more intricate interactions between the mesothelial and cancer cells at the levels of proliferation, cytokines activity, immune modulation and nutrition may provide the answer to the exact mechanisms of malignant pleural effusion formation in lung cancer.

Imaging

A chest radiograph may detect around 200 ml in a volume of pleural effusion with CT scan and thoracic ultrasound being more sensitive as these imaging modalities can identify much smaller amounts of pleural fluid, quantify and characterise it and allow to distinguish pleural effusion from other pathologies such as consolidation, lung collapse, raised hemi-diaphragm or diaphragmatic hernia all of which can mimic pleural effusion [61]. There are certain characteristics that both the CT scan and the thoracic ultrasound can categorize that may suggest malignant pathology, namely pleural thickening greater than 1 cm, diaphragmatic thickening of more or equal to 7 mm or pleural nodularity or [65]. CT scan may also help in identifying mediastinal pleural nodularity, circumferential pleural thickening or mediastinal involvement, which in the context of malignancy were reported to have a specificity of 88-94% [66]. However, as CT was reported to have a relatively low sensitivity of 36% to 51% and PET scan in the recent meta-analysis was shown to have moderate accuracy with a sensitivity of 81% and specificity of 74% for differentiation between malignant and benign pleural effusions, and for this reason, a third of the cases of malignant pleural effusion may require further more invasive evaluation [66, 67].

Thoracic ultrasound has become a valuable tool in the evaluation of patients with malignant pleural effusion not only from imaging aspects but also when guiding pleural procedures including thoracentesis, which all according to the current guidelines should be performed under the thoracic ultrasound guidance [68]. When pleural procedures are performed without image guidance, complications can occur in around 30% of cases with pneumothorax being reported in one in ten of cases compared to around 4% when imaging is used as evidenced by the findings from a large meta-analysis of over 6,600 pleural fluid aspiration procedures [69]. Similarly, a recent large retrospective study of over 62,000 of pleural fluid aspirations revealed that the use of thoracic ultrasound reduced the risk of pneumothorax by 19% [70]. Thoracic ultrasound training has become an integral part of the respiratory medicine curriculum in the UK and many other countries. The pleural fluid sampling may provide a relatively rapid cytological diagnosis with reported success rates around 60% [60]. However, in the current era of personalized therapy where not only sub-typing but also cancer genotyping are required, many patients would require pleural biopsy either under image guidance or using techniques such as thoracoscopy. There is evidence from a randomised trial that CT guided pleural biopsy in patients with cytology negative pleural effusion of exudate type had an overall sensitivity of 87.5% compared with that of medical thoracoscopy of 94.1%, which was not statistically different [71]. The sensitivity of medical thoracoscopy was 100% for the smooth less than 1 cm in thickness compared to that of 73% for the CT guided biopsy [71]. The decision, whether to undertake invasive pleural procedures would depend on the patients' symptoms as well as the need for obtaining biopsy samples for diagnosis. Clearly, medical thoracoscopy or CT guided biopsy should be undertaken in patients in whom histological diagnosis will change the management and in those who are expected to have a reasonable survival time [72].

Recent guidelines recommend that patients with malignant pleural effusion who remain asymptomatic may not necessarily require any intervention. For example, a small study reported that none of the 13 patients with lung cancer and malignant pleural effusion followed up for a period of over 3 months required any interventions [73]. Similarly, a larger study found that none of the 20% of patients with lung cancer who developed small pleural effusion required any intervention over the 10 months follow up period [74]. More controversial is the issue of surgery for patients with lung cancer and malignant pleural effusion but without extra-thoracic involvement for whom usual therapeutic options include palliative chemotherapy. There is limited evidence that in this subgroup of patients extra-pleural pneumonectomy may improve 5-year survival from 22% to 33.7% [75]. Arietta et al. reported progression free survival of 15.9 months for 6 patients with lung cancer and malignant pleural effusion but without extra-thoracic involvement who underwent chemotherapy followed by surgery [76]. However, at present, due to the paucity of data no formal recommendations can be made in this subgroup of patients with regards to surgical options in addition to systemic treatment.

Medical Thoracoscopy

Thoracoscopy involves the insertion of an endoscope into the pleural cavity through a small incision and allows for examination and sampling of the pleura [72, 77]. Medical thoracoscopy is performed with patients in the lateral position, breathing spontaneously under the local anaesthesia and awake sedation [78]. There are absolute contra-indications for medical thoracoscopy, which include circumferential adherent pleura, uncontrollable coagulopathy, hypercapnia, the poor cardiopulmonary reserve to tolerate pneumothorax and intractable cough. Thoracoscopy is a relatively safe procedure with a reported mortality of 0.09% to [79, 80]. The most common serious complications of thoracoscopy included empyema and haemorrhage, which were reported in 3 out of 652 procedures [79, 80]. The risk of intra-pleural bleeding can be reduced by not performing a biopsy of any of the pulsatile lesions or making sure that during the biopsy, forceps are supported by the underlying rib. Low oxygen saturation occurs in 2% of procedures and other less common complications include surgical emphysema, persistent air leak, pulmonary oedema and arrhythmia. Therefore, cardiac and oxygen monitoring is recommended during the procedure. The patients may develop early complications such as vaso-vagal syncope, which commonly occurs at the time of insertion of the trocar. Pain may occur at the time of the insertion of the trocar or the thoracoscope as well as during the biopsy and this may be alleviated by the use of local anaesthetic subcutaneously and intra-pleurally. However, it is important to use the local anaesthetic such as lidocaine within the recommended dose to avoid serious central nervous system side effects. When the pleural fluid is drained the patients may develop cough, which usually improves once the air enters the pleural space. Similarly, some patients may develop broncho-spasm, which normally can be controlled with nebulised bronchodilators.

It is recommended that the trocar insertion is performed under the ultrasound guidance in order to locate pleural effusion and to reduce the risk of complications and to avoid areas where there are adhesions or septations [72]. The most commonly used entry point is in the mid-axillary line in the fourth of fifth intercostal space as it allows for a good examination of the thoracic cavity. Once the appropriate area is located, it is infiltrated with the local anaesthetic, an incision is made through the skin and subcutaneous tissue and then the trocar is inserted into the pleural cavity. Subsequently, the trocar is removed leaving the cannula within the pleural cavity, which allows for the pleural fluid to be drained, but this should not be undertaken too fast so to avoid the re-expansion pulmonary oedema, and to make sure that the air enters in to the pleural cavity replacing the removed fluid and allowing for the lung to collapse. Subsequently, a rigid, usually 9 mm in diameter thoracoscope, which is an optic telescope connected to a xenon light source allowing for the images to be transmitted onto a screen, is introduced into the pleural cavity through the cannula [81]. A smaller 3 mm rigid thoracoscope may be used and was shown to have a diagnostic yield of around 93% [82]. The thoracoscope allows for the pleural cavity to be examined in a systematic manner and to locate any abnormal areas for biopsy. In the single port technique following the pleural space examination, the scope is removed and an optical biopsy forceps are introduced and pleural biopsies are performed. In the double port technique, the biopsy forceps are introduced through a second smaller trocar and the biopsy is performed under the direct guidance and visualisation from the thoracoscope. At the end of the procedure, a chest drain is inserted to remove the remaining air and fluid. The chest drain is removed once the air leak is ceased and the fluid drainage either stops or is less than 150 ml in 24 hours. There are alternative options for inserting an indwelling pleural catheter rather than a chest drain at the end of the procedure. Another technique involves the use of a semi-rigid scope, which has controls similar to those in a flexible bronchoscope and advantage of an easier manoeuvrability within the plural cavity [83]. Its main disadvantages are related to the smaller size of the biopsies resulting in between 4% and 9.5% non-diagnostic procedures [83]. In addition to the white light thoracoscopy the technology allows the use of autofluorescence, which has been shown in a large series of 491 pleural biopsies to have 100% sensitivity for identifying pleural lesions compared to that of 92.8% for the white light thoracoscopy [84]. Similarly, narrow band imaging, which allows for capturing light wavelength corresponding to oxyhaemoglobin absorption can be used during thoracoscopy with benefits of identifying irregular vascular patterns of areas where the tumour is growing [85]. Although the precise role of the narrow band imaging in the context of medical thoracoscopy is not currently clear.

Pleurodesis

One of the advantages of thoracoscopy is the fact that in patients with pleural effusion during the procedure, the fluid can be drained, a biopsy of the pleura undertaken and talc poudrage pleurodesis can be performed. The main interventional use of medical thoracoscopy is for talc poudrage pleurodesis. The current guidelines define pleurodesis as a procedure during which a drug or a material is administered into the pleural space to cause adhesions between the parietal and visceral pleura and prevention of pleural fluid re-accumulation [59, 68, 72]. During pleurodesis, an agent is administered into the pleural space resulting in chemical irritation leading to pleuritis, and ultimately to pleural fibrosis and obliteration of the pleural space, however the exact molecular mechanisms of this process are not fully understood [68]. It is possible, using thoracic ultrasound to assess whether the pleural apposition occurred following the pleurodesis. A meta-analysis of 36 randomized controlled studies that included 1499 patients reported on a number of different sclerosing agents used for pleurodesis of which talc was shown to have the highest efficacy [86]. There was no evidence for any increase in mortality following talc pleurodesis. Talc pleurodesis can be performed through thoracoscopic poudrage or as talc slurry instillation through an intercostal chest drain or, more recently, through an indwelling pleural catheter.

The guidelines for managing malignant pleural effusion following re-accumulation after the initial thoracocentesis recommend that the patients should undergo a definitive pleural procedure resulting in improvement of patients' symptoms and reduction in pleural, including unplanned, procedures and associated complications [59, 68, 72]. A large retrospective study revealed that only less than a quarter of patients after the fluid re-accumulation underwent a definitive pleural procedure rather than repeat thoracocentesis [87]. The options of the definitive procedure include a chest drain insertion with pleural fluid drainage and talc slurry pleurodesis, indwelling pleural catheter insertion with an option of talc slurry pleurodesis, medical or surgical thoracoscopy with talc poudrage pleurodesis or with indwelling pleural catheter insertion [59, 88]. The studies have shown that a fifth of patients who had talc slurry pleurodesis using a chest drain required further pleural procedures [68]. For this reason, thoracoscopy with talc poudrage pleurodesis may be a better option in a proportion of the patients. In a randomised study, thoracoscopic talc poudrage pleurodesis was shown to be superior to pleurodesis with doxycycline through an intercostal chest drain [89]. In another large randomised trial of over 480 patients with expandable lung, thoracoscopy and talc insufflation had a 78% success rate for pleurodesis at 1 months compared to that of 72% for intercostal chest drain insertion and talc slurry, which did not reach statistical significance [86]. In patients with lung cancer the thoracoscopic talc poudrage pleurodesis was reported to have a higher success rate of 82% with no cases of acute respiratory distress syndrome following the procedure [90]. A recent meta-analysis included 62 randomised controlled studies that involved different pleurodesis agents as well as the use of indwelling pleural catheters showed that talc pleurodesis was effective in reducing pleural fluid re-accumulation but with no difference between talc poudrage or talc slurry [91]. For patients with longer survival, bedside pleurodesis was the least expensive and thoracoscopic pleurodesis the most effective treatment option. The current guidelines recommend that in patients with recurrent malignant pleural effusion and expandable lung; chest drain insertion with talc slurry or thoracoscopy with talc poudrage can be undertaken and that based on currently available evidence both interventions have similar success rates.

Indwelling Pleural Catheters

The presence of an un-expandable lung is one of the potential contraindications for pleurodesis. The guidelines suggest that a large volume thoracocentesis may be used to assess for the presence of un-expandable lung [59]. During the procedure, the effect of pleura fluid drainage on the symptoms may be assessed as well as the time for the fluid to re-accumulate. The presence of an un-expandable lung, which develops in a proportion of patients with lung cancer and malignant pleural effusion, may require a different interventional strategies. For patients with expected survival of around 3 months a repeat thoracocentesis may be the most appropriate and the least expensive treatment option [91]. For patients with a longer expected survival, an indwelling pleural catheter may be more cost effective and thoracoscopic pleurodesis being the most effective treatment option [92]. The indwelling pleural catheters can be inserted in the ambulatory settings. The drain is inserted using a needle and guide wire technique. A subcutaneous tunnel is created through which the catheter is advanced and subsequently introduced into the pleural space through a pull away sheath. The indwelling pleural catheter is secured and can be kept long term allowing for intermittent pleural fluid drainage by attaching a negative pressure bottle through then one way system. Indwelling pleural catheters were reported to improve symptoms in 95% of cases and 45% of patients had spontaneous pleurodesis [93]. The indwelling pleural catheters are relatively safe with a small number of complications, of which the most concerning are cellulitis and malfunction of the catheter. Recent guidelines recommend that cellulitis can be managed using antibiotics without the need from the removal of the drain. Although indwelling pleural catheters were initially used for the patients with pleural effusion and un-expandable lung or those with failed pleurodesis and there is evidence to support their use as first line treatment where there were shown to have good symptoms control and 70% spontaneous pleurodesis to 90 days [94]. Demmy et al. in the CALGB randomised trial, of patients with malignant pleural effusion of which 63% had lung cancer, showed that the group who had the indwelling pleural catheters inserted compared with that who underwent pleurodesis had better 30-day effusion control 82% and 52% respectively and activity without dyspnoea [95]. The NVALT-14 randomised study showed that compared to talc pleurodesis indwelling pleural catheters were not superior in improving breathless in symptomatic patients with malignant pleural effusion but resulted in lower hospital stay, fewer admissions and re-interventions [96]. The Ample-2 study showed no difference in daily or symptom guided drainage regimens for indwelling pleural catheters in controlling dyspnoea, but daily drainage was more effective for spontaneous pleurodesis [97]. In TIME 2 study, the patients were randomised to indwelling pleural catheter insertion or chest drain insertion and talc slurry pleurodesis and the results showed no difference between the two interventions in improving dyspnoea in symptomatic patients with malignant pleural effusion but the indwelling pleural catheter group had a shorter hospital stay and needed fewer number of subsequent pleural procedures [98]. In a recent study, patients with malignant pleural effusion had an indwelling pleural catheter inserted and after 10 days of drainage, if there was no evidence of un-expandable lung, had talc slurry pleurodesis through the indwelling pleural catheter showing a significantly higher at 35 days 43% successful pleurodesis compared with that of 23% in those who had drainage alone [99]. There is also evidence that indwelling pleural catheters may be inserted at medical thoracoscopy with this approach being reported to be safe within outpatient settings and allowing for the patients to be discharged earlier, reducing hospital length of stay [100]. Therefore, based on currently available data, indwelling pleural catheters can be used in patients with un-expandable lung or those with failed pleurodesis as well as in carefully selected patients as a first line treatment for malignant pleural effusion and as an alternative to chest drain at thoracoscopy. Moreover, there is more evidence emerging to suggest that talc slurry pleurodesis may be a feasible option to manage malignant pleural effusion.

INVESTIGATIONAL PATHWAY

The investigational and diagnostic pathways for lung cancer will differ depending on individual cases. The aim is to provide a rapid diagnosis of lung cancer using the most appropriate investigations that would offer staging and histological information. There are some common aspects of the diagnostic protocols for patients with suspected lung cancer. All patients with suspected lung cancer should be assessed through a rapid access specialist clinic as a part of a multidisciplinary team structure. Imaging in the form of a chest radiograph, CT scan and, if appropriate, a PET scan should be undertaken as this would allow for non invasive staging of the disease. Patients, especially those considered for radical treatment, with enlarged more than 10 mm in short axis or PET avid hilar or mediastinal lymph nodes would require staging with an EBUS, EUS or a mediastinoscopy. Other investigations such as image guided biopsy with the CT or the ultrasound may be required depending on the individual cases. All patients with suspected lung cancer should have performance status assessed as well as spirometry performed. Patients considered for radical treatment should have formal fitness testing, including pulmonary function and exercise assessment, including CPET, if appropriate. Histological confirmation should ideally be achieved prior to the radical treatments such as surgery as it allows to confirm the diagnosis and plan surgery, *e.g.*, lobectomy or sub-lobar resection. Therefore, CT guided biopsy or newer techniques, including radial EBUS or navigational bronchoscopy should be available within the investigational pathways. Finally, once all the required information is available a multidisciplinary team decision for the best therapeutic approach should be undertaken.

CONCLUSION

Investigation of patients with suspected lung cancer should be undertaken within a specialist team that allows for patients to have access to all potential investigational procedures. All patients should have access to imaging investigations such as CT and PET scan, which form an important aspect of the staging of the disease. Moreover, access to EBUS and EUS as well as mediastinoscopy is required as nodal staging affects the therapeutic options. The technological improvements have resulted in new novel procedures available for diagnosing lung cancer. Therefore, access to all required investigational technologies should be available within the centres involved in investigations and management of patients with lung cancer. This is important from the aspects of timely diagnosis and staging of lung cancer, which affect therapeutic options and prognosis.

CONSENT FOR PUBLICATION

Not applicable.

CONFLICT OF INTEREST

The author declares that there is no conflict of interest in this chapter.

ACKNOWLEDGEMENTS

Declared none.

REFERENCES

[1]   NICE Guidelines Updates Team (UK). Lung cancer: diagnosis and management 2019.

[2]   Lim E, Baldwin D, Beckles M, *et al.* Guidelines on the radical management of patients with lung cancer. Thorax 2010; 65 (Suppl. 3): iii1-iii27.
[http://dx.doi.org/10.1136/thx.2010.145938] [PMID: 20940263]

[3]   Ramnath N, Dilling TJ, Harris LJ, *et al.* Treatment of stage iii non-small cell lung cancer: Diagnosis and management of lung cancer, 3rd ed: American college of chest physicians evidence-based clinical

practice guidelines. Chest 2013; 143: e314S-e340S.

[4]   Postmus PE, Kerr KM, Oudkerk M, *et al.* Early and locally advanced non-small-cell lung cancer (nsclc): ESMO clinical practice guidelines for diagnosis, treatment and follow-up. Ann Oncol 2017; 28: iv1-iv21.
[http://dx.doi.org/10.1093/annonc/mdx222]

[5]   Vansteenkiste J, De Ruysscher D, Eberhardt WE, *et al.* Early and locally advanced non-small-cell lung cancer (NSCLC): ESMO Clinical Practice Guidelines for diagnosis, treatment and follow-up. Ann Oncol 2013; 24 (Suppl. 6): vi89-98.
[http://dx.doi.org/10.1093/annonc/mdt241] [PMID: 23860613]

[6]   Walter FM, Rubin G, Bankhead C, *et al.* Symptoms and other factors associated with time to diagnosis and stage of lung cancer: a prospective cohort study. Br J Cancer 2015; 112 (Suppl. 1): S6-S13.
[http://dx.doi.org/10.1038/bjc.2015.30] [PMID: 25734397]

[7]   Smith SM, Campbell NC, MacLeod U, *et al.* Factors contributing to the time taken to consult with symptoms of lung cancer: a cross-sectional study. Thorax 2009; 64(6): 523-31.
[http://dx.doi.org/10.1136/thx.2008.096560] [PMID: 19052045]

[8]   Kennedy MPT, Cheyne L, Darby M, *et al.* Lung cancer stage-shift following a symptom awareness campaign. Thorax 2018; 73(12): 1128-36.
[http://dx.doi.org/10.1136/thoraxjnl-2018-211842] [PMID: 29950525]

[9]   Smith SM, Murchie P, Devereux G, *et al.* Developing a complex intervention to reduce time to presentation with symptoms of lung cancer. Br J Gen Pract 2012; 62(602): e605-15.
[http://dx.doi.org/10.3399/bjgp12X654579] [PMID: 22947581]

[10]   Emery JD, Murray SR, Walter FM, *et al.* The Chest Australia Trial: a randomised controlled trial of an intervention to increase consultation rates in smokers at risk of lung cancer. Thorax 2019; 74(4): 362-70.
[http://dx.doi.org/10.1136/thoraxjnl-2018-212506] [PMID: 30630891]

[11]   Neal RD, Tharmanathan P, France B, *et al.* Is increased time to diagnosis and treatment in symptomatic cancer associated with poorer outcomes? Systematic review. Br J Cancer 2015; 112 (Suppl. 1): S92-S107.
[http://dx.doi.org/10.1038/bjc.2015.48] [PMID: 25734382]

[12]   Maconachie R, Mercer T, Navani N, McVeigh G. Lung cancer: diagnosis and management: summary of updated NICE guidance. BMJ 2019; 364: l1049.
[http://dx.doi.org/10.1136/bmj.l1049] [PMID: 30923038]

[13]   Navani N, Nankivell M, Lawrence DR, *et al.* Lung cancer diagnosis and staging with endobronchial ultrasound-guided transbronchial needle aspiration compared with conventional approaches: an open-label, pragmatic, randomised controlled trial. Lancet Respir Med 2015; 3(4): 282-9.
[http://dx.doi.org/10.1016/S2213-2600(15)00029-6] [PMID: 25660225]

[14]   http://www.cancerresearchuk.org/sites/default/files/national_optimal_lung_pathway_aug_2017.pdf

[15]   Taylor SA, Mallett S, Ball S, *et al.* Diagnostic accuracy of whole-body MRI versus standard imaging pathways for metastatic disease in newly diagnosed non-small-cell lung cancer: the prospective Streamline L trial. Lancet Respir Med 2019; 7(6): 523-32.
[http://dx.doi.org/10.1016/S2213-2600(19)30090-6] [PMID: 31080129]

[16]   Schmidt-Hansen M, Baldwin DR, Hasler E, *et al.* PET-CT for assessing mediastinal lymph node involvement in patients with suspected resectable non-small cell lung cancer. Cochrane Database Syst Rev 2014; 13(11)CD009519
[http://dx.doi.org/10.1002/14651858.CD009519.pub2] [PMID: 25393718]

[17]   Annema JT, van Meerbeeck JP, Rintoul RC, *et al.* Mediastinoscopy vs endosonography for mediastinal nodal staging of lung cancer: a randomized trial. JAMA 2010; 304(20): 2245-52.
[http://dx.doi.org/10.1001/jama.2010.1705] [PMID: 21098770]

[18]   Yasufuku K, Pierre A, Darling G, *et al.* A prospective controlled trial of endobronchial ultrasound-guided transbronchial needle aspiration compared with mediastinoscopy for mediastinal lymph node staging of lung cancer. J Thorac Cardiavsc Surg 2011; 142: 1393-1400 e1391.

[19]   von Bartheld MB, van Breda A, Annema JT. Complication rate of endosonography (endobronchial and endoscopic ultrasound): a systematic review. Respiration 2014; 87(4): 343-51.
[http://dx.doi.org/10.1159/000357066] [PMID: 24434575]

[20]   Hammoud ZT, Anderson RC, Meyers BF, *et al.* The current role of mediastinoscopy in the evaluation of thoracic disease. J Thorac Cardiovasc Surg 1999; 118(5): 894-9.
[http://dx.doi.org/10.1016/S0022-5223(99)70059-0] [PMID: 10534695]

[21]   Groth SS, Andrade RS. Endobronchial ultrasound-guided transbronchial needle aspiration for mediastinal lymph node staging in non-small cell lung cancer. Semin Thorac Cardiovasc Surg 2008; 20(4): 274-8.
[http://dx.doi.org/10.1053/j.semtcvs.2008.11.004] [PMID: 19251164]

[22]   Zhang R, Ying K, Shi L, Zhang L, Zhou L. Combined endobronchial and endoscopic ultrasound-guided fine needle aspiration for mediastinal lymph node staging of lung cancer: a meta-analysis. Eur J Cancer 2013; 49(8): 1860-7.
[http://dx.doi.org/10.1016/j.ejca.2013.02.008] [PMID: 23481511]

[23]   Herth FJ, Eberhardt R, Vilmann P, Krasnik M, Ernst A. Real-time endobronchial ultrasound guided transbronchial needle aspiration for sampling mediastinal lymph nodes. Thorax 2006; 61(9): 795-8.
[http://dx.doi.org/10.1136/thx.2005.047829] [PMID: 16738038]

[24]   Herth FJ, Ernst A, Eberhardt R, *et al.* Endobronchial ultrasound-guided transbronchial needle aspiration of lymph nodes in the radiologically normal mediastinum. Eur Respir J 2006; 28(5): 910-4.
[http://dx.doi.org/10.1183/09031936.06.00124905] [PMID: 16807262]

[25]   Um SW, Kim HK, Jung SH, *et al.* Endobronchial ultrasound versus mediastinoscopy for mediastinal nodal staging of non-small-cell lung cancer. J Thorac Oncol 2015; 10(2): 331-7.
[http://dx.doi.org/10.1097/JTO.0000000000000388] [PMID: 25611227]

[26]   Dong X, Qiu X, Liu Q, Jia J. Endobronchial ultrasound-guided transbronchial needle aspiration in the mediastinal staging of non-small cell lung cancer: a meta-analysis. Ann Thorac Surg 2013; 96(4): 1502-7.
[http://dx.doi.org/10.1016/j.athoracsur.2013.05.016] [PMID: 23993894]

[27]   Liberman M, Sampalis J, Duranceau A, *et al.* Endosonographic mediastinal lymph node staging of lung cancer. Chest 2014; 146(2): 389-97.
[http://dx.doi.org/10.1378/chest.13-2349] [PMID: 24603902]

[28]   Herth FJ, Annema JT, Eberhardt R, *et al.* Endobronchial ultrasound with transbronchial needle aspiration for restaging the mediastinum in lung cancer. J Clin Oncol 2008; 26(20): 3346-50.
[http://dx.doi.org/10.1200/JCO.2007.14.9229] [PMID: 18519953]

[29]   Manhire A, Charig M, Clelland C, *et al.* Guidelines for radiologically guided lung biopsy. Thorax 2003; 58(11): 920-36.
[http://dx.doi.org/10.1136/thorax.58.11.920] [PMID: 14586042]

[30]   Damhuis RA, Schütte PR. Resection rates and postoperative mortality in 7,899 patients with lung cancer. Eur Respir J 1996; 9(1): 7-10.
[http://dx.doi.org/10.1183/09031936.96.09010007] [PMID: 8834326]

[31]   Thomas DC, Blasberg JD, Arnold BN, *et al.* Validating the thoracic revised cardiac risk index following lung resection. Ann Thorac Surg 2017; 104(2): 389-94.
[http://dx.doi.org/10.1016/j.athoracsur.2017.02.006] [PMID: 28499655]

[32]   Wotton R, Marshall A, Kerr A, *et al.* Does the revised cardiac risk index predict cardiac complications following elective lung resection? J Cardiothorac Surg 2013; 8: 220.
[http://dx.doi.org/10.1186/1749-8090-8-220] [PMID: 24289748]

[33]   Brunelli A, Charloux A, Bolliger CT, *et al.* ERS/ESTS clinical guidelines on fitness for radical therapy in lung cancer patients (surgery and chemo-radiotherapy). Eur Respir J 2009; 34(1): 17-41.
[http://dx.doi.org/10.1183/09031936.00184308] [PMID: 19567600]

[34]   Brunelli A, Charloux A, Bolliger CT, *et al.* The European Respiratory Society and European Society of Thoracic Surgeons clinical guidelines for evaluating fitness for radical treatment (surgery and chemoradiotherapy) in patients with lung cancer. Eur J Cardiothorac Surg 2009; 36(1): 181-4.
[http://dx.doi.org/10.1016/j.ejcts.2009.04.022] [PMID: 19477657]

[35]   Charloux A, Brunelli A, Bolliger CT, *et al.* Lung function evaluation before surgery in lung cancer patients: how are recent advances put into practice? A survey among members of the European Society of Thoracic Surgeons (ESTS) and of the Thoracic Oncology Section of the European Respiratory Society (ERS). Interact Cardiovasc Thorac Surg 2009; 9(6): 925-31.
[http://dx.doi.org/10.1510/icvts.2009.211219] [PMID: 19752152]

[36]   BTS guidelines: guidelines on the selection of patients with lung cancer for surgery. Thorax 2001; 56(2): 89-108.
[http://dx.doi.org/10.1136/thorax.56.2.89] [PMID: 11209097]

[37]   Brunelli A, Refai MA, Salati M, Sabbatini A, Morgan-Hughes NJ, Rocco G. Carbon monoxide lung diffusion capacity improves risk stratification in patients without airflow limitation: evidence for systematic measurement before lung resection. Eur J Cardiothorac Surg 2006; 29(4): 567-70.
[http://dx.doi.org/10.1016/j.ejcts.2006.01.014] [PMID: 16481190]

[38]   Brunelli A, Belardinelli R, Pompili C, *et al.* Minute ventilation-to-carbon dioxide output (VE/VCO2) slope is the strongest predictor of respiratory complications and death after pulmonary resection. Ann Thorac Surg 2012; 93(6): 1802-6.
[http://dx.doi.org/10.1016/j.athoracsur.2012.03.022] [PMID: 22560968]

[39]   Brunelli A, Kim AW, Berger KI, Addrizzo-Harris DJ. Physiologic evaluation of the patient with lung cancer being considered for resectional surgery: Diagnosis and management of lung cancer, 3rd ed: American college of chest physicians evidence-based clinical practice guidelines. Chest 2013; 143: e166S-e190S.

[40]   Rami-Porta R. Staging manual in thoracic oncology. 2nd ed. North Fort Myers, FL: Editorial RX Press 2017; pp. 81-132.

[41]   Rami-Porta R, Asamura H, Travis WD, Rusch VW. Lung cancer - major changes in the American Joint Committee on Cancer eighth edition cancer staging manual. CA Cancer J Clin 2017; 67(2): 138-55.
[http://dx.doi.org/10.3322/caac.21390] [PMID: 28140453]

[42]   Oudkerk M, Devaraj A, Vliegenthart R, *et al.* European position statement on lung cancer screening. Lancet Oncol 2017; 18(12): e754-66.
[http://dx.doi.org/10.1016/S1470-2045(17)30861-6] [PMID: 29208441]

[43]   Baldwin D, Callister M, Akram A, *et al.* British Thoracic Society quality standards for the investigation and management of pulmonary nodules. BMJ Open Respir Res 2018; 5(1)e000273
[http://dx.doi.org/10.1136/bmjresp-2017-000273] [PMID: 29682290]

[44]   Aberle DR, Adams AM, Berg CD, *et al.* Reduced lung-cancer mortality with low-dose computed tomographic screening. N Engl J Med 2011; 365(5): 395-409.
[http://dx.doi.org/10.1056/NEJMoa1102873] [PMID: 21714641]

[45]   de Koning HJ, van der Aalst CM, de Jong PA, *et al.* Reduced lung-cancer mortality with volume CT screening in a randomized trial. N Engl J Med 2020; 382(6): 503-13.
[http://dx.doi.org/10.1056/NEJMoa1911793] [PMID: 31995683]

[46]   Field JK, Duffy SW. Lung cancer CT screening: are we ready to consider screening biennially in a subgroup of low-risk individuals? Thorax 2018; 73(11): 1006-7.
[http://dx.doi.org/10.1136/thoraxjnl-2018-211814] [PMID: 29954858]

[47] Walter JE, Heuvelmans MA, Ten Haaf K, *et al.* Persisting new nodules in incidence rounds of the NELSON CT lung cancer screening study. Thorax 2019; 74(3): 247-53.
[http://dx.doi.org/10.1136/thoraxjnl-2018-212152] [PMID: 30591535]

[48] Henschke CI, Naidich DP, Yankelevitz DF, *et al.* Early lung cancer action project: initial findings on repeat screenings. Cancer 2001; 92(1): 153-9.
[http://dx.doi.org/10.1002/1097-0142(20010701)92:1<153::AID-CNCR1303>3.0.CO;2-S] [PMID: 11443621]

[49] Henschke CI, Yankelevitz DF, Libby DM, *et al.* Survival of patients with stage I lung cancer detected on CT screening. N Engl J Med 2006; 355(17): 1763-71.
[http://dx.doi.org/10.1056/NEJMoa060476] [PMID: 17065637]

[50] Belanger AR, Akulian JA. An update on the role of advanced diagnostic bronchoscopy in the evaluation and staging of lung cancer. Ther Adv Respir Dis 2017; 11(5): 211-21.
[http://dx.doi.org/10.1177/1753465817695981] [PMID: 28470104]

[51] Steinfort DP, Khor YH, Manser RL, Irving LB. Radial probe endobronchial ultrasound for the diagnosis of peripheral lung cancer: systematic review and meta-analysis. Eur Respir J 2011; 37(4): 902-10.
[http://dx.doi.org/10.1183/09031936.00075310] [PMID: 20693253]

[52] Steinfort DP, Vincent J, Heinze S, Antippa P, Irving LB. Comparative effectiveness of radial probe endobronchial ultrasound versus CT-guided needle biopsy for evaluation of peripheral pulmonary lesions: a randomized pragmatic trial. Respir Med 2011; 105(11): 1704-11.
[http://dx.doi.org/10.1016/j.rmed.2011.08.008] [PMID: 21875783]

[53] Khan KA, Nardelli P, Jaeger A, *et al.* Navigational bronchoscopy for early lung cancer: A road to therapy. Adv Ther 2016; 33(4): 580-96.
[http://dx.doi.org/10.1007/s12325-016-0319-4] [PMID: 27084723]

[54] Asano F, Shinagawa N, Ishida T, *et al.* Virtual bronchoscopic navigation improves the diagnostic yield of radial-endobronchial ultrasound for peripheral pulmonary lesions with involved bronchi on CT. Intern Med 2015; 54(9): 1021-5.
[http://dx.doi.org/10.2169/internalmedicine.54.3497] [PMID: 25948341]

[55] Asano F, Eberhardt R, Herth FJ. Virtual bronchoscopic navigation for peripheral pulmonary lesions. Respiration 2014; 88(5): 430-40.
[http://dx.doi.org/10.1159/000367900] [PMID: 25402610]

[56] Khandhar SJ, Bowling MR, Flandes J, *et al.* Electromagnetic navigation bronchoscopy to access lung lesions in 1,000 subjects: first results of the prospective, multicenter NAVIGATE study. BMC Pulm Med 2017; 17(1): 59-68.
[http://dx.doi.org/10.1186/s12890-017-0403-9] [PMID: 28399830]

[57] Evison MMF, Batchelor T. What is the role of surgery in potentially resectable N2 non-small cell lung cancer? Thorax 2018; 73: 1105-9.
[http://dx.doi.org/10.1136/thoraxjnl-2018-212287]

[58] Eberhardt WE, De Ruysscher D, Weder W, *et al.* 2nd ESMO consensus conference in lung cancer: Locally advanced stage iii non-small-cell lung cancer. Annal Oncol 2015; 26: 1573-1588.

[59] Feller-Kopman DJ, Reddy CB, DeCamp MM, *et al.* Management of Malignant Pleural Effusions. An Official ATS/STS/STR Clinical Practice Guideline. Am J Respir Crit Care Med 2018; 198(7): 839-49.
[http://dx.doi.org/10.1164/rccm.201807-1415ST] [PMID: 30272503]

[60] Bibby AC, Dorn P, Psallidas I, *et al.* ERS/EACTS statement on the management of malignant pleural effusions. Eur Respir J 2018; 52(1)1800349
[http://dx.doi.org/10.1183/13993003.00349-2018] [PMID: 30054348]

[61] Kastelik JA. Management of malignant pleural effusion. Lung 2013; 191(2): 165-75.
[http://dx.doi.org/10.1007/s00408-012-9445-1] [PMID: 23315213]

[62]   Morgensztern D, Waqar S, Subramanian J, Trinkaus K, Govindan R. Prognostic impact of malignant pleural effusion at presentation in patients with metastatic non-small-cell lung cancer. J Thorac Oncol 2012; 7(10): 1485-9.
[http://dx.doi.org/10.1097/JTO.0b013e318267223a] [PMID: 22982649]

[63]   Clive AO, Kahan BC, Hooper CE, *et al.* Predicting survival in malignant pleural effusion: development and validation of the LENT prognostic score. Thorax 2014; 69(12): 1098-104.
[http://dx.doi.org/10.1136/thoraxjnl-2014-205285] [PMID: 25100651]

[64]   Psallidas I, Kanellakis NI, Gerry S, *et al.* Development and validation of response markers to predict survival and pleurodesis success in patients with malignant pleural effusion (PROMISE): a multicohort analysis. Lancet Oncol 2018; 19(7): 930-9.
[http://dx.doi.org/10.1016/S1470-2045(18)30294-8] [PMID: 29908990]

[65]   Qureshi NR, Rahman NM, Gleeson FV. Thoracic ultrasound in the diagnosis of malignant pleural effusion. Thorax 2009; 64(2): 139-43.
[http://dx.doi.org/10.1136/thx.2008.100545] [PMID: 18852159]

[66]   Leung AN, Müller NL, Miller RR. CT in differential diagnosis of diffuse pleural disease. AJR Am J Roentgenol 1990; 154(3): 487-92.
[http://dx.doi.org/10.2214/ajr.154.3.2106209] [PMID: 2106209]

[67]   Porcel JM, Pardina M, Bielsa S, González A, Light RW. Derivation and validation of a CT scan scoring system for discriminating malignant from benign pleural effusions. Chest 2015; 147(2): 513-9.
[http://dx.doi.org/10.1378/chest.14-0013] [PMID: 25255186]

[68]   Reddy CB, DeCamp MM, Diekemper RL, *et al.* Summary for Clinicians: Clinical Practice Guideline for Management of Malignant Pleural Effusions. Ann Am Thorac Soc 2019; 16(1): 17-21.
[http://dx.doi.org/10.1513/AnnalsATS.201809-620CME] [PMID: 30516394]

[69]   Gordon CE, Feller-Kopman D, Balk EM, Smetana GW. Pneumothorax following thoracentesis: a systematic review and meta-analysis. Arch Intern Med 2010; 170(4): 332-9.
[http://dx.doi.org/10.1001/archinternmed.2009.548] [PMID: 20177035]

[70]   Mercaldi CJ, Lanes SF. Ultrasound guidance decreases complications and improves the cost of care among patients undergoing thoracentesis and paracentesis 2013.
[http://dx.doi.org/10.1378/chest.12-0447]

[71]   Metintas M, Ak G, Dundar E, *et al.* Medical thoracoscopy vs CT scan-guided Abrams pleural needle biopsy for diagnosis of patients with pleural effusions: a randomized, controlled trial. Chest 2010; 137(6): 1362-8.
[http://dx.doi.org/10.1378/chest.09-0884] [PMID: 20154079]

[72]   Rahman NM, Ali NJ, Brown G, *et al.* Local anaesthetic thoracoscopy: British Thoracic Society Pleural Disease Guideline 2010. Thorax 2010; 65 (Suppl. 2): ii54-60.
[http://dx.doi.org/10.1136/thx.2010.137018] [PMID: 20696694]

[73]   Tremblay A, Robins S, Berthiaume L, Michaud G. Natural history of asymptomatic pleural effusion in lung cancer patients. J Bronchol 2007; 14(98): 98-100.
[http://dx.doi.org/10.1097/LBR.0b013e31804f5aa6]

[74]   Porcel JM, Gasol A, Bielsa S, *et al.* Clinical features and survival of lung cancer patients with pleural effusions. Respirology 2015; 20(4): 654-9. [eng.].
[http://dx.doi.org/10.1111/resp.12496] [PMID: 25706291]

[75]   Fukui T, Yokoi K. The role of surgical intervention in lung cancer with carcinomatous pleuritis. J Thorac Dis 2016; 8 (Suppl. 11): S901-7.
[http://dx.doi.org/10.21037/jtd.2016.06.36] [PMID: 27942413]

[76]   Arrieta O, Escamilla-López I, Lyra-González I, *et al.* Radical aggressive treatment among non-small cell lung cancer patients with malignant pleural effusion without extra-thoracic disease. J Thorac Dis 2019; 11(2): 595-601.

[http://dx.doi.org/10.21037/jtd.2019.01.36] [PMID: 30963004]

[77] Bhatnagar R, Corcoran JP, Maldonado F, *et al.* Advanced medical interventions in pleural disease. Eur Respir Rev 2016; 25(140): 199-213.
[http://dx.doi.org/10.1183/16000617.0020-2016] [PMID: 27246597]

[78] Rodriguez-Panadero F, Janssen JP, Astoul P. Thoracoscopy: general overview and place in the diagnosis and management of pleural effusion. Eur Respir J 2006; 28(2): 409-22.
[http://dx.doi.org/10.1183/09031936.06.00013706] [PMID: 16880371]

[79] Viskum K. Contraindications and complications to thoracoscopy. Pneumologie 1989; 43(2): 55-7.
[PMID: 2717557]

[80] Viskum K, Enk B. Complications of thoracoscopy. Poumon Coeur 1981; 37(1): 25-8.
[PMID: 7019876]

[81] Tassi GF, Marchetti GP, Aliprandi PL. Advanced medical thoracoscopy. Monaldi Arch Chest Dis 2011; 75(1): 99-101.
[PMID: 21627005]

[82] Tassi GF, Marchetti GP, Pinelli V. Minithoracoscopy: a complementary technique for medical thoracoscopy. Respiration 2011; 82(2): 204-6.
[http://dx.doi.org/10.1159/000324072] [PMID: 21447932]

[83] Mohan A, Chandra S, Agarwal D, Naik S, Munavvar M. Utility of semirigid thoracoscopy in the diagnosis of pleural effusions: a systematic review. J Bronchology Interv Pulmonol 2010; 17(3): 195-201.
[http://dx.doi.org/10.1097/LBR.0b013e3181e6a2e7] [PMID: 23168883]

[84] Wang F, Wang Z, Tong Z, *et al.* A pilot study of autofluorescence in the diagnosis of pleural disease. Chest 2015; 147(5): 1395-400.
[http://dx.doi.org/10.1378/chest.14-1351] [PMID: 25411951]

[85] Ishida A, Ishikawa F, Nakamura M, *et al.* Narrow band imaging applied to pleuroscopy for the assessment of vascular patterns of the pleura. Respiration 2009; 78(4): 432-9.
[http://dx.doi.org/10.1159/000247335] [PMID: 19844135]

[86] Dresler CM, Olak J, Herndon JE II, *et al.* Phase III intergroup study of talc poudrage vs talc slurry sclerosis for malignant pleural effusion. Chest 2005; 127(3): 909-15.
[http://dx.doi.org/10.1378/chest.127.3.909] [PMID: 15764775]

[87] Ost DE, Niu J, Zhao H, Grosu HB, Giordano SH. Quality gaps and comparative effectiveness of management strategies for recurrent malignant pleural effusions. Chest 2018; 153(2): 438-52.
[http://dx.doi.org/10.1016/j.chest.2017.08.026] [PMID: 28864054]

[88] Bhatnagar R, Kahan BC, Morley AJ, *et al.* The efficacy of indwelling pleural catheter placement versus placement plus talc sclerosant in patients with malignant pleural effusions managed exclusively as outpatients (IPC-PLUS): study protocol for a randomised controlled trial. Trials 2015; 16: 48.
[http://dx.doi.org/10.1186/s13063-015-0563-y] [PMID: 25880969]

[89] Putnam JB Jr, Light RW, Rodriguez RM, *et al.* A randomized comparison of indwelling pleural catheter and doxycycline pleurodesis in the management of malignant pleural effusions. Cancer 1999; 86(10): 1992-9.
[http://dx.doi.org/10.1002/(SICI)1097-0142(19991115)86:10<1992::AID-CNCR16>3.0.CO;2-M] [PMID: 10570423]

[90] Shaw P, Agarwal R. Pleurodesis for malignant pleural effusions. Cochrane Database Syst Rev 2004; (1): CD002916
[PMID: 14973997]

[91] Clive AO, Jones HE, Bhatnagar R, Preston NJ, Maskell N. Interventions for the management of malignant pleural effusions: a network meta-analysis. Cochrane Database Syst Rev 2016; 8(5)CD010529

[http://dx.doi.org/10.1002/14651858.CD010529.pub2] [PMID: 27155783]

[92] Puri V, Pyrdeck TL, Crabtree TD, *et al.* Treatment of malignant pleural effusion: a cost-effectiveness analysis. Ann Thorac Surg 2012; 94(2): 374-9.
[http://dx.doi.org/10.1016/j.athoracsur.2012.02.100] [PMID: 22579398]

[93] Van Meter ME, McKee KY, Kohlwes RJ. Efficacy and safety of tunneled pleural catheters in adults with malignant pleural effusions: a systematic review. J Gen Intern Med 2011; 26(1): 70-6.
[http://dx.doi.org/10.1007/s11606-010-1472-0] [PMID: 20697963]

[94] Tremblay A, Mason C, Michaud G. Use of tunnelled catheters for malignant pleural effusions in patients fit for pleurodesis. Eur Respir J 2007; 30(4): 759-62.
[http://dx.doi.org/10.1183/09031936.00164706] [PMID: 17567670]

[95] Demmy TL, Gu L, Burkhalter JE, *et al.* Optimal management of malignant pleural effusions (results of CALGB 30102). J Natl Compr Canc Netw 2012; 10(8): 975-82.
[http://dx.doi.org/10.6004/jnccn.2012.0102] [PMID: 22878823]

[96] Boshuizen RC, Vd Noort V, Burgers JA, *et al.* A randomized controlled trial comparing indwelling pleural catheters with talc pleurodesis (NVALT-14). Lung Cancer 2017; 108: 9-14.
[http://dx.doi.org/10.1016/j.lungcan.2017.01.019] [PMID: 28625655]

[97] Muruganandan S, Azzopardi M, Fitzgerald DB, *et al.* Aggressive versus symptom-guided drainage of malignant pleural effusion via indwelling pleural catheters (AMPLE-2): an open-label randomised trial. Lancet Respir Med 2018; 6(9): 671-80.
[http://dx.doi.org/10.1016/S2213-2600(18)30288-1] [PMID: 30037711]

[98] Davies HE, Mishra EK, Kahan BC, *et al.* Effect of an indwelling pleural catheter vs chest tube and talc pleurodesis for relieving dyspnea in patients with malignant pleural effusion: the TIME2 randomized controlled trial. JAMA 2012; 307(22): 2383-9.
[http://dx.doi.org/10.1001/jama.2012.5535] [PMID: 22610520]

[99] Bhatnagar R, Keenan EK, Morley AJ, *et al.* Outpatient Talc Administration by Indwelling Pleural Catheter for Malignant Effusion 2018.
[http://dx.doi.org/10.1056/NEJMoa1716883]

[100] Kyskan R, Li P, Mulpuru S, Souza C, Amjadi K. Safety and performance characteristics of outpatient medical thoracoscopy and indwelling pleural catheter insertion for evaluation and diagnosis of pleural disease at a tertiary center in Canada. Can Respir J 2017; 20179345324
[http://dx.doi.org/10.1155/2017/9345324] [PMID: 28951662]

CHAPTER 6

Bronchoscopy: Diagnostic & Therapeutic

Keyvan Moghissi[1,*] and **Jack Kastelik**[2]

¹ The Yorkshire Laser Centre, Goole & District Hospital, Goole, UK

² Castle Hill Hospital & Hull Royal Infirmary, Hull University Teaching Hospitals, Hull, UK

Abstract: This chapter consists of two sections. In the first section, bronchoscopy and its contribution in diagnosis of central lung cancer are discussed. Particular emphasis is made on autofluorescence bronchoscopy and endobronchial sonography. Therapeutic bronchoscopy discusses the various methods with particular emphasis on the role of Nd Yag laser and Photodynamic Therapy.

Keywords: Autofluorescence bronchoscopy, Bronchoscopy, Endobronchial sonography EBUS, Laser and PDT in the bronchus, Therapeutic Bronchoscopy.

BRONCHOSCOPY

Bronchoscopy is an important method of investigation and, in conjunction with radiology, is the most helpful diagnostic procedure for bronchopulmonary neoplasm.

DIAGNOSTIC BRONCHOSCOPY

Even in the presence of a normal chest radiograph and CT scan, patients suffering from persistent bronchopulmonary symptoms, particularly haemoptysis, should have a screening bronchoscopy. A lesion may be in its early development in the bronchial tree without apparent radiological abnormalities.

For diagnostic purposes, in order to detect early lesions (high grade dysplasia and carcinoma in site), AutoFluorescence Bronchoscopy (AFB) is an indispensable companion to "White Light Bronchoscopy" (WLB).

* **Corresponding author Keyvan Moghissi:** The Yorkshire Laser Centre, Goole & District Hospital, Goole UK; Tel: 01724 290456; E-mail: kmoghissi@yorkshirelasercentre.org

Keyvan Moghissi, Jack Kastelik, Philip Barber & Peyman Sardari Nia (Eds.)

Bronchoscopy for diagnosis allows:

Acquisition of samples of bronchial secretion for:

i. Identification of pathogenic micro-organisms and sensitivity to anti-microbial chemotherapy.
ii. Cytological examination, notably identification of malignant cells.

Biopsy material for histological examination.

Instrumentation

There are basically two types of bronchoscopes:

Rigid Bronchoscope (RB)

In 1920, Chevalier Jackson [1] introduced a bronchoscope and bronchoscopy describing the range of procedures which could be carried out with its use, in addition to the visual examination of the airway. His instrument, with a few modifications, became what is basically the rigid bronchoscope (RB) of today. By the 1950's, bronchoscopy became a well-established procedure and every trainee thoracic surgeon had to be proficient in diagnostic and therapeutic bronchoscopy. Accessory devices include a range of forceps for grasping, provision of biopsy and/or punching/coring out tumors, dilators and diathermy probes. In addition, operative bronchoscopes have been designed for specific interventions, such as laser-therapy [2, 3]. Rigid Bronchoscopy is generally performed under general anaesthesia during which controlled ventilation is provided most effectively by hand operated (Sander's)injectors or jet ventilation. In Emergency, rigid bronchoscopy may be performed under topical anesthesia or no anesthesia as the aim is provision of the clear airway which becomes a lifesaving necessity.

Flexible Fibreoptic Bronchoscope (FFB)

The FFB was developed in the 1960's, the first instrument designed by the Japanese, Shigeto Ikeda [4]. Its flexibility allowed examination of segmental bronchi in more detail than through a telescope inserted in the rigid instrument.

There are now a number of FFB's available with various accessory devices, such as biopsy forceps, needles for injection, aspirators, and dilators. FFB offers a recording system and monitor for live viewing and storing of bronchoscopic events. It can also incorporate fluorescence imaging system for Auto Fluorescence

Bronchoscopy (AFB). FFB is essentially a diagnostic tool, which is used under local/topical anaesthetics and sedation. Some models provide facilities for delivery devices for some of the therapeutic endoscopic methods.

Fluorescence Bronchoscopy [5 - 7]

The meaning and principle of fluorescence imaging has been discussed in different parts of the book (Chapter 4: Imaging for Lung Cancer). At this juncture, it is worth recalling that the manner in which an incident light interacts with a tissue, such as mucosa of the bronchial lumen, is governed by the optical characteristics of the tissue (cell with their matrix), notably their chromophore and the parameter of the light, such as its wave length and fluence.

The manifestation of the interaction is dependent, essentially on absorption and scattering. The latter can be straight reflexion, which is emission of the light with similar characteristics as the incident light in terms of wavelength, or alternatively, the re-emitted light can be at a different but usually a higher wavelength, which is a fluorescent light.

In practical terms, the interaction between tissues and an incident light, within a visible spectrum, results in fluorescence re-emission within the visible spectrum. This is precisely the basis of the Autofluorescence Bronchoscopy (AFB) that when a light with the wavelength in the region of Ultra Violet – Blue (blue region 400-440 nm) is projected on to the normal bronchial mucosa, its fluorescence emission will also be in the region of green (500-530 nm).

Differential fluorescence emission from the normal versus abnormal tissue on the basis of photo diagnosis in AFB is presented in Fig. (**1**). In physics terms, Fluorescence is a reflected light by a substance that has absorbed an incident light and emit a light of a different wavelength (usually higher than the incident light).

Endobronchial Ultrasound

Indications

Bronchoscopic evaluation of mediastinal lymph nodes was initially undertaken using a blind transbronchial fine needle aspiration. This technique is not recommended anymore due to its poor and less predictable diagnostic yield ranging from 40 to 75% and the fact that there are better procedures for sampling mediastinal and hilar lymph nodes, such as EBUS (Groth and Andrade 2008). There are two types of endobronchial ultrasound convex (EBUS) and radial (rEBUS). EBUS allows for examination and sampling of the Study of Lung Cancer (IASLC) Lymph Node Map stations 2, 3, 4, 7, 10, 11 and mediastinoscopy stations 1, 2, 3, 4, 7 [8]. A radial probe EBUS, which allows localization of the lymph nodes but not for real time biopsies is not widely used for mediastinal lymph node staging, although it has its role for sampling of the peripheral lung lesions.

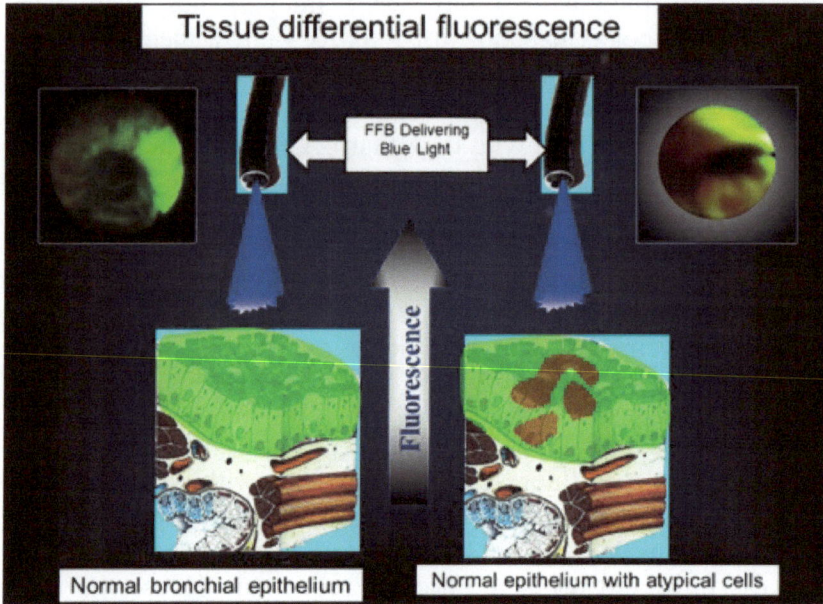

Fig. (1). Differential autofluorescence between normal and early neoplastic lesions Left: Normal fluorescence. Right: Early neoplastic. Notice the patch of brownish red of abnormal fluorescence in the early neoplastic endobronchial lesion.

Safety

EBUS can be performed under general anaesthesia with an 8.5 mm or larger endotracheal tube, with main advantages being better control of oxygenation and possibly improved sampling of smaller lymph nodes with disadvantages related to potential side effects of the anaesthetic agents and a longer recovery time. Conversely, EBUS can be undertaken under awake sedation and local anaesthesia. EBUS is a safe procedure which has mainly self-limiting complications, such as sore throat, mild hypoxia, cough and pyrexia, and relatively uncommon reported serious complications, such as pneumothorax of 0.05% to 1.43% [9, 10].

Equipment

Endobronchial Ultrasound, similar to a flexible fibreoptic bronchoscopes, are composed of glass fibres, which transmit white light and images and a working channel allowing for suctioning and introduction of biopsy instruments. The EBUS allows visualization at 35rather than direct visualization of fibreoptic bronchoscope and therefore, the both procedures differ in the technique applied. An EBUS has an ultrasound probe at its tip, which is a convex probe and a 7.5 MHz transducer, which allows real time visualization and biopsy of the lymph nodes (Fig. **2**). EBUS has a working channel through which four sizes of biopsy (19, 21, 22 and 25 gauge) can be inserted [11]. The biopsy is undertaken under the real time and allows to visualize the lymph node and the movement of the biopsy needle within, assuring that the needle does not pass through the lymph node, therefore, avoiding potential damage to the surrounding structures and assuring that the adequate technique biopsy is achieved. It is recommended that three or more needle-passes are required per lymph node (2 passes if presence of core tissue) or ROSE are performed and on each occasion, 10 to 15 needle passes are undertaken [9 - 12].

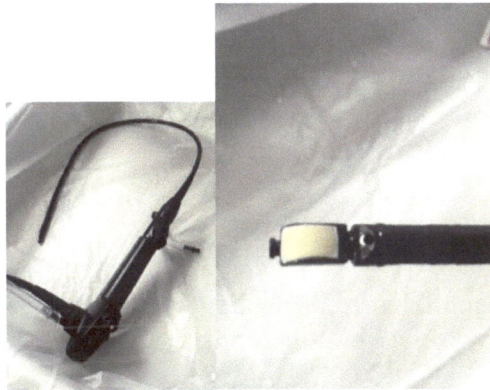

Fig. (2). Convex endobronchial ultrasound scope.

Learning Curve

The learning curve for EBUS may vary and may depend on the sampled stations and the size of the lymph nodes, as usually station 7 and station 4 may be easier to master to sample than smaller hilar lymph nodes, but reports suggest that after around 50 procedures, a 90% diagnostic yield can be achieved [13]. The American Thoracic Society (ATS) and the European Respiratory Society (ERS) recommend that before proficiency in EBUS is achieved, at least 40 procedures under supervision should be undertaken with the American College of Chest

Physicians (ACCP) recommending at least 50 procedures [14, 15]. Similar to learning bronchoscopy skills, simulation training can speed up the learning curve for EBUS skills [16].

Advances in EBUS Technology

There are newer modified instruments, which have been developed, including a hybrid EBUS scope and a thin convex probe EBUS bronchoscope. The hybrid EBUS scope has 10° angle of view and 130° of anterior flexion resulting in better visualization of airways, especially lower lobes but with no additional benefit in the diagnostic yield, when compared with conventional EBUS [10]. Similarly, thin convex probe EBUS has thinner diameter 5.9 mm and 170° viewing angle, and 20° oblique view which allows for better manoeuvrability through the bronchial tree, but it has a smaller 1.7 mm working channel allowing a 25 gauge needle biopsy whose diagnostic yield has not yet been compared to that of conventional EBUS. This may be of particular importance as in the current context of individualized therapy samples are tested for mutations, such as EGFR, ALK and PD-L1, ROS-1. EBUS may also be of use in diagnosing non-neoplastic conditions, such as sarcoidosis or tuberculosis. Another new technique involves the use of elastography, which is the measurement of tissue stiffness, which may have some role in selection of malignant nodes for biopsy [17].

THERAPEUTIC/INTERVENTIONAL BRONCHOSCOPY

Introduction

Bronchoscopy is frequently carried for diagnostic and sampling purposes, under topical anaesthesia using a flexible fibreoptic instrument (FFB).

Therapeutic/Interventional Bronchoscopy refers to methods in which bronchoscopic instrumentation and the airway are used to access bronchial trees or the lungs for therapeutic procedures.

Interventional Bronchoscopy (IB), Instrumentation and General Principles

Most therapeutic interventional bronchoscopies require either the use of a metallic rigid bronchoscope or the combination of the rigid and the FFB. Nevertheless, many interventional respiratory physicians prefer the use of FFB alone under local/topical aesthesia.

The use of FFB alone for interventional bronchoscopy is uncomfortable for both patient and operator. Also, it can prove hazardous if there is bleeding, which requires rapid clearance or control and it can hinder a procedure when there are copious bronchial secretions which, in some patients, make the bronchoscopic vision blurred and the operation area looking like an "under water" field. Furthermore, for some interventions, such as the application of thermal laser, the procedure cannot be safely performed when FFB is used on its own.

For many IB methods, the combined use of RB-FFB (Fig. **3**) under general anaesthesia (GA) is the ideal method of practice. This allows comfort for patient and operator, efficient visualization of the lesion using white light and fluorescence bronchoscopy. Moreover, precise targeting and application of the delivery device will be undisturbed by cough or bronchial secretion. It is important to note that such a method is not incompatible with treatment being undertaken as a day case procedure [18].

INTERVENTIONAL BRONCHOSCOPY (IB), INSTRUMENTATIONS, GENERAL PRINCIPLES AND METHODS

It is unrealistic to describe all the currently available methods of IB. It is equally unrealistic to expect that a thoracic surgeon or a respiratory physician can master all of the methods. It is nevertheless important that a regional centre for Respiratory Medicine and Thoracic surgery have the equipment and expertise to carry out commonly used methods of IBS.

Therefore, it is proposed to describe the most frequently used methods, particularly those which offer future rather than those that adhere to the traditional past.

Many or some of the methods may not be practiced in some countries due to financial constraints and/or bias attitude, but they are still discussed. On the other hand, some other method could be in use because in some hospitals, they have no chance of introducing costly methods.

It is convenient to group the various methods.

The following classification is proposed for Therapeutic/Interventional Bronchoscopy Methods.

1. Mechanical: *Cleaning of bronchial tree, Foreign Body removal and Bronchial Lavage*
2. Thermal: *Cryotherapy, Electro-Cautery, Argon Plasma Coagulator, Radio-Frequency, CO2 Laser, Nd YAG Laser*
3. Biological: Cancer Specific Methods Brachytherapy Photodynamic Therapy

(PDT)

4. Stents

The basis for selecting a method for a given patient is governed by:

- The topography and morphology of the lesion within the airway
- The histopathology of the lesion
- The objective of therapy.
- The experience of the operator

Only those methods which are applicable in lung cancer will be discussed.

Mechanical Methods

Bronchoscopic Clearing of the Airway

This is one of the simplest procedures, commonly practiced by thoracic surgeons in patients with retention of secretions after pulmonary resection.

In the 1970s and 1980s, the method was practiced using the rigid bronchoscope with the patient sitting up in bed. Bronchoscopies were performed under sedation and an endotracheal injection of lignocaine 4%.

Currently, this is performed by FFB. Bronchoscopy and suction of copious secretions in patients with collapse (atelectasis) of the residual lobe or even the whole lung is attended by immediate expansion of the lung if sputum retention is recognized early enough before pneumonic consolidation sets in.

Foreign Body (FB) Retrieval

Bronchoscopy allows visualization, identification, and extraction of the foreign body within the airway. Other than for extreme emergency situations, this is best carried out by a practitioner (either a thoracic surgeon or respiratory physician) who has experience. The rigid instrument has the advantage of method control of accidental bleeding and clearing the airway. On the other hand, the FFB has a certain simplicity and in the hands of an experienced operator can be used just as effectively as the RB.

Bronchial Lavage/Whole Lung Lavage

The use of bronchial lavage as a therapeutic method is now only for cases of alveolar proteinosis [19, 20]. Basically, the method consists of injecting a large volume (several litres) of normal saline into the bronchial tree and aspirated. A precise volume of aspirated fluid (with debris) should be checked in order to equal the injected volume.

In the past modification of the method that has been used in patients with bronchiectasis and those with cystic fibrosis and copious volumes of secretion resistant bacteria or fungal organisms resistant to most antibiotics. For this, up to a litre of fluid is injected, 50 ml at a time, followed by aspiration. This method was used by thoracic surgeons and is now practically abandoned.

Thermal Methods

Diathermy Assisted Piecemeal Excision of Endobronchial Tumor

"Piecemeal" Excision of the tumor with Electrodiathermie probe passed through a rigid bronchoscope was an option which was used frequently by many surgeons, in the 1950s through to 1980s, as a way of palliation of patients suffering from inoperable lung cancer.

Haemoptysis and/or main bronchial tumor obstruction of a tumor constituted the major indication. The procedure needs to be repeated, in order to expand the lung giving the patient an extra functioning pulmonary capacity.

This method almost became extinguished with the advances of thermal laser (CO2 and NdYAG Lasers) in the 1980s.

With a recent lack of funding in the UK and some other countries, the method could well have found its way back.

Bleeding can be an intra-operative hazard, in addition to post bronchoscopic resection complication, related to clot obstruction of the lumen which, in turn, will require bronchoscopic suction.

Cryotherapy

Cryotherapy employs freezing to achieve necrosis of pathological tissues by rapid freezing followed by slow thawing, leading to the destruction of the target tissue [21 - 24]. Ice crystals are formed, both within the cells and in the extra-cellular compartment. Additionally, there are vascular effects in terms of vasoconstriction followed by vasodilatation and vascular thrombosis. This effect is achieved via a probe delivering nitrous oxide (N_2O), which is passed through the bronchoscope.

There are a variety of flexible and rigid cryoprobes to match FFB or RB.

Cryotherapy may be used for:

- Locally advanced endobronchial tumors, either benign or malignant. In malignancy, the aim is palliation of dyspnoea or haemoptysis.
- Superficial endobronchial malignant tumors. The treatment is undertaken with curative intent, in patients ineligible for surgical resection.
- In association with chemo/radiation [18].

Eight to ten days post-therapy bronchoscopy should be performed for:

- Evaluation of the extent of tissue damage/destruction
- Removing of debris/slough
- Additional treatment if required.

Argon Plasma Coagulator (APC) [25 - 27]

APC is a process involving emission of a jet of argon gas, which is ionized by a high voltage discharge. High-frequency electrical current is conducted through the gas jet resulting in thermal coagulation of only a few millimetres without physical contact with the lesion.

It is of particular use with FFB under topical anaesthesia and sedation.

Indications

- Coagulation of lesions where electro diathermy probes or catheters are unable to reach [27].
- Disposal of superficial and obstructing endoluminal tumors [26, 27]. In bulkier lesions, APC needs to be used in conjunction with manual removal.

Result

97% control of haemoptysis [24], though long-term complete response is rare; recurrence is to be expected in cases of malignancy.

Although APC is relatively safe with few complications, haemorrhage, perforation, fire, and gas embolism have been reported [28].

Radiofrequency Ablation (RFA)

Radiofrequency ablation (RFA) is a minimally invasive modality, which employs an electromagnetic wave of the same frequency as the electric scalpel commonly used in surgery. By inserting the radiofrequency electrode into a tumor, heat is generated, thus inducing coagulative necrosis and cell death. Though it has been used in hepatic tumors and peripheral lung tumors under CT guidance [29], bronchoscopic use has not undergone a thorough clinical evaluation.

Lasers (see also Chapter 14: Lasers and Photodynamic Therapy (PDT) in Lung Cancer)

LASER: Light Amplification by Stimulated Emission of Radiation.

The term refers to devices producing specific wavelengths of light with characteristics which are:

- Monochromatic: denoting that the emitted light comprises a single wavelength.
- Coherent: there is a close phase relationship between all components of the emitted light.
- Collimated: radiation propagation is a narrow beam with low divergence.

There is a variety of lasers, which can generate / emit light across a broad range of wavelengths; only those within the range of ultraviolet, visible light and infrared have found clinical application.

Laser Classification

- According to wavelength.
- Based on their effect on tissue e.g. thermal/non-thermal
- Depending on the element which generates the laser light.

Bronchoscopic thermal laser therapy is usually performed with the use of a Neodymium Yttrium Aluminium Garnet (Nd-YAG) machine, though the D60 diode laser is effective for contact work; Co2 Laser is used by Head & Neck and Ear Nose and Throat Surgeons for the upper airway.

Nd-YAG laser emits light of 1064nm (infra-red). Since the emitted light is colorless, it is coupled with a Helium-Neon aiming beam, emitting 630nm red light. Thus, the light can be directed, via an optical fiber, to the treatment area. A cooling mechanism, incorporated within the delivery system, renders the machine suitable for both contact and non-contact work.

Indications [30 - 34]

- Locally advanced primary endobronchial malignant tumor - central lung cancer - allowing anatomical and functional integrity of the airway to be rapidly restored

following the treatment. Many hundreds of publications, reporting results in several thousands of patients, attest to the safety and efficacy of the method.
- Primary early central lung cancer. This is not a generally accepted indication in that the target area is ablated, whether it is benign or malignant.
- Secondary malignant endoluminal airway lesions. As above, the Nd YAG will destroy any target, regardless whether it is malignant or benign.

Method

Nd YAG treatment is best carried out under GA with the use of a rigid bronchoscope - RB-FFB - as previously described. Following the visual assessment of topography and extent of the lesion, the delivery fiber is introduced through the biopsy channel of the FFB instrument, being careful that the distal end of the delivery fiber is protruding at least 1cm beyond the end of the FFB; intense heat produced will damage the FFB. The pilot He-Ne beam - a red circle – will indicate the aiming target of the laser light (Fig. **3**).

Bursts of 4-10 seconds at between 30-50 Watts are delivered over the tumor. The resulting debris and charred tissue may be removed using biopsy forceps. Treatment pulses are continued until the lesion is ablated before bronchial lavage using warm normal saline.

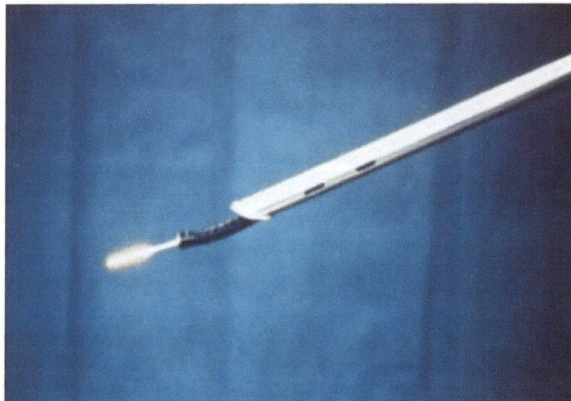

Fig. (3). This shows an FFB within the RB. Note the optical fibre for delivery of the laser light.

Results

Nd-YAG laser brings immediate relief of benign and malignant exophytic tumors (Figs. **4** and **5**). It is safe and effective and can be used in a day surgery setting. However, in malignant obstructive lesions it will need to be repeated every 4-6 weeks [33, 34].

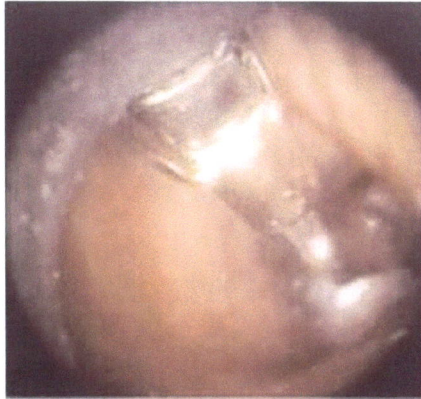

Fig. (4). Laser device targeting the tumor (Note the red circle of neon helium laser light).

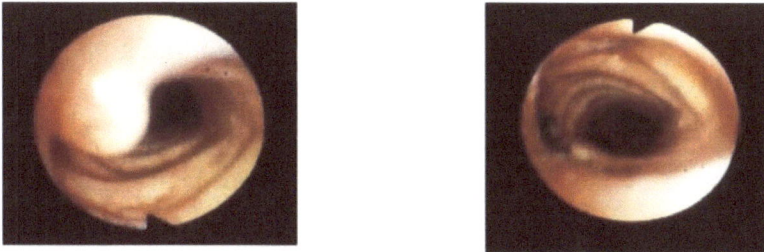

Fig. (5). Nd-YAG Photo radiation for excision of a main stem bronchial tumor Left: Pre-laser radiation Right Post Laser treatment.

Complications are rare in experienced hands. Rarely, haemorrhage, perforation, and (very rarely) fire in the airway have been reported [30, 35].

Therapeutic Bronchoscopy; Cancer Specific Methods (CSM), Mechanical and thermal bronchoscopic therapies are designed to eliminate blockage, malignant or benign, within the lumen of the bronchi; the lesion is targeted with the aim: VIEW, TARGET and ZAP (VITZ). CSMs target and destroy only malignant tissue. They are endowed with a double targeting mechanism; VITZ in where the operator views the lesion and targets it under vision but, also, they have the ability to specifically and preferentially target the malignant lesions independent of visual and imaging systems.

There are 2 bronchoscopic CSMs - Brachytherapy and Photodynamic Therapy (PDT). For either method, definite histological proof of malignancy is mandatory.

Brachytherapy (BT) [34 - 36]

In brachytherapy, a radioactive source (iridium-192) is placed within the bronchus involved in malignant tumor, enabling local radiotherapy [36].

Treatment requires the participation of a radiation oncologist to undertake planning of the radiation dose and number of sessions/fractions to achieve an optimal outcome. This multi-speciality input may, sometimes, be difficult to achieve.

The mechanism involved concerns DNA damage resulting in accelerated apoptosis and decrease in cell proliferation. BT can be performed as a day case procedure, using the fibreoptic instrument and with the patient under topical/local anaesthesia.

Indications and Results

Brachytherapy may be employed for palliation or with curative intent though, in either indication, it is important to evaluate extent and topography of the tumor, taking all previous treatments into account, particularly External Beam Radiotherapy.

In its palliative role, BT achieves its objective of improved ventilation, and relief of haemoptysis [36, 37]. In its curative intent role, BT provides a long-lasting complete response in over 25% of patients [24, 38].

Brachytherapy, under topical anaesthesia, is not well tolerated by patients with profuse secretion and in patients with COPD. Following treatment, pleuritic pain may sometimes be experienced and, infrequently, pneumothorax, radiation bronchitis, haemoptysis and bronchial fistula may occur.

Photodynamic Therapy (PDT)

PDT is a treatment modality which has three components:

- A chemical photosensitizer.
- A wavelength of light matching the absorption band of the photosensitizer.
- Molecular oxygen.

The interaction between the drug and the light, in the presence of oxygen, releases cytotoxic species, notably singlet oxygen, bringing about necrosis of the targeted cells and tissues.

The mechanism of tissue destruction in PDT involves direct cellular damage, through injury to cell membranes and sub-cellular structures and also by vascular ischemic action through vasoconstriction and endothelial damage [37, 38]. There are also indications that PDT can enhance immunological competence. Bronchoscopically, PDT is used principally for endobronchial malignancies [39, 40].

Bronchoscopic PDT is undertaken as a two-phase process [31]:

1. Pre-sensitization: the photosensitizer (PS) is administered intravenously and time is allowed for the uptake and retention of the PS, predominantly in the neoplastic tissue. This latent period is variable, according to the chemical structure of the PS.
2. Illumination: when the lesion is exposed to light - usually laser light.

The drug most commonly used in bronchoscopic PDT is Photofrin (Porfimer Sodium), which is licenced in most countries, including the UK and EU. It is activated by red light of around 630 nm wavelength.

Following pre-sensitization using Photofrin and a latent period of between 24-72 h, bronchoscopic illumination is carried out.

There are 2 types of delivery fibers:

- Diffuser - the distal fiber tip has a cylindrical diffuser for interstitial illumination; *i.e.* insertion into the tumor mass. (Fig. **6**).
- Microlens - for forward firing illumination (Fig. **7**).

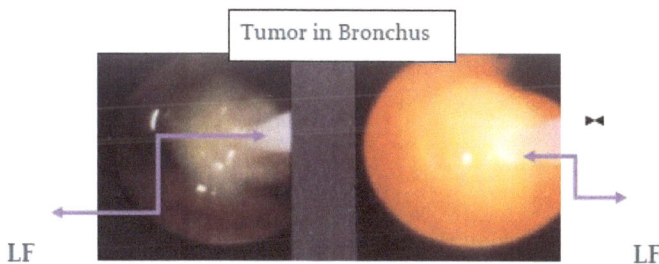

Fig. (6). Interstitial illumination with the laser diffuser within the mass of the tumor (T). LF = Laser fiber.

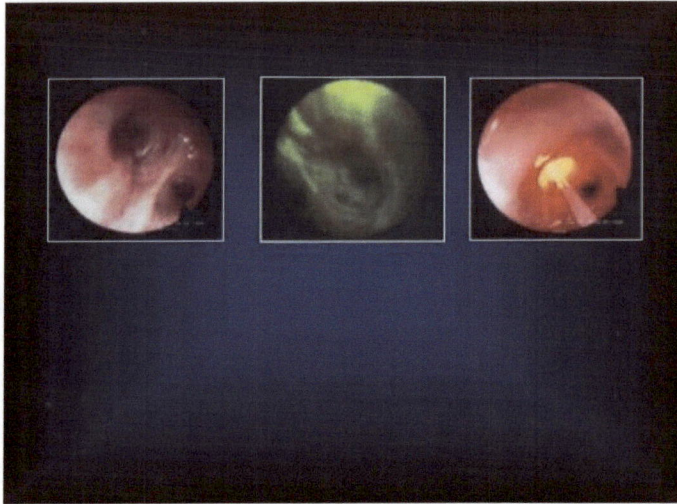

Fig. (7). Surface illumination Left: WLB view. Middle: AFB view showing the extent of the lesion for illumination Right: Surface illumination. Note laser delivery fibre. Bronchoscopic PDT for early endobronchial cancer.

Either method employs bronchoscopic illumination under GA using RB-FFB combination [40, 41].

Following illumination, debridement is undertaken. Experience shows that this is important in locally advanced tumors with a mass obstructing main and lobar bronchi, though it may not be required in early, superficial lesions.

Indications [39 - 41]

- PDT has been extensively used in a variety of bronchoscopically accessible lung cancers. The aim in these cases is palliation with survival advantage and improved quality of life.
- In early superficial endobronchial carcinoma, PDT is used with curative intent [42 - 46]. An important cohort is those patients who are ineligible for surgical resection on account of high co-morbidity and poor general and cardio-pulmonary function.
- Multifocal and Metachronous lesions, the latter after major previous resection.
- Salvage PDT in patients unresponsive to chemotherapy.
- In airway stent, the elimination of over and undergrowth of neoplastic tissue.

Results

In locally advanced diseases, PDT is used with the aim of symptom palliation [39 - 41]. Breathing and performance status improves and malignant bronchial obstruction is substantially (>60%) relieved with lung expansion. Additionally, there is an improvement in ventilation and spirometry.

Other than the potential for photosensitivity skin reaction, complications are few in bronchoscopic PDT. Literature review [33] shows 2% haemorrhage, 3-4% respiratory complications and 11% photosensitivity skin reaction. The latter, in centres which are doing PDT fairly routinely, is between 0-5% [37]. owing to rigorous patient counselling.

In early stage diseases; PDT can achieve total response and clearance for long periods; statistics show 60% 5 years survival [42 - 44]. In patients with small superficial or occult bronchial lesions, 80% 5 years survival has been recorded [35]. In such early disease, Auto Fluorescence Bronchoscopy (AFB) may be required for detection [45, 46].

Stents

These devices are fitted within the airway to maintain luminal opening. They act as an internal splint, having no effect on the pathology of the lesion. There are a variety of stents available.

Indications

Primarily, stenting is used in stenosis of the major airways, caused by extrinsic compression by the malignant tumour. Other indications are:

- Endoluminal malignant obstruction.
- Bypassing of malignant fistula, the covering of bronchial dehiscence in cases of bronchopleural fistula though, in the opinion of this author, stenting in such circumstances should only be used for short term palliation.

Instrumentation and Methods

General anaesthesia is used with rigid bronchoscopy for insertion of many stents. However, the bronchial stent can be inserted using FFB under topical anaesthetics.

Types of Stent

1. Plastic, usually silicone
2. Metallic
3. Combination of plastic and metal

Stents are either tracheal, tracheobronchial or bronchial. They can be invaluable in an emergency situation and when the trachea and its bifurcation is the start of the obstruction. They do, however, have drawbacks such as migration, obstruction, ulceration, and extrusion.

The stents should be selected based on the following criteria:

• Remain in place with no or low migration potential.
• Flexible yet firm enough to maintain the lumen.
• Tissue inert.
• Designed to prevent tumor ingrowth and granulation tissue.
• Not easily blocked.
• Not cause ulceration and/or perforation.
• Easily removable and re-insertable.

There is no stent which can incorporate all the above attributes. The commonly used stents are:

• Montgomery type (T-Tube) and its variants [47, 48] for trachea and its bifurcation. This maintains its position well.
• Dumon stent, and its modified subtypes [49, 50], with external studs for major airway; the studs reduce the chance of migration.
• Expandable metallic stents (Gianturco) with a single zig zag loop of stainless-steel coil [51, 52]; both covered and uncovered types are available. It is possible to place these stents using FFB [53].
• Of note is a stent developed by Frietag; this is plastic with loops of metal antero-laterally [54].

Comparable degrees of expertise of authors reporting on all categories of stent make comparison problematic.

Aftercare and Complications

All patients with stents require regular follow up and check bronchoscopy with inspection and cleaning. Migration, extrusion, granulation tissue formation, bleeding, ingrowth in particular and undergrowth by neoplastic tissue have been reported with variable frequency.

CONCLUSION

Bronchoscopy remains an indispensable diagnostic procedure in lung cancer. Many investigators and authors do not seem to consider the necessity of bronchoscopy in peripheral lung cancer. This, however, is not based on conclusive evidence provided by cytology or fluorescence imaging.

Fluorescence bronchoscopy should be part of the package of diagnostic bronchoscopy and not be thought of as an added "luxury".

Interventional bronchoscopy covers a range of procedures. however, experience shows that Respiratory Units or Regional Thoracic Surgery Centres in Britain and many European countries neither have the equipment nor the expertise to carry the range which is mentioned in this chapter.

Bronchoscopic Nd Yag lasers have consistently shown to be useful within the palliative care of patients with central lung cancer. The expense of the equipment and the need for expertise have excluded its use, in recent years, for it to become a universal practice.

PDT has the advantage that it is cancer specific. Its usefulness, particularly in patients with early endobronchial cancer, has been universally agreed. Nevertheless, in many countries, early stage cancer patients are preferably and rightly (in the opinion of the senior author of this chapter) treated by surgery. On the other hand, locally advanced endobronchial cancers benefit from PDT, particularly, if combined with another modality of treatment, such as Nd Yag laser or radiotherapy.

In future, the major indication of PDT should be within multi modal global treatment of lung cancer.

FURTHER READING

Bolliger CT, Mathur PN, Beamis JF et al. ERS/EACTS statement on interventional pulmonary. Eur Resp Society/American Thoracic Society. Euro Respiratory J 2002; 19: 356

British Thoracic Society guideline for advanced diagnostic and therapeutic flexible bronchoscopy in adults. November 2011 Vol 66 Supple 3

CONSENT FOR PUBLICATION

Not applicable.

CONFLICT OF INTEREST

The author declares that there is no conflict of interest in this chapter.

ACKNOWLEDGEMENTS

Kate Dixon & Janet Melvin.

REFERENCES

[1]　Jackson C. Bronchoscopy, Past, Present, and Future. N Engl J Med 1928; 199: 759-63.
[http://dx.doi.org/10.1056/NEJM192810181991603]

[2]　Bryan-Dumon Rigid Bronchoscope. www.Bryancorp.com/therpeutic-endoscopy.cfm

[3]　Moghissi K, Jessop T, Dench M. A new bronchoscopy set for laser therapy. Thorax 1986; 41(6): 485-6.
[http://dx.doi.org/10.1136/thx.41.6.485] [PMID: 3787525]

[4]　Ikeda S, Tsuboi E. ONO R Flexible Bronchofiberscope JPN. J Clin Oncol 1971; 1: 55-65.

[5]　Stringer M, Moghissi K. Photodiagnosis and fluorescence imaging in clinical practice. Photodiagn Photodyn Ther 2004; 1(1): 9-12.
[http://dx.doi.org/10.1016/S1572-1000(04)00004-3] [PMID: 25048059]

[6]　Lam S, MacAulay C, Hung J, LeRiche J, Profio AE, Palcic B. Detection of dysplasia and carcinoma in situ with a lung imaging fluorescence endoscope device. J Thorac Cardiovasc Surg 1993; 105(6): 1035-40.
[http://dx.doi.org/10.1016/S0022-5223(19)33775-4] [PMID: 8501931]

[7]　Moghissi K, Dixon K, Stringer MR. Current indications and future perspective of fluorescence bronchoscopy: a review study. Photodiagn Photodyn Ther 2008; 5(4): 238-46.
[http://dx.doi.org/10.1016/j.pdpdt.2009.01.008] [PMID: 19356663]

[8]　Chansky K, Detterbeck FC, Nicholson AG, *et al.* The IASLC Lung Cancer Staging Project: External Validation of the Revision of the TNM Stage Groupings in the Eighth Edition of the TNM Classification of Lung Cancer. J Thorac Oncol 2017; 12(7): 1109-21.
[http://dx.doi.org/10.1016/j.jtho.2017.04.011] [PMID: 28461257]

[9]　Gompelmann D, Eberhardt R, Herth FJ. Endobronchial ultrasound. Endosc Ultrasound 2012; 1(2): 69-74.
[http://dx.doi.org/10.7178/eus.02.003] [PMID: 24949340]

[10]　Belanger AR, Akulian JA. An update on the role of advanced diagnostic bronchoscopy in the evaluation and staging of lung cancer. Ther Adv Respir Dis 2017; 11(5): 211-21.
[http://dx.doi.org/10.1177/1753465817695981] [PMID: 28470104]

[11]　Fuso L, Varone F, Magnini D, *et al.* Ultrasonography of the mediastinum: Techniques, current practice, and future directions. Respir Care 2018; 63(11): 1421-38. [doi].
[http://dx.doi.org/10.4187/respcare.06047] [PMID: 30065076]

[12]　Kang HJ, Hwangbo B. Technical aspects of endobronchial ultrasound-guided transbronchial needle aspiration. Tuberc Respir Dis (Seoul) 2013; 75(4): 135-9.
[http://dx.doi.org/10.4046/trd.2013.75.4.135] [PMID: 24265641]

[13]　Izumo T, Sasada S, Chavez C, Matsumoto Y, Tsuchida T. Endobronchial ultrasound elastography in the diagnosis of mediastinal and hilar lymph nodes. Jpn J Clin Oncol 2014; 44(10): 956-62.
[http://dx.doi.org/10.1093/jjco/hyu105] [PMID: 25121724]

[14]　Bellinger CR, Chatterjee AB, Adair N, *et al.* Training in and experience with endobronchial ultrasound. Respiration 2014; 88(6): 478-83.
[http://dx.doi.org/10.1159/000368366] [PMID: 25402619]

[15]　Bolliger CT, Mathur PN, Beamis JF, *et al.* ERS/ATS statement on interventional pulmonology. Eur Respir J 2002; 19(2): 356-73.
[http://dx.doi.org/10.1183/09031936.02.00204602] [PMID: 11866017]

[16]   Ernst A, Silvestri GA, Johnstone D. Interventional pulmonary procedures: Guidelines from the american college of chest physicians. Chest 2003; 123(5): 1693-717.
[http://dx.doi.org/10.1378/chest.123.5.1693] [PMID: 12740291]

[17]   Stather DR, MacEachern P, Chee A, Dumoulin E, Tremblay A. Evaluation of clinical endobronchial ultrasound skills following clinical versus simulation training. Respirology 2012; 17(2): 291-9.
[http://dx.doi.org/10.1111/j.1440-1843.2011.02068.x] [PMID: 21943051]

[18]   Homasson JP, Pecking A, Roden S, Angebault M, Bonniot JP. Tumor fixation of bleomycin labeled with 57 cobalt before and after cryotherapy of bronchial carcinoma. Cryobiology 1992; 29(5): 543-8.
[http://dx.doi.org/10.1016/0011-2240(92)90059-B] [PMID: 1385037]

[19]   Ramirez-Rivera J, Schultz RB, Dutton RE. Pulmonary alveolar proteinosis: A new technique and rational for treatment. Arch Intern Med 1963; 112: 173-85.

[20]   Lippmann M, Mok MS. Anesthetic management of pulmonary lavage in adults. Anesth Analg 1977; 56(5): 661-8.
[http://dx.doi.org/10.1213/00000539-197709000-00012] [PMID: 562090]

[21]   Homasson JP, Renault P, Angebault M, Bonniot JP, Bell NJ. Bronchoscopic cryotherapy for airway strictures caused by tumors. Chest 1986; 90(2): 159-64.
[http://dx.doi.org/10.1378/chest.90.2.159] [PMID: 2426045]

[22]   Maiwand MO, Homasson JP. Cryotherapy for tracheobronchial disorders. Clin Chest Med 1995; 16(3): 427-43.
[PMID: 8521698]

[23]   Vergnon JM. Cryothérapie endobronchique: techniques et indications. Rev Mal Respir 1999; 16(4 Pt 2): 619-23.
[PMID: 10897824]

[24]   Vergnon JM, Huber RM, Moghissi K. Place of cryotherapy, brachytherapy and photodynamic therapy in therapeutic bronchoscopy of lung cancers. Eur Respir J 2006; 28(1): 200-18.
[http://dx.doi.org/10.1183/09031936.06.00014006] [PMID: 16816349]

[25]   Sutedja T. Bolliger CT, Endobronchia. Electrocautery and Argon Plasma Coagulation.Bolligher CT and Mathur PN. Basel: Karger 2000; pp. PP120-32.

[26]   Bolliger CT, Sutedja TG, Strausz J, Freitag L. Therapeutic bronchoscopy with immediate effect: laser, electrocautery, argon plasma coagulation and stents. Eur Respir J 2006; 27(6): 1258-71.
[http://dx.doi.org/10.1183/09031936.06.00013906] [PMID: 16772389]

[27]   Morice RC, Ece T, Ece F, Keus L. Endobronchial argon plasma coagulation for treatment of hemoptysis and neoplastic airway obstruction. Chest 2001; 119(3): 781-7.
[http://dx.doi.org/10.1378/chest.119.3.781] [PMID: 11243957]

[28]   Reddy C, Majid A, Michaud G, et al. Gas embolism following bronchoscopic argon plasma coagulation: a case series. Chest 2008; 134(5): 1066-9.
[http://dx.doi.org/10.1378/chest.08-0474] [PMID: 18988782]

[29]   Carrafiello G, Mangini M, Fontana F, Lagana D. et al.. Radiofrequency ablation for single lung tumours not suitable for surgery: seven years experience. Radiol Med 2012; 117: 1320-32.

[30]   Personne C, Colchen A, Leroy M, Vourc'h G, Toty L. Indications and technique for endoscopic laser resections in bronchology. A critical analysis based upon 2,284 resections. J Thorac Cardiovasc Surg 1986; 91(5): 710-5.
[http://dx.doi.org/10.1016/S0022-5223(19)35991-4] [PMID: 3009998]

[31]   Cavaliere S, Foccoli P, Farina PL. Nd:YAG laser bronchoscopy. A five-year experience with 1,396 applications in 1,000 patients. Chest 1988; 94(1): 15-21.
[http://dx.doi.org/10.1378/chest.94.1.15] [PMID: 3383627]

[32]   Moghissi K, Dixon K. Bronchoscopic NdYAG laser treatment in lung cancer, 30 years on: an

institutional review. Lasers Med Sci 2006; 21(4): 186-91.
[http://dx.doi.org/10.1007/s10103-006-0400-3] [PMID: 17003957]

[33]   Casey KR, Fairfax WR, Smith SJ, Dixon JA. Intratracheal fire ignited by the Nd-YAG laser during treatment of tracheal stenosis. Chest 1983; 84(3): 295-6.
[http://dx.doi.org/10.1378/chest.84.3.295] [PMID: 6688392]

[34]   Macha HN, Freitag L. The role of brachytherapy in the treatment and control of central bronchial carcinoma. Monaldi Arch Chest Dis 1996; 51(4): 325-8.
[PMID: 8909019]

[35]   Macha HN, Wahlers B, Relchele G, vonZwehl D. Endobronchial radiation therapy for obstructing malignancies; ten years experience with Irridium-192 high- dose. Lung 1995; 173: 871-80.
[http://dx.doi.org/10.1007/BF00176890]

[36]   Saito M, Yokoyama A, Kurita Y, Uematsu T, *et al.* Treatment of roengenologically occult endobronchial carcinoma with external beam radiotherapy and Intraluminal low dose brachytherapy. Int J radiat Oncol Bio Phys 1996; 34: 1029-35.

[37]   Castano AP, Demidova TN, Hamblin MR. Mechanisms in photodynamic therapy: part two-cellular signaling, cell metabolism and modes of cell death. Photodiagn Photodyn Ther 2005; 2(1): 1-23.
[http://dx.doi.org/10.1016/S1572-1000(05)00030-X] [PMID: 25048553]

[38]   Allison RR, Moghissi K. Photodynamic Therapy (PDT): PDT Mechanisms. Clin Endosc 2013; 46(1): 24-9.
[http://dx.doi.org/10.5946/ce.2013.46.1.24] [PMID: 23422955]

[39]   Moghissi K, Dixon K. Is bronchoscopic photodynamic therapy a therapeutic option in lung cancer? Eur Respir J 2003; 22(3): 535-41.
[http://dx.doi.org/10.1183/09031936.03.00005203] [PMID: 14516148]

[40]   Moghissi K, Dixon K, Thorpe JAC, Oxtoby C, Stringer MR. Photodynamic therapy (PDT) for lung cancer: the Yorkshire Laser Centre experience. Photodiagn Photodyn Ther 2004; 1(3): 253-62.
[http://dx.doi.org/10.1016/S1572-1000(04)00047-X] [PMID: 25048340]

[41]   Moghissi K, Dixon K, Stringer M, *et al.* The place of bronchoscopic photodynamic therapy in advanced unresectable lung cancer: experience of 100 cases. Eur J Cardiothorac Surg 1999; 15(1): 1-6.
[http://dx.doi.org/10.1016/S1010-7940(98)00295-4] [PMID: 10077365]

[42]   Moghissi K, Dixon K, Thorpe J A, Stringer M R, Oxtoby C. Photodynamic therapy in early central lung cancer: a treatment option for patients ineligible for surgical resection. Thorax 2007; 5: 391.5.
[http://dx.doi.org/10.1136/thx.2006.061143]

[43]   Hayata Y, Kato H, Furuse K, Kusunoki Y, Suzuki S, Mimura S. Photodynamic Therapy of 169 early stage cancer of the lung and oesophagus: a Japanese multi-centre study. Lasers Med Sci 1996; 11: 255-9.
[http://dx.doi.org/10.1007/BF02134916]

[44]   Cortese DA, Edell ES, Kinsey JH. Photodynamic therapy for early stage squamous cell carcinoma of the lung. Mayo Clin Proc 1997; 72(7): 595-602.
[http://dx.doi.org/10.1016/S0025-6196(11)63563-5] [PMID: 9212759]

[45]   Moghissi K, Dixon K. Update on the current indications, practice and results of photodynamic therapy (PDT) in early central lung cancer (ECLC). Photodiagn Photodyn Ther 2008; 5(1): 10-8.
[http://dx.doi.org/10.1016/j.pdpdt.2007.11.001] [PMID: 19356631]

[46]   Endo C, Miyamoto A, Sakurada A, *et al.* Results of long-term follow-up of photodynamic therapy for roentgenographically occult bronchogenic squamous cell carcinoma. Chest 2009; 136(2): 369-75.
[http://dx.doi.org/10.1378/chest.08-2237] [PMID: 19318660]

[47]   Montgomery WW. T-tube tracheal stent. Arch Otolaryngol 1965; 82: 320-1.
[http://dx.doi.org/10.1001/archotol.1965.00760010322023] [PMID: 14327039]

[48]   Westaby S, Jackson JW, Pearson FG. A bifurcated silicone rubber stent for relief of tracheobronchial obstruction. J Thorac Cardiovasc Surg 1982; 83(3): 414-7.
[http://dx.doi.org/10.1016/S0022-5223(19)37277-0] [PMID: 7062752]

[49]   Dumon JF. A dedicated tracheobronchial stent. Chest 1990; 97(2): 328-32.
[http://dx.doi.org/10.1378/chest.97.2.328] [PMID: 1688757]

[50]   Tayama K, Eriguchi N, Futamata Y, *et al.* Modified dumon stent for the treatment of a bronchopleural fistula after pneumonectomy. Ann Thorac Surg 2003; 75(1): 290-2.
[http://dx.doi.org/10.1016/S0003-4975(02)04282-0] [PMID: 12537239]

[51]   Wallace MJ, Charnsangavej C, Ogawa K, *et al.* Tracheobronchial tree: expandable metallic stents used in experimental and clinical applications. Work in progress. Radiology 1986; 158(2): 309-12.
[http://dx.doi.org/10.1148/radiology.158.2.3941857] [PMID: 3941857]

[52]   Ushida BT, Putman JS, Rasch J. Modification of Gianturco expandable wire stent. Am J Roentergenol 1988; 150: 1185-7.
[http://dx.doi.org/10.2214/ajr.150.5.1185]

[53]   Saad CP, Murthy S, Krizmanich G, Mehta AC. Self-expandable metallic airway stents and flexible bronchoscopy: long-term outcomes analysis. Chest 2003; 124(5): 1993-9.
[http://dx.doi.org/10.1378/chest.124.5.1993] [PMID: 14605078]

[54]   Freitag L, Tekolf E, Stamatis G, Greschuchna D. Clinical evaluation of a new bifurcated dynamic airway stent: a 5-year experience with 135 patients. Thorac Cardiovasc Surg 1997; 45(1): 6-12.
[http://dx.doi.org/10.1055/s-2007-1013675] [PMID: 9089967]

Frontiers in Lung Cancer, 2020, Vol. 1, 137-151   137

Three-Dimensional Reconstruction and Printing in Surgical Treatment of Lung Cancer

Samuel Heuts and Peyman Sardari Nia*

Department of Cardiothoracic Surgery, Maastricht University Medical Center, Maastricht, the Netherlands

Abstract: The application of VATS (Video-Assisted Thoracic Surgery) for a variety of thoracic surgical procedures has increased the technical complexity of these procedures, especially in long-sparing oncological resections. Pre-operative assessment of procedural feasibility is imperative for these new techniques and approaches, making imaging modalities increasingly important for the diagnosis and treatment of lung cancer. Three-dimensional (3D) reconstructions of these two-dimensional images can aid in a better visuospatial understanding of thoracic anatomy. Using this method, tumors can be localized precisely with respect to their anatomical borders, possibly leading to an increase in the use of sublobar resections. Furthermore, deviant vascular anatomy can be detected pre-operatively, potentially facilitating the procedures. In order to create a tangible model, rapid prototyping (more commonly known as 3D printing) can facilitate a better understanding of pulmonary vascular anatomy and anatomical relations to the tumor. Additionally, these models can be used to improve patient counseling and result in higher patient knowledge scores. We foresee these techniques to evolve rapidly in the nearby future, with the introduction of whole-slide scanning, 3D scanning and bioprinting. For diagnosis and treatment of thoracic disease, these methods will undoubtedly prove useful for many processes.

Keywords: Computed tomography, Imaging, Lung cancer, Lung surgery, Lobectomy, Preoperative planning, Rapid prototyping, Segmentectomy, Surgical simulation, Three-dimensional printing, Three-dimensional reconstruction.

INTRODUCTION

Since the first laparoscopic appendectomy was performed by German gynecologist Kurt Semm in Kiel in 1981 [1], a trend towards less invasive procedures for the treatment of common surgical pathologies has been observed [2]. By standardizing endoscopic techniques, the superiority of minimally invasive surgical (MIS) techniques has been proven over conventional surgical

---

* **Corresponding author Peyman Sardari Nia, MD, PhD:** Department of Cardiothoracic Surgery, Maastricht University Medical Center, Maastricht, the Netherlands; Tel: +31433875070; Fax: +31433875075; E-mail: peyman.sardarinia@mumc.nl

Keyvan Moghissi, Jack Kastelik, Philip Barber & Peyman Sardari Nia (Eds.)

treatment in general (*e.g.* abdominal) surgery, whereafter MIS became the gold standard for a variety of procedures [3, 4].

For pulmonary oncological surgical procedures, thoracotomy was the most accepted approach before the introduction of video-assisted thoracoscopic surgery (VATS). Although this thoracoscopic technique was already initiated in 1910 by Jacobaeous for treatment of tuberculosis induced pneumothorax *via* a cystoscope [5], this approach has only been widely adopted since 1992 for anatomical oncological resections [6]. Generally, entrance in the thorax is achieved through three stab-wound incisions, measuring approximately 1cm, and a utility port, without rib-spreading [7]. Since standardization of this technique, superiority has been proven in terms of complications, blood loss and length of hospital stay, while maintaining similar surgical results in terms of resection radicality and survival [8, 9]. Still, this technique remains more challenging than an open procedure, as surgeons need to maneuver through small working ports with long-shafted instruments and have to rely on thoracoscopic images. Furthermore, it is more challenging to manipulate and palpate the deflated lung, whilst maintaining optimal visual exposure. These challenges become even greater with the recent introduction of uniportal VATS (uVATS), in which the surgeon uses only one port for instrumental, camera and utility access [10].

In the meantime, the use of anatomical sublobar resections (*i.e.* segmentectomy) for surgical treatment of stage IA lung cancer has emerged. In these early stages of lung cancer, this technique has proven to be equal in terms of operating times, complications and recurrence rates [11, 12]. As a benefit, this technique could offer improved pulmonary function preservation than lobectomy.

Both the introduction of less invasive procedures (VATS, uVATS), combined with the minimalization of pulmonary resection volume (segmentectomy in early stage lung cancer), requires technically more demanding skills of the thoracic surgeon. Firstly, it is imperative to more adequately plan such procedures, as pre-operative assessment of the various available imaging modalities determines whether such an approach and anatomical resection are feasible in the patient. In this light, high-quality computed tomography imaging with subsequent semi-automated three-dimensional (3D) reconstruction of anatomical structures is more important than ever. Furthermore, physical realization (*i.e.* 3D printing) of these structures could enhance understanding of the visuospatial relationships and could help in patient's counselling. Secondly, the acquisition of such specific surgical skills is more time-consuming, while surgical exposure in the operating room is actually getting more limited for current residents with the introduction of the European working time directive. Therefore, we believe pre-operative planning and surgical simulation will become an indispensable cornerstone in the thoracic surgical training program of residents.

In the following chapter, we will discuss conventional methods of planning for lung surgery and upcoming techniques, including 3D reconstruction and printing.

PLANNING OF MINIMALLY INVASIVE LUNG SURGERY

Conventional Methods

Chest X-ray

Chest X-ray (CXR) is the most commonly used screening modality for detection of skeletal, cardiac and pulmonary abnormalities. However, in 90% of cases, errors in the diagnosis of lung cancer occur on CXR. Therefore, this modality is of limited use in the detection and staging of cancer. Still, as it is a cost- and time-effective first method of choice, CXR can be used in surgical planning. First of all, diaphragm level can adequately be assessed on CXR, potentially avoiding abdominal entrance upon trocar placement in patients with phrenic nerve palsy. Secondly, although normally visible on physical examination, the extent of skeletal deformations (scoliosis, pectus excavatum, pectus carinatum) can be evaluated on CXR.

Computed Tomography

Computed Tomography (CT) technology relies on the stacking of multiple axial CXR's, enabling the assessor to 'scroll' through the patients' anatomy. Traditionally, slice thicknesses were limited to 5mm or more, leading to false negative results in diagnostic scans for lung cancer. With recent technological advances, such as automated tube voltage selection, tube current modulation and ultra-fast scan acquisition, the radiation dose can be reduced markedly, while slice thickness can be improved [13, 14]. Currently, most scans for detection of lung cancer are performed at low radiation risk with slice thicknesses of 1.5mm, almost eliminating false-negative results. On the contrary, these more specific imaging possibilities can lead to more false-positive results, potentially leading to unnecessary follow-up and sometimes even treatment.

Diagnostic and follow-up CT's are nowadays indispensable in lung cancer treatment. The need for contrast enhancement depends on specific clinical indications. Routinely, in malignancy work-up, contrast is used as it facilitates a delineation of the hilum, chest wall, vascular margins and tumour [15].

In staging of cancer, radiological assessment gives an insight into the invasiveness of the tumour (T-stadium in TNM classification). Stage 1A cancers (*i.e.* T1a, T1b) and tumours are amenable to segmentectomy (still ensuring adequate resection margins) and could potentially be planned for such a procedure. As conventional CT traditionally remains a two-dimensional modality, visual understanding of physiological and deviant pulmonary vascularization remains interpreter-dependent. Three-dimensional reconstruction of these images could aid in a better understanding of these visuospatial relations.

Three-dimensional Anatomical Reconstructions

Imaging Modalities

As described earlier, several techniques have been used in imaging of pulmonary anatomy, mostly relying on high-energy electromagnetic radiation (CXR, CT). For 3D reconstruction purposes, a variety of modalities have been proposed to realize anatomical models of vascular and abdominal pathologies, such as CT, echography and magnetic resonance imaging (MRI). Although useful in other (non-skeletal caged) body parts, echography is of limited use in pulmonary assessment as it is hampered by acoustic shadowing of the ribs. For MRI, the lung remains a difficult organ because of the high susceptibility to motion artifacts and the decrease in signal intensity due to air-soft tissue interfaces [16].

Therefore, in this subchapter on 3D anatomical reconstructions, we focus on the realization of these models based on CT technology.

Three-dimensional Reconstruction Principal

Several open-source, commercially available, and vendor-available software packages exist, enabling the anatomical 3D reconstruction of CT images (Table **1**).

The first principle of acquisition of adequate reconstructions is the availability of high quality, contrast-enhanced CT images with thin slice thickness (1.5mm or less). In most of the existing software packages, the use of contrast agent, in combination with the right timing of the contrast, allows the system to automatically perform 3D reconstructions of the pulmonary arteries and veins. Additionally, extraction of the tumor with volume calculation, and definition of the thoracic cage and virtual simulation of pulmonary resections can be performed to visualize the resection surface and the extent of the presumed surgical margin [20].

Table 1. Open-source, commercially available, and vendor-available software packages for anatomical three-dimensional reconstruction based on computed tomography imaging.

	Software Package/Reconstruction Techniques	Company	Reference
Open source	*Osirix*	Pixmeo, Geneva, Switzerland	[17]
Commercially available	*Visible patient*	Visible patient, Strasbourg, France	[18]
	Vesalius3D	PS-Medtech, Amsterdam, the Netherlands	[19]
	Synapse Vincent	FujiFilm, Tokyo, Japan	[20, 21]
	Velocity AI	Varian medical systems, Palo Alto, CA, USA	[22]
	Apollo	Vida diagnostics, Coralville, IA, USA	[23]
CT vendors	*VEO, ASIR20*	GE Healthcare	[24, 25]
	SAFIRE3	Siemens	[24, 26]
	Routine, Sharp+, iDose2	Philips	[24, 27]
	AIDR 3D	Toshiba	[24, 28]

3D Anatomical Reconstructions in Surgical Planning

The aforementioned 3D anatomical reconstructions can be used for a variety of reasons in pre-operative planning of lung resection. First, it is of great use to identify potential vascular deviations in the pre-operative phase, as this can influence procedural outcome and complication rates [29, 30]. An example of deviating pulmonary vasculature, is presented in Fig. (**1**).

Secondly, by use of 3D reconstruction and subsequent tumor localization and its relation to segmental borders, feasibility of segmentectomy (adequate resection margins) can already be assessed in the pre-operative stage (Fig. **2**).

With recent technological advances, these reconstructions can even be taken into the operating room, either on an iPad/tablet [17], or in a .pdf-file [20], enabling the surgeon to revisit the images intra-operatively. Furthermore, some software packages enable the surgeon to reduce the visual intensity of the various pulmonary structures, in order to obtain an optimal understanding of the involved lobe or segment (Fig. **3**).

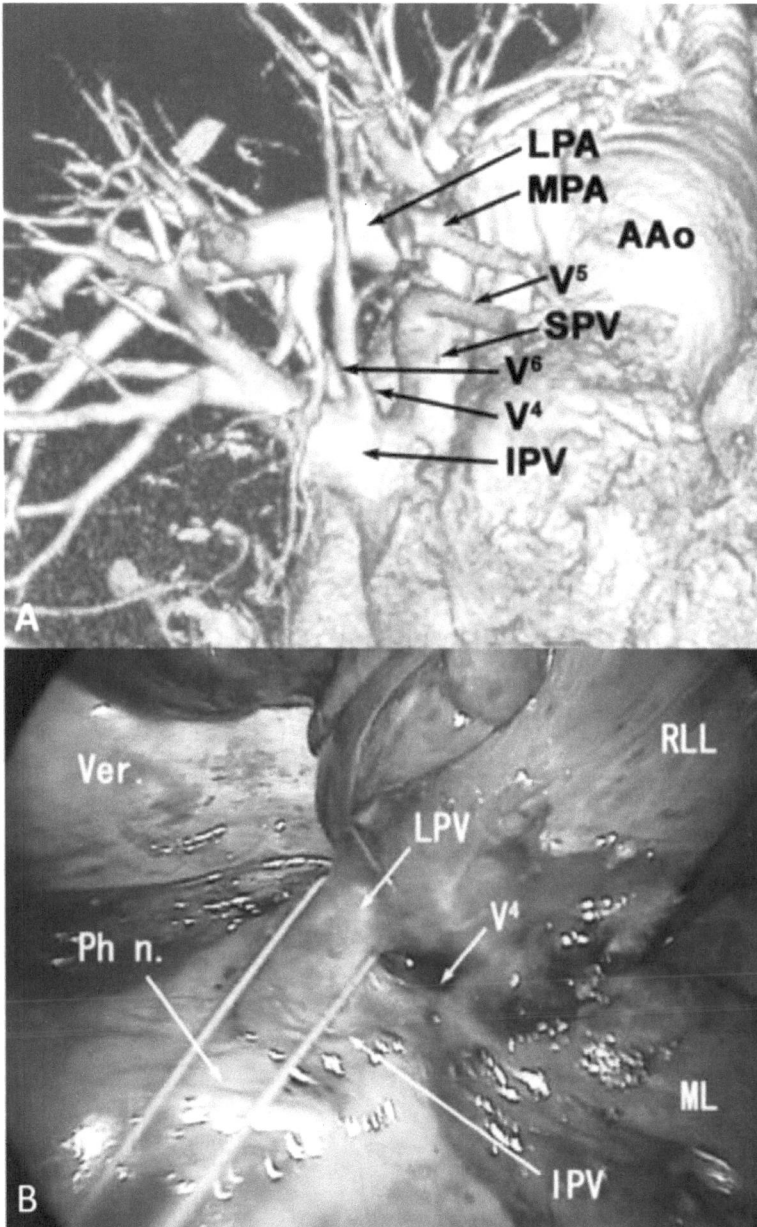

Fig. (1). A: Anterior caudal view of the right hilar region shows the superior and inferior pulmonary veins. The lateral part of the middle lobe vein (V4) drains into the inferior pulmonary vein (IPV), and the medial part of the middle lobe vein (V5) drains into the superior pulmonary vein (SPV). LPA, lower lobe artery of the right lung; MPA, middle lobe artery of the right lung; AAo, ascending aorta; V6, superior segment of the inferior pulmonary vein. B: Thoracoscopic view. Right lower lobe (RLL) and middle lobe (ML) are retracted toward the apex. The lateral part of the middle lobe vein (V4) drains into the inferior pulmonary vein (IPV). LPV, lower lobe vein; Ver., thoracic vertebra; Ph n., phrenic nerve. (reproduced with permission) [31].

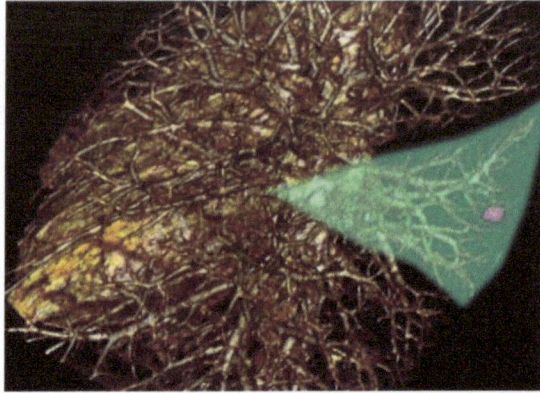

Fig. (2). Left lateral view of reconstructed bronchial and vascular 3D images with the tumor in the upper left segment (reproduced with permission) [17].

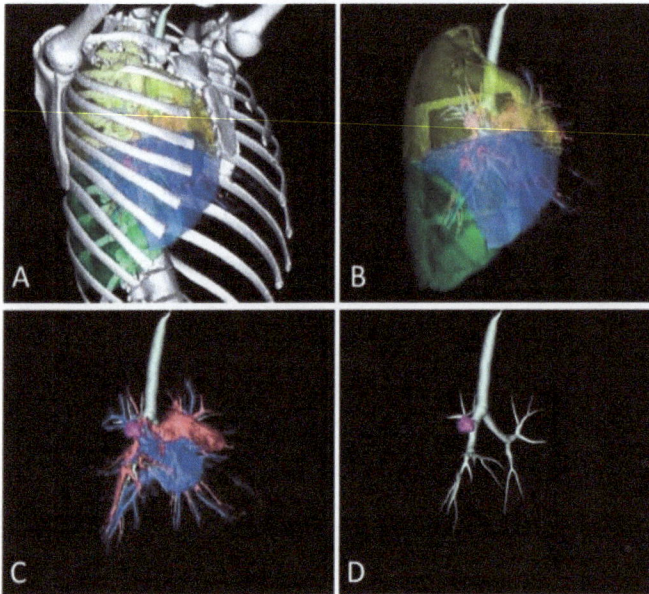

Fig. (3). Some software packages enable the surgeon to reduce the visual intensity of the various pulmonary structures, in order to obtain an optimal understanding of the involved lobe or segment. Reconstructions are based on the same patient, at the same angle of view. A: Full view of right upper lobe tumor with skeletal structures, B: Transparent lobes without skeletal interference, C: Relation of the tumor to the arterial and venous vascular tree, D: Relation of the tumor to the bronchial tree.

Three-dimensional Printing

Printing Process

In the early 1980's, the concept of Rapid Prototyping (RP) was introduced (*i.e.* 3D-printing). Its first application was seen in the industrial sector, in which 3D-printing was used to manufacture a tangible prototype before initiation of large-scale production [32]. A decade later, 3D-printing was introduced in the medical field with its first application in maxillofacial surgery, manufacturing a model of cranial bone anatomy [33]. Since then, RP has become more cost-effective and subsequently more widely available [34]. Currently, its use has spread to almost all medical specialties, of which orthopedics and maxillofacial surgery are the most predominant ones. Its applications range from manufacturing patient-specific implants or prostheses to anatomical models for surgical preparation [35 - 39]. Future directives for further investigation even aim at bio-printing tissues and organs [40, 41].

For thoracic oncological surgery, in depth understanding of the complex pulmonary and vascular anatomy and pathology is mandatory. Conventional CT imaging can help to comprehend these aspects, but relies on the interpreter's ability to extract 3D structures from a two-dimensional (2D) screen, even when this includes a 3D reconstruction.

Generally, 2D acquired data (*i.e.* CT-images) are stacked into digital imaging and communication in medicine (DICOM)-files and converted into surface tessellation language (.stl)-files. These .stl files possess the capability to fuse successive 2D layers of material and create a 'digitally tangible model' [42]. All 3D printers use data encoded in these .stl files. However, the method of printing differs between these modalities displayed in Table **2**. The first method, *vat photopolymerization*, more widely known as *stereolithography*, is the most widely used printing method in medicine.

Table 2. Different techniques for three-dimensional printing with their corresponding commercially available printer, with references.

Technique	Printer	Reference
Vat photopolymerization (stereolithography)	ProJet 7000, 3D Systems, Rock Hill, SC, USA	[43, 44]
Material jetting	Objet500 Connex printer, Statasys, Eden Prairie, MN, USA	[45]
Binder jetting	ProJet 660Pro, 3D Systems, Rock Hill, SC, USA	[46]
Material extrusion	Fortus 400MC, Statasys, Eden Prairie, MN, USA	[47]
Powder bed fusion		[48]

Three-dimensional Printing in Surgical Planning

After realization of 3D anatomical structures, these can be used for a variety of purposes. First, as recently described, 3D printed models can aid in patient information and patient understanding of surgery for lung cancer, even resulting in higher patient knowledge scores [49] (Fig. **4**).

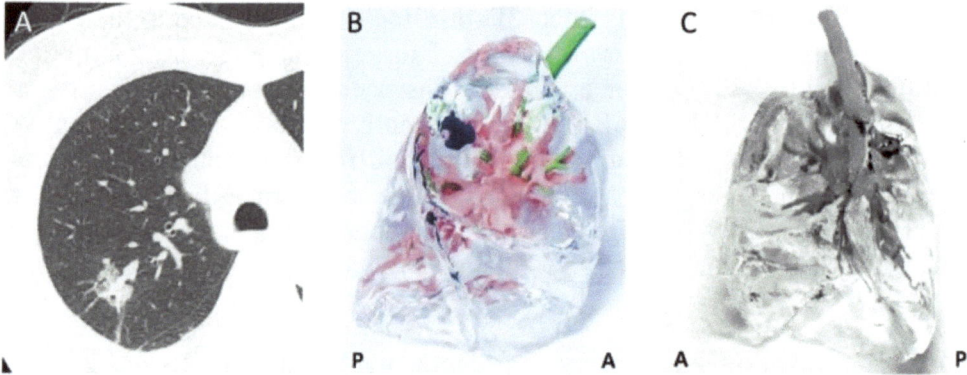

Fig. (4). Representative computed tomography and 3D-printed model images of a 54-year-old woman with primary lung adenocarcinoma (T1cN0M0). (A) A computed tomography image shows a 2.1-cm part-solid ground glass nodule in the posterior segment of the right upper lobe. A subsegmental pulmonary vein passes through the nodule. (B, C) A 3D-printed model shows the nodule (dark blue) within transparent flexible lung parenchyma. The pulmonary vessel passing through the nodule (pink) is located at the center of the tumor and the tracheobronchial structures are colored in green. A: anterior, P: posterior. (Reproduced with permission) [49].

This application can also be used in the process of understanding the relation between the tumor and the bronchial and vascular tree (Fig. **5**), and the visuospatial comprehension of thoracic wall infiltration (Fig. **6**).

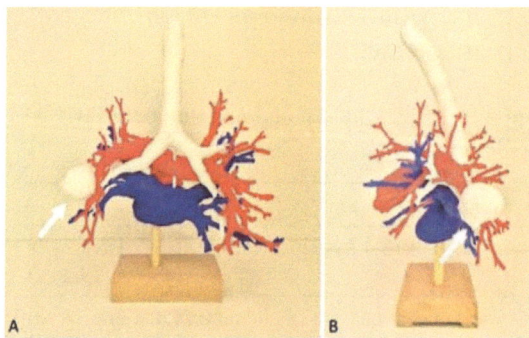

Fig. 5. 3D printed model of a left lower lobe tumor (white arrow) and its relation to pulmonary vasculature and the bronchial tree. A: frontal view, B: sagittal view. (authors own work).

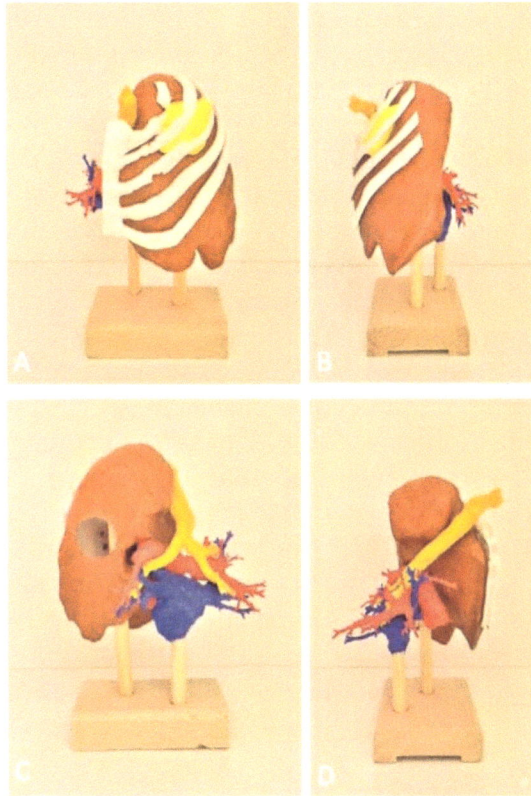

Fig. (6). Three-dimensional printed model of a patient with Stage IV cancer (thoracic wall infiltration). A: frontal, B: sagittal, C: dorsal, D: medial view. (authors own work).

Pre-operative Planning Specified to Robotic Lung Surgery

Robotic lung surgery is an evolution of VATS that is becoming increasingly popular [50]. In contrast to VATS, this approach facilitates 3D vision coupled with optimal instrument maneuverability. In recent literature, however scarce, direct comparisons between these techniques suggest similar results [51].

With regard to the planning of robotic procedures, the aforementioned planning methods can be used to determine patient placement on the operating table and ideal robotic port placement, based on CT derived reconstructions [18]. A highly expected future development in the field of robotic surgery, is the integration of augmented reality into the real-time 3D vision.

FUTURE PERSPECTIVES

Although realization of 3D reconstructions is becoming more time-efficient (it used to take hours, now minutes), conversion of 2D to 3D images remains laborious. Therefore, we foresee the emerge of 'whole-slide' 3D scanning, a technique which already has been introduced on small scale [52]. Three-dimensional scanning is already relatively prevalent across many non-medical domains. High-end commercial scanners are used by archeologists and preservationists to acquire models of remains, historical artifacts and large excavations [53]. In the medical field, its use is not yet widespread and still limited to the planning of maxillofacial and reconstructive surgery [54]. For thoracic disease, this method would undoubtedly prove useful for many processes, including tumor staging, margin assessment, pathologic-radiologic correlation, macro-microscopic correlation, and better insights into disease processes [55]. Although currently merely used for diagnostic and educational purposes, we expect 3D printing techniques to evolve in such a way, that it can actually be the basis of patient treatment. In several other medical fields, 3D printed prostheses are already accepted as a standard approach, as it facilitates a personalized, patient-specific, custom made experience [56]. The next step in this fascinating process will be the use of actual bio-prints, meaning the direct printing of biological materials [57]. In thoracic surgery, such implants could be used to reconstruct airways and potentially even lung tissue. In the foreseeable future however, the use of therapeutic 3D printing in thoracic surgery is limited to the reconstruction of the rib cage after thoracic wall resection [58].

CONCLUSION

Minimally invasive techniques are becoming the standard of care in almost all surgical fields. Still, these techniques remain technically more challenging and require extensive pre-operative planning. Three-dimensional anatomical reconstruction of CT derived images is a promising technique which facilitates a more widely adaptation of these minimally invasive techniques. Using this method, the feasibility of a minimally invasive approach, in combination with a minimal pulmonary resection volume, can already be assessed and determined in the pre-operative phase. For thoracic surgery, 3D printing is still in its infancy and its use has been limited to diagnostic and educational purposes, but we foresee an explosion in the use of these techniques in the near future.

CONSENT FOR PUBLICATION

Not applicable.

CONFLICT OF INTEREST

Peyman Sardari Nia, MD, PhD, is a consultant to Fujifilm Corp., Tokyo, Japan

ACKNOWLEDGEMENTS

Declared none.

REFERENCES

[1]   Bhattacharya K. Kurt Semm: A laparoscopic crusader. J Minim Access Surg 2007; 3(1): 35-6.
       [http://dx.doi.org/10.4103/0972-9941.30686] [PMID: 20668618]

[2]   Kelley WE Jr. The evolution of laparoscopy and the revolution in surgery in the decade of the 1990s.
       JSLS 2008; 12(4): 351-7.
       [PMID: 19275847]

[3]   Steiner CA, Bass EB, Talamini MA, Pitt HA, Steinberg EP. Surgical rates and operative mortality for
       open and laparoscopic cholecystectomy in Maryland. N Engl J Med 1994; 330(6): 403-8.
       [http://dx.doi.org/10.1056/NEJM199402103300607] [PMID: 8284007]

[4]   Frazee RC, Roberts JW, Symmonds RE, *et al.* A prospective randomized trial comparing open versus
       laparoscopic appendectomy. Ann Surg 1994; 219(6): 725-8.
       [http://dx.doi.org/10.1097/00000658-199406000-00017] [PMID: 8203983]

[5]   Jacobaeus H. Ueber die Möglichkeit die Zystoskopie bei Untersuching seröser Höhlungen
       anzuwenden. Munch Med Wochschr 1910; pp. 2090-2.

[6]   Landreneau RJ, Mack MJ, Hazelrigg SR, *et al.* Video-assisted thoracic surgery: basic technical
       concepts and intercostal approach strategies. Ann Thorac Surg 1992; 54(4): 800-7.
       [http://dx.doi.org/10.1016/0003-4975(92)91040-G] [PMID: 1417251]

[7]   Mitchell JD. Techniques of VATS lobectomy. J Thorac Dis 2013; 5 (Suppl. 3): S177-81.
       [PMID: 24040520]

[8]   Flores RM, Park BJ, Dycoco J, *et al.* Lobectomy by video-assisted thoracic surgery (VATS) versus
       thoracotomy for lung cancer. J Thorac Cardiovasc Surg 2009; 138(1): 11-8.
       [http://dx.doi.org/10.1016/j.jtcvs.2009.03.030] [PMID: 19577048]

[9]   Kirby TJ, Mack MJ, Landreneau RJ, Rice TW. Thoracoscopic segmentectomy for T1 classification of
       non-small cell lung cancer: a single center experience. Eur J Cardiothorac Surg 1995; 42(1): 83-8.

[10]   Gonzalez-Rivas D. VATS lobectomy: surgical evolution from conventional VATS to uniportal
       approach. ScientificWorldJournal 2012; 2012780842
       [http://dx.doi.org/10.1100/2012/780842] [PMID: 23346022]

[11]   Yamashita S, Tokuishi K, Anami K, *et al.* Thoracoscopic segmentectomy for T1 classification of non-
       small cell lung cancer: a single center experience. Eur J Cardiothorac Surg 2012; 42(1): 83-8.
       [http://dx.doi.org/10.1093/ejcts/ezr254] [PMID: 22228839]

[12]   Zhong C, Fang W, Mao T, Yao F, Chen W, Hu D. Comparison of thoracoscopic segmentectomy and
       thoracoscopic lobectomy for small-sized stage IA lung cancer. Ann Thorac Surg 2012; 94(2): 362-7.
       [http://dx.doi.org/10.1016/j.athoracsur.2012.04.047] [PMID: 22727321]

[13]   Kok M, Mihl C, Seehofnerová A, *et al.* Automated tube voltage selection for radiation dose reduction
       in CT angiography using different contrast media concentrations and a constant iodine delivery rate.
       AJR Am J Roentgenol 2015; 205(6): 1332-8.
       [http://dx.doi.org/10.2214/AJR.14.13957] [PMID: 26587942]

[14]   Kok M, Mihl C, Hendriks BM, *et al.* Optimizing contrast media application in coronary CT
       angiography at lower tube voltage: Evaluation in a circulation phantom and sixty patients. Eur J Radiol
       2016; 85(6): 1068-74.
       [http://dx.doi.org/10.1016/j.ejrad.2016.03.022] [PMID: 27161054]

[15]   Bae KT. Intravenous contrast medium administration and scan timing at CT: considerations and
       approaches. Radiology 2010; 256(1): 32-61.

[http://dx.doi.org/10.1148/radiol.10090908] [PMID: 20574084]

[16]   Müller NL. Computed tomography and magnetic resonance imaging: past, present and future. Eur Respir J Suppl 2002; 35: 3s-12s.
[http://dx.doi.org/10.1183/09031936.02.00248202] [PMID: 12064679]

[17]   Volonté F, Robert JH, Ratib O, Triponez F. A lung segmentectomy performed with 3D reconstruction images available on the operating table with an iPad. Interact Cardiovasc Thorac Surg 2011; 12(6): 1066-8.
[http://dx.doi.org/10.1510/icvts.2010.261073] [PMID: 21388979]

[18]   Le Moal J, Peillon C, Dacher JN, Baste JM. Three-dimensional computed tomography reconstruction for operative planning in robotic segmentectomy: a pilot study. J Thorac Dis 2018; 10(1): 196-201.
[http://dx.doi.org/10.21037/jtd.2017.11.144] [PMID: 29600049]

[19]   Heuts S, Maessen JG, Sardari Nia P. Preoperative planning of left-sided valve surgery with 3D computed tomography reconstruction models: sternotomy or a minimally invasive approach? Interact Cardiovasc Thorac Surg 2016; 22(5): 587-93.
[http://dx.doi.org/10.1093/icvts/ivv408] [PMID: 26826714]

[20]   Sardari Nia P, Olsthoorn JR, Heuts S, Maessen JG. Interactive 3D reconstruction of pulmonary anatomy for preoperative planning, virtual simulation, and intraoperative guiding in video-assisted thoracoscopic lung surgery. Innovations (Phila) 2019; 14(1): 17-26.
[http://dx.doi.org/10.1177/1556984519826321] [PMID: 30848710]

[21]   Ikeda N, Yoshimura A, Hagiwara M, Akata S, Saji H. Three dimensional computed tomography lung modeling is useful in simulation and navigation of lung cancer surgery. Ann Thorac Cardiovasc Surg 2013; 19(1): 1-5.
[http://dx.doi.org/10.5761/atcs.ra.12.02174] [PMID: 23364234]

[22]   Chan EG, Landreneau JR, Schuchert MJ, *et al.* Preoperative (3-dimensional) computed tomography lung reconstruction before anatomic segmentectomy or lobectomy for stage I non-small cell lung cancer. J Thorac Cardiovasc Surg 2015; 150(3): 523-8.
[http://dx.doi.org/10.1016/j.jtcvs.2015.06.051] [PMID: 26319461]

[23]   Iyer KS, Newell JD Jr, Jin D, *et al.* Quantitative dual-energy computed tomography supports a vascular etiology of smoking-induced inflammatory lung disease. Am J Respir Crit Care Med 2016; 193(6): 652-61.
[http://dx.doi.org/10.1164/rccm.201506-1196OC] [PMID: 26569033]

[24]   Andersen HK, Völgyes D, Martinsen ACT. Image quality with iterative reconstruction techniques in CT of the lungs-A phantom study. Eur J Radiol Open 2018; 5: 35-40.
[http://dx.doi.org/10.1016/j.ejro.2018.02.002] [PMID: 29719856]

[25]   Rodriguez A, Ranallo FN, Judy PF, Fain SB. The effects of iterative reconstruction and kernel selection on quantitative computed tomography measures of lung density. Med Phys 2017; 44(6): 2267-80.
[http://dx.doi.org/10.1002/mp.12255] [PMID: 28376262]

[26]   Young S, Kim HJ, Ko MM, *et al.* Variability in CT lung-nodule volumetry: Effects of dose reduction and reconstruction methods. Med Phys 2015; 42(5): 2679-89.
[http://dx.doi.org/10.1118/1.4918919] [PMID: 25979066]

[27]   Willemink MJ, Leiner T, Budde RP, *et al.* Systematic error in lung nodule volumetry: effect of iterative reconstruction versus filtered back projection at different CT parameters. AJR Am J Roentgenol 2012; 199(6): 1241-6.
[http://dx.doi.org/10.2214/AJR.12.8727] [PMID: 23169714]

[28]   Seki S, Koyama H, Ohno Y, *et al.* Adaptive iterative dose reduction 3D (AIDR 3D) *vs.* filtered back projection: radiation dose reduction capabilities of wide volume and helical scanning techniques on area-detector CT in a chest phantom study. Acta Radiol 2016; 57(6): 684-90.
[http://dx.doi.org/10.1177/0284185115603418] [PMID: 26339037]

[29]   Cory RA, Valentine EJ. Varying patterns of the lobar branches of the pulmonary artery. A study of 524 lungs and lobes seen at operation of 426 patients. Thorax 1959; 14: 267-80.
[http://dx.doi.org/10.1136/thx.14.4.267] [PMID: 13812149]

[30]   Watanabe S, Arai K, Watanabe T, Koda W, Urayama H. Use of three-dimensional computed tomographic angiography of pulmonary vessels for lung resections. Ann Thorac Surg 2003; 75(2): 388-92.
[http://dx.doi.org/10.1016/S0003-4975(02)04375-8] [PMID: 12607645]

[31]   Akiba T, Marushima H, Harada J, Kobayashi S, Morikawa T. Anomalous pulmonary vein detected using three-dimensional computed tomography in a patient with lung cancer undergoing thoracoscopic lobectomy. Gen Thorac Cardiovasc Surg 2008; 56(8): 413-6.
[http://dx.doi.org/10.1007/s11748-008-0258-3] [PMID: 18696208]

[32]   Lindstrom A. Selective laser sintering, birth of an industry http://www.me.utexas.edu/news/news/selective-laser-sintering-birth-of-an-industry

[33]   Kim MS, Hansgen AR, Wink O, Quaife RA, Carroll JD. Rapid prototyping: a new tool in understanding and treating structural heart disease. Circulation 2008; 117(18): 2388-94.
[http://dx.doi.org/10.1161/CIRCULATIONAHA.107.740977] [PMID: 18458180]

[34]   Ventola CL. Medical applications for 3D printing: current and projected uses. P&T 2014; 39(10): 704-11.
[PMID: 25336867]

[35]   D'Urso PS, Earwaker WJ, Barker TM, *et al.* Custom cranioplasty using stereolithography and acrylic. Br J Plast Surg 2000; 53(3): 200-4.
[http://dx.doi.org/10.1054/bjps.1999.3268] [PMID: 10738323]

[36]   Fink DJ, DiNovo ST, Ward TJ. Rapid, customized bone prosthesis. Google Patents 1994.

[37]   Kurenov SN, Ionita C, Sammons D, Demmy TL. Three-dimensional printing to facilitate anatomic study, device development, simulation, and planning in thoracic surgery 2015.
[http://dx.doi.org/10.1016/j.jtcvs.2014.12.059]

[38]   Nia PS, Heuts S, Daemen J, *et al.* Preoperative planning with three-dimensional reconstruction of patient's anatomy, rapid prototyping and simulation for endoscopic mitral valve repair. Interact Cardiovasc Thorac Surg 2016.: ivw308.

[39]   Nocerino E, Remondino F, Uccheddu F, Gallo M, Gerosa G. 3D modelling and rapid prototyping for cardiovascular surgical planning–two case studies. Lung 2016; 1000: 800.

[40]   Billiet T, Vandenhaute M, Schelfhout J, Van Vlierberghe S, Dubruel P. A review of trends and limitations in hydrogel-rapid prototyping for tissue engineering. Biomaterials 2012; 33(26): 6020-41.
[http://dx.doi.org/10.1016/j.biomaterials.2012.04.050] [PMID: 22681979]

[41]   Landers R, Pfister A, Hübner U, John H, Schmelzeisen R, Mülhaupt R. Fabrication of soft tissue engineering scaffolds by means of rapid prototyping techniques. J Mater Sci 2002; 37(15): 3107-16.
[http://dx.doi.org/10.1023/A:1016189724389]

[42]   Mitsouras D, Liacouras P, Imanzadeh A, *et al.* Medical 3D Printing for the Radiologist. Radiographics 2015; 35(7): 1965-88.
[http://dx.doi.org/10.1148/rg.2015140320] [PMID: 26562233]

[43]   Sardari Nia P, Heuts S, Daemen J, *et al.* Preoperative planning with three-dimensional reconstruction of patient's anatomy, rapid prototyping and simulation for endoscopic mitral valve repair. Interact Cardiovasc Thorac Surg 2017; 24(2): 163-8.
[PMID: 27677879]

[44]   Tumbleston JR, Shirvanyants D, Ermoshkin N, *et al.* Additive manufacturing. Continuous liquid interface production of 3D objects. Science 2015; 347(6228): 1349-52.
[http://dx.doi.org/10.1126/science.aaa2397] [PMID: 25780246]

[45]   Kurenov SN, Ionita C, Sammons D, Demmy TL. Three-dimensional printing to facilitate anatomic study, device development, simulation, and planning in thoracic surgery. J Thorac Cardiovasc Surg 2015; 149(4): 9-973.

[46]   Ju SG, Kim MK, Hong CS, *et al.* New technique for developing a proton range compensator with use of a 3-dimensional printer. Int J Radiat Oncol Biol Phys 2014; 88(2): 453-8.
[http://dx.doi.org/10.1016/j.ijrobp.2013.10.024] [PMID: 24315564]

[47]   Kim SW, Shin HJ, Kay CS, Son SH. A customized bolus produced using a 3-dimensional printer for radiotherapy. PLoS One 2014; 9(10)e110746
[http://dx.doi.org/10.1371/journal.pone.0110746] [PMID: 25337700]

[48]   Norman J, Madurawe RD, Moore CM, Khan MA, Khairuzzaman A. A new chapter in pharmaceutical manufacturing: 3D-printed drug products. Adv Drug Deliv Rev 2017; 108: 39-50.
[http://dx.doi.org/10.1016/j.addr.2016.03.001] [PMID: 27001902]

[49]   Yoon SH, Park S, Kang CH, *et al.* Personalized 3D-Printed Model for Informed Consent for Stage I Lung Cancer: A Randomized Pilot Trial. Semin Thorac Cardiovasc Surg 2019; 31(2): 316-8.
[http://dx.doi.org/10.1053/j.semtcvs.2018.10.017] [PMID: 30412772]

[50]   Morgan JA, Ginsburg ME, Sonett JR, *et al.* Advanced thoracoscopic procedures are facilitated by computer-aided robotic technology. Eur J Cardiothorac Surg 2003; 23(6): 883-7.
[http://dx.doi.org/10.1016/S1010-7940(03)00160-X] [PMID: 12829062]

[51]   Nakamura H. Systematic review of published studies on safety and efficacy of thoracoscopic and robot-assisted lobectomy for lung cancer. Ann Thorac Cardiovasc Surg 2014; 20(2): 93-8.
[http://dx.doi.org/10.5761/atcs.ra.13-00314] [PMID: 24583699]

[52]   Farahani N, Braun A, Jutt D, *et al.* Three-dimensional imaging and scanning: Current and future applications for pathology. J Pathol Inform 2017; 8: 36.
[http://dx.doi.org/10.4103/jpi.jpi_32_17] [PMID: 28966836]

[53]   Yu MC, Nien HL, Wu TC. Application of 3D laser scanning technology in historical building preservation: a case study of a Chinese temple. Optical Methods for Arts and Archaeology 2005; p. 5857.

[54]   Bottino A, De Simone M, Laurentini A, Sforza C. A new 3-D tool for planning plastic surgery. IEEE Trans Biomed Eng 2012; 59(12): 3439-49.
[http://dx.doi.org/10.1109/TBME.2012.2217496] [PMID: 22968204]

[55]   Prakash S, Venkataraman S, Slanetz PJ, *et al.* Improving patient care by incorporation of multidisciplinary breast radiology-pathology correlation conference. Can Assoc Radiol J 2016; 67(2): 122-9.
[http://dx.doi.org/10.1016/j.carj.2015.07.003] [PMID: 26632099]

[56]   Gretsch KF, Lather HD, Peddada KV, Deeken CR. Development of novel 3D-printed robotic prosthetic for transradial amputees. Prosthet Orthot Int 2016; 40(3): 400-3.
[http://dx.doi.org/10.1177/0309364615579317] [PMID: 25934422]

[57]   Cui H, Nowicki M, Fisher JP, Zhang LG. 3D bioprinting for organ regeneration. Adv Healthc Mater 2017; 6(1)
[http://dx.doi.org/10.1002/adhm.201601118] [PMID: 27995751]

[58]   Wu Y, Chen N, Xu Z, *et al.* Application of 3D printing technology to thoracic wall tumor resection and thoracic wall reconstruction. J Thorac Dis 2018; 10(12): 6880-90.
[http://dx.doi.org/10.21037/jtd.2018.11.109] [PMID: 30746234]

CHAPTER 8

Thoracic Incisions – Surgical Access to the Thoracic Cavity for Operations on the Lung

Keyvan Moghissi*

The Yorkshire Laser Centre, Goole & District Hospital, Goole, UK

Abstract: In standard and conventional surgery of the lung, there are a variety of incisions allowing access to the chest cavity. The common feature to all is to place the incision in a way which allows better surgical treatment for the lesion. The commonest approach is postero-lateral thoracotomy through the fifth inter space, with the patient placed on the operating table in an appropriate lateral position. This allows exploration of the lungs as well as the mediastinum. A prone position/face down also allows good exploration of the lungs and the postero mediastinum. All the anterior and antero-lateral incisions allow limited exploration of the lungs and arterial mediastinum. In this chapter, the variety of incisions for the approach to the lung at different angles have been briefly described and illustrated. Important advantages of standard thoracotomy incisions and approaches to the thoracic cavity for lung cancer operations are: Firstly, ample visual inspection with/without optical technology assistance. Secondly, to enable the surgeon to use the palpation method, which is an important attribute not endowed by the minimal access VATS methods.

Keywords: Antero-Lateral, Anterior Thoracotomies, Median Sternotomy, Postero-Lateral, Standard Pulmonary Resection For Cancer.

GENERAL PRINCIPLES OF THE SURGICAL INCISION AND ACCESS TO THE THORACIC CAVITY

The intrathoracic part of the airway, lungs and mediastinum may be surgically approached anteriorly, antero-laterally, postero-laterally and posteriorly. The thoracotomy incision is planned according to operative requirements and the topography of the lesion, which is the surgical target. There are, however, some general principles which apply to all "standard" thoracotomies aimed to approach the thoracic cavity and its structure within, as opposed to thoracoscopic access to the chest cavity.

---

* **Corresponding author Keyvan Moghissi:** The Yorkshire Laser Centre, Goole, UK; Tel 01724 290456; E-mail: kmoghissi@yorkshirelasercentre.org

Keyvan Moghissi, Jack Kastelik, Philip Barber & Peyman Sardari Nia (Eds.)

- The incision is usually made along skin creases and following the line of a rib.
- Incisions for exposure of the anterior mediastinum are carried over the sternum with transverse or vertical sternotomy if a wider exposure is needed.
- The chest wall muscles are incised or split into layers.
- Posteriorly, the trapezius and latissimus dorsi are divided in continuation. Between the two, the triangle of auscultation is bare of muscles and is covered only by fascia. The incision through this fascia exposes the rhomboids and indicates the direction of the underlying ribs.
- The serratus anterior should be cut nearer to its costal digitation rather than near to the scapula.
- Excision of a rib, once a common practice, is, as a rule, unnecessary.
- The chest is usually entered through an intercostal space by incising and stripping the costal periosteum together with the intercostal muscles from the upper border of a rib, thus gaining access to the thoracic cavity. This is done using the periosteum elevator and proceeding from the posterior to the anterior end of the upper border of the rib.
- A wider space may be created by incising the posterior end of the rib using a costotome or, alternatively, dislocating the costo-transverse joint.
- In anterior thoracotomy, the perichondrium is stripped, and the costal cartilages may be incised in order to provide a wider space.
- In all cases, a self-retaining rib spreader is inserted between two adjacent ribs and the space widened as required for surgical manoeuvres within the chest.
- Before closure and repair of thoracotomy wounds, the chest is usually drained using a tube(s) connected to an underwater sealed drainage system.

STANDARD POSTEROLATERAL THORACOTOMY TECHNIQUE (FIG. 1)

This is the most frequently used thoracotomy and is the standard approach for pulmonary surgery.

- Posterolateral thoracotomy is usually carried out with the patient in the lateral position. Very occasionally, postero-lateral thoracotomy is carried out with the patient placed in a prone position.
- For lateral position thoracotomy, the hemithorax to be entered is placed uppermost. To obtain a good lateral position, the spine should be parallel to the longitudinal axis of the operating table. To facilitate surgical manipulation and manoeuvres, the patient's back is placed near to the edge of the operating table. The uppermost leg is extended and the lower leg flexed beneath it to about 90°. A pillow is placed between the legs protecting the bony prominence of knees. The diathermy pad is then placed and fixed around the uppermost leg.

- Various accessory devices are used to obtain firm fixation of the patient to the table and prevent movement during operation.

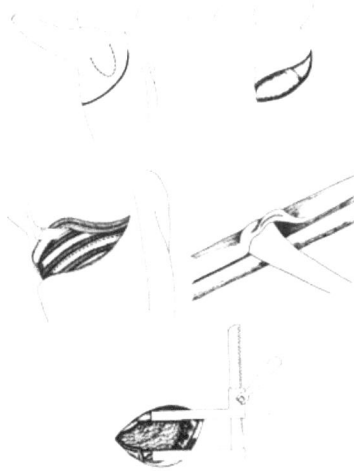

Fig. (1). Standard posterolateral thoracotomy technique.

Devices for monitoring and anaesthetic requirements appropriate for the type of the operation are planned in consultation with the anaesthetic team.

The incision is made parallel to the line of the obliquity of the ribs starting in front, lateral to the sternocostal junction running backwards 3-4 cm below the angle of the scapula, then upwards between the vertebral border of the scapula and the spine for a variable distance, according to the selected thoracotomy site, but not higher than the upper border of the scapula. The skin incision is made with a scalpel, but the flat muscles of the chest are divided by cutting diathermy.

THORACOTOMY – PRONE POSITION (OVERHOLT AND SELLORS-BROWN POSITION)

Prone position thoracotomy was used in the past for patients with copious bronchial secretions, *e.g.*, bronchiectasis. This approach has been largely superseded by the advent of double lumen tube intubation. Nevertheless, the position is useful for children and when double lumen tubes are not available or cannot be placed.

The patient is placed on the table lying flat and face down (Fig. 2). The upper part of the thorax and the pelvis are lifted off the table by pads and padded rests, so that the upper abdomen and the lower chest (diaphragmatic area) are away from the table. Slight Trendelenburg tilt is made, and the head is turned to one side. On the thoracotomy side, the arm hangs down but with no pressure on the axilla. The essence of this position is that the lungs and trachea are placed higher than the mouth, allowing free passage of a secretion from the lungs into a large endotracheal tube, which can be aspirated by the anaesthetist. This position prevents the spillover of bronchial secretion from the diseased into the healthy side.

General principles of repair of thoracotomy:

Before proceeding to the thoracotomy closure;

- Haemostasis is carried out.

- One or more drains are inserted through a lower intercostal space into the pleural cavity and connected to an underwater sealed drainage system.

- Closure of the thoracotomy wound requires layer by layer stitching. Five anatomical planes can be recognised and should be stitched.

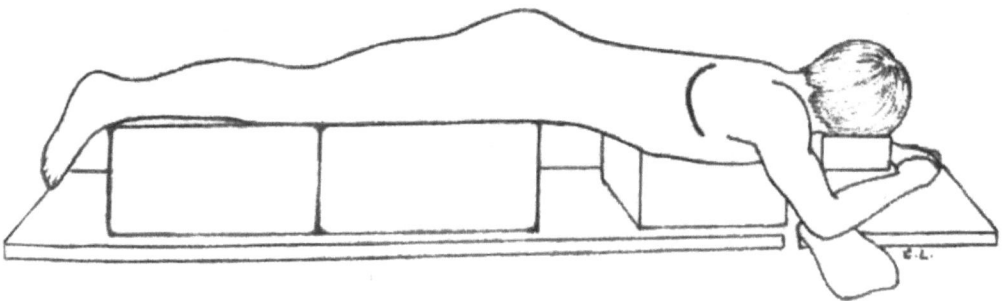

Fig. (2). Thoracotomy-prone position.

- Intercostal layers, including the parietal pleura. A rib approximator usually required to facilitate repair of this layer.
- Closure of the intercostal layer has to be airtight. This can be achieved using continuous running stitching.
- Deep muscular layer consists of a serratus anterior and the rhomboids muscles.
- Superficial muscular layer. The muscles in this layer consist of trapezius and latissimus dorsi in the posterolateral and pectoralis muscles in anterior and antero-lateral thoracotomies.
- Subcutaneous layer.

ANTERO-LATERAL THORACOTOMY (FIG. 3)

This approach is not particularly convenient for accessing all segments of the lung, but it is useful in some cases for metastatectomies. The patient is placed supine on the operating table and the operative side is elevated about 30 degrees or more. To achieve this, pads are placed behind the buttock and back, preventing the pelvis from falling back. The upper shoulder is rotated backwards for about 30 degrees and the elbow is flexed. The position is secured by tapes, table-rests and supports. A sub-mammary incision is made from the lateral border of the sternum anteriorly, extending for a variable length posteriorly and laterally along the line of the rib curve. In this position, the pectoralis major and sometimes the pectoralis minor, according to the level of the incision, are divided.

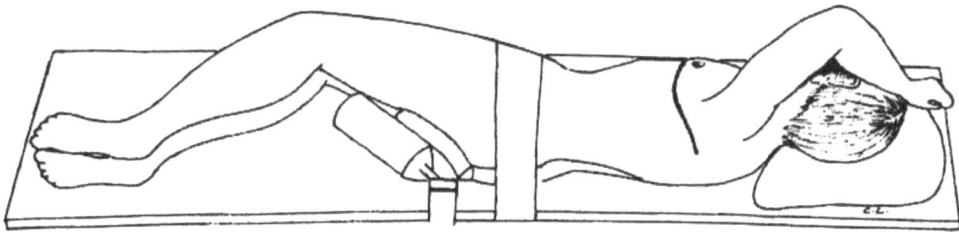

Fig. (3). Antero-lateral Thoracotomy.

ANTERIOR THORACOTOMY (FIG. 4)

The patient is placed in a supine position and surgical drapes laid in a manner to expose a square area of the upper abdomen above the umbilicus and the whole of hemithorax below the clavicle. Inclusion of the angle of Louis and the 2nd costal cartilage in the exposed area facilitates the identification of ribs and the accurate position of the incision.

A sub-mammary incision is made along the rib, starting from the lateral border of the sternum and extending laterally for a variable distance. The underlying muscles are divided. In emergency situations, the intercostal muscles and the pleura are incised directly, otherwise, the periosteum is elevated from the upper border of the rib together with the intercostal muscles. In either case, a chest spreader is introduced, and the opening widened by winding up the retractor. Closure of an anterior thoracotomy wound is similar to that of antero-lateral thoracotomy.

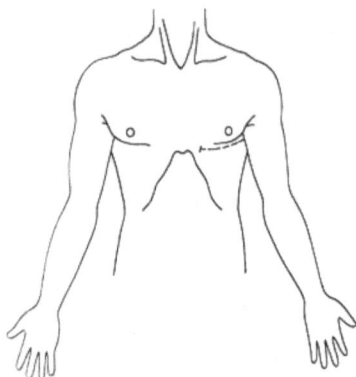

Fig. (4). Left anterior sub-mammary incision -dotted line.

Anterior Thoracotomy with Trans-sternal Extension

When further exposure of the mediastinum becomes necessary, the transverse section of the sternum is carried out in continuation with the anterior end of the incision. It is important to secure the internal mammary vessels or protect them.

MEDIAN STERNOTOMY (FIG. 5)

This approach is most commonly used for all types of open-heart surgical operations. In pulmonary operations, it is ideal for bilateral pulmonary metastatectomies, particularly those placed in the anterior, apical and medial segments of either of the lungs. It is also a choice incision for access to anterior mediastinal lymphatic chains.

The patient is placed in the supine position. A vertical midline incision is made extending from the suprasternal notch to a point midway between the xiphoid process and the umbilicus. Below the skin, subcutaneous tissue, pectoralis major fascia (and sometimes muscle fibres) and periosteum are incised with diathermy. The sternum is next divided using an electric saw (with a substernal protection guard), or other available devices for the sternal section. It is important to be aware of one or two veins around the xiphoid, which can cause bleeding. Whilst sternal division is proceeding, the lungs are hyperventilated to avoid the accidental opening of mediastinal pleura.

Once the sternum is divided, the strong interclavicular ligament, situated just above the suprasternal notch, requires division with scissors. The upper part of the linea alba also needs incising to allow wide separation of the two components of the sternum.

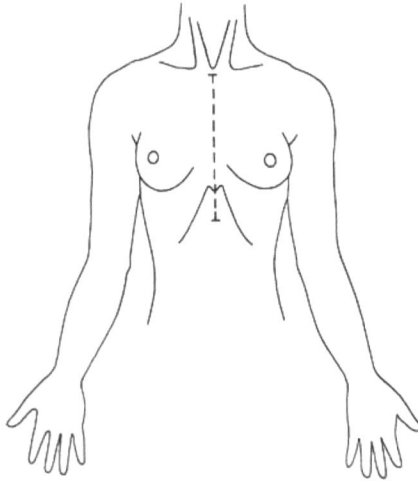

Fig. (5). Median sternotomy.

On completion of the operation, drains are placed and are led out through a stab incision placed below and lateral to the incision. All drains are connected to an underwater sealed system. The approximation of the two divided edges of the sternum is achieved, usually with 5 heavy stainless-steel wires or strong absorbable sutures. The wire may be placed through the bone or at the extreme anterior end of the intercostal spaces, i.e., around the sternum. Care should be taken to avoid injury to internal mammary vessels. The wires are crossed and twisted, bringing the sternal edges together. The excess length of each wire is cut, and the twisted portion is buried in the bone. The periosteum, together with fascia and the linea alba, the subcutaneous tissue and the skin are closed in sequence. The skin is closed with subcuticular stitches or otherwise as desired.

TRANS-STERNAL BILATERAL THORACOTOMY (FIG. 6)

Syn Clamshell Thoracotomy/Transverse Sternotomy

The 'clamshell' incision can be useful in some cases of bilateral pulmonary metastatectomies and when simultaneous bilateral pleural space access is required.

The patient is placed in the supine position on the operating table, with both arms abducted on support boards. A bilateral submammary incision is made from one mid axillary line to follow the curvature of the 4th and/or 5th ribs and, in continuation, transversely over the sternum. The incision is carried down to reach the intercostal spaces bilaterally. It is necessary to incise the fascia over the pectoralis major and to divide digitations of serratus anterior to reach intercostal spaces and muscles. These muscles and endothoracic fascia are divided next to reach the pleura. Positive pressure ventilation is best discontinued in order to incise the pleura without the risk of injuring the underlying lung. The internal mammary vessels are identified and tied securely or stitched and then divided. The sternum is now divided transversally.

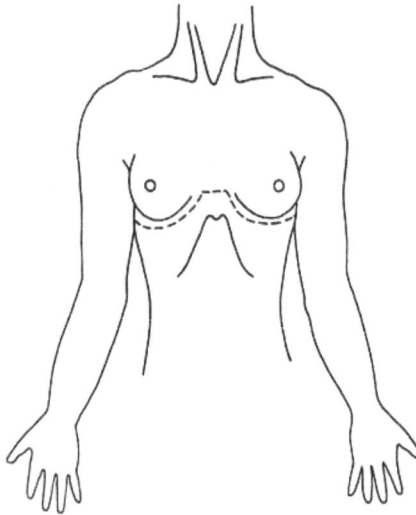

Fig. (6). Trans-sternal bilateral thoracotomy.

Closure of the wound is carried out as per anterior and antero-lateral thoracotomy with an approximation of sternal "moieties" by 2 wire sutures.

EXTENDED ANTERO-LATERAL THORACOTOMY (HEMI-CLAMSHELL - TRAP DOOR INCISION) (FIG. 7)

This approach provides access to the superior mediastinum and structures of the root of the neck. It is also a convenient approach to access the great vessels of the root of the neck and thoracic outlet tumours. The patient is placed more favourably in the supine position and the arm on the operating side is abducted.

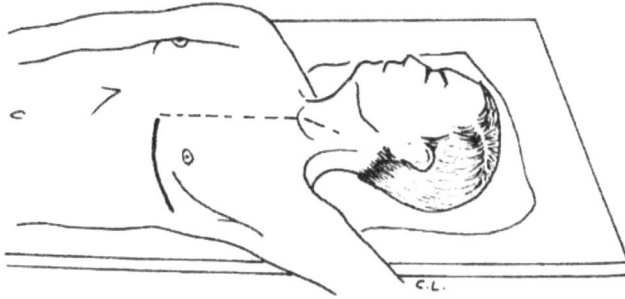

Fig. (7). Extended Antero-lateral thoracotomy (Hemiclamshell - trap door incision).

The incision has 3 components:

a. Cervical which can be oblique along the anterior border of the sterno-mastoid 4-5 cm above the suprasternal notch. Alternatively, this part of the incision can be more horizontal above the clavicle for 4-5 cm lateral to the sterno-clavicular joint.
b. Sternal part, which is a midline incision over the manubrium and the upper part of the body of the sternum to 2nd or 3rd costal cartilage.
c. The anterior thoracotomy component is a curved incision following the line of the 3rd rib anteriorly towards the anterior axillary line.

The three components of this composite incision are carried down; platysma and deep cervical fascia are incised, and the sterno-mastoid muscle can be divided if necessary. The sternum is divided into the mid-line Anterior thoracotomy that necessitates the division of the pectoralis major fascia and muscle-and some fibres of pectoralis minor. This approach provides a flap which, like a trap door, can be lifted upwards and laterally to expose structures in the root of the neck and superior-mediastinum.

Modifications of Antero-lateral Thoracotomy

Anterior-Cervico – Thoracic

In order to obtain a good exposure in cases of pancoast tumours, Dartevelle and colleagues (1994) proposed access through an L shaped incision, which provides an anterior trans-cervical approach. The vertical limb of the incision follows the anterior border of sterno-mastoid to sterno-clavicular joint. The horizontal part of the incision turns laterally under the medial half of the inferior border of the clavicle. This part of the bone is excised and the sternal attachment of sternum mastoid detached, providing access to the root of the neck. The incision is particularly useful in more unusual cases of Pancoast, which extends anteriorly and upwards.

LIMITED AND MUSCLE SPARING THORACOTOMIES

Introduction

Standard thoracotomies with a wide exposure of the intrathoracic structures may not be necessary for a number of cases in which excision of a nodular lesion by laser or wedge resection could be carried out. In such and similar cases, limited and muscle sparing thoracotomies may be used with great advantage. Currently, this incision is supplanted

The basic principle of these thoracotomies is to gain access to the thoracic cavity through intercostal spaces which are not covered by large chest wall muscles. Appraisal of the anatomical arrangement of the chest wall and its muscular covering indicates two such zones:

- A postero-lateral triangular area known as the triangle of auscultation is situated below the inferior angle of the scapula, between the lower border of the trapezius and the upper border of the latissimus dorsi muscle. Space is covered by fascia overlying the ribs and intercostal muscle.
- Sub axillary space: This is the area between the upwards rising postero lateral border of the pectoralis major anteriorly and the anterior border of the latissimus dorsi muscle. The floor is covered by the digitation of the serratus anterior. Incision over this area, together with detachment or division of some of the fibres of serratus anterior, provides easy access to the chest.

Taking these anatomical arrangements into account, the following muscle sparing thoracotomies are currently in use:

Limited/postero-lateral (Para Scapular) Thoracotomy

This incision is largely superseded by the advent of Minimal Access operations using VATS with the patient in a lateral thoracotomy position and the arm extended forward, the skin incision is made over the triangle of auscultation. The incision is carried along the medial border of the scapula and is extended downwards and forward for 8-10 cm below the inferior angle of the scapula. The fascia covering the floor of the triangle is opened to expose a portion of ribs 5-7 and their intercostal spaces. Elevation of the angle of the scapula by an assistant helps this exposure. The trapezius and the latissimus muscles are retracted posterior-medially and anterior inferiorly, respectively in order to gain better intra thoracic exposure. Entry to the chest is made through the 5th or 6th intercostal space as in standard postero-lateral thoracotomy. The closure is carried out in layers.

Axillary and Sub-axillary Thoracotomies

The patient is placed either in a lateral decubitus or oblique position. The arm is at 90 degrees abduction. In either case, there are options for:

a. Oblique incision (Fig. **8**).
b. Horizontal incision.
c. Vertical incision (Fig. **9**); In all cases, the incision is made in such a way as to avoid the posterior border of the pectoralis major and the anterior border of the latissimus dorsi. The latter muscle is retracted posteriorly and the digitations of the serratus are divided anteriorly in order to reach ribs and intercostal muscles.

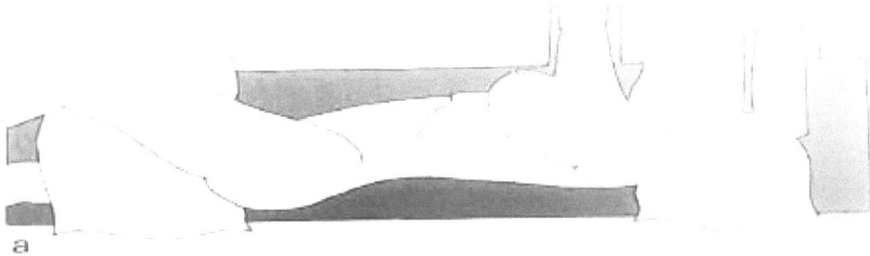

Fig. (8). Axillary Thoracotomy, Oblique incision.

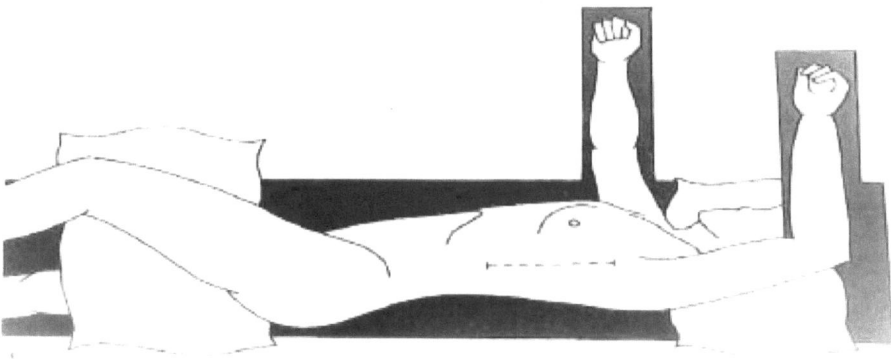

Fig. (9). Axillary Thoracotomy Vertical Incision.

Indications for muscle sparing thoracotomies:

1. Limited lung resection.
2. Exploratory thoracotomy with the possibility of extending the incision allowing better access to the posterior mediastinum and nodal dissection for broncho-plastic procedures.
3. As a 'utility incision' in conjunction with Video Assisted Thoracoscopic Surgery (VATS).

Advantages/Disadvantages of Muscle Sparing Thoracotomies

Advantages of Muscle Sparing Thoracotomies

1. Reduction of post-operative pain.
2. Partial reduction of post-operative complications (*e.g.*, pulmonary collapse).
3. Reduction of morbidity.

Disadvantages of Muscle Sparing Thoracotomies

1. Limitation of exposure.
2. Limitation for extensive lymph node excision in cancer surgery.
3. Difficulty of undertaking complicated surgery such as broncho-vascular plastic operations.
4. Difficulty in dealing speedily with major vascular accidental haemorrhage in complicated dissections.
5. Difficulty in identifying sources of bleeding on re-opening in cases of early post-operative clot retention and haemothorax.

Some of these disadvantages may be eliminated by combining such incisions and accesses with video-thoracoscopic surgery.

INCISIONS AND APPROACHES FOR MINIMALLY INVASIVE (MINIMAL ACCESS) SURGERY; VIDEO ASSISTED THORACIC SURGERY (VATS)

The Thoracoscope was adapted from a Cystoscope at the turn of the 20th C by Jacobaeus who wanted to use it in the pleural space, to section adhesions in order to maintain artificial pneumothorax. Collapse therapy method of employing "Induction pneumothorax" was a method which was used in the pre- antibiotics as well as pre-surgical era for treating pulmonary tuberculosis.

The 1950s and 1960s were the epoque of surgical resection for tuberculosis of the lung which usually affected apical and posterior segments of the upper lobes. However, in many of the Sanatoria, the Physiologists continued with thoracoscopic section of adhesion for the maintenance of the previously induced pneumothorax.

Towards the end of the 20th century, thoracoscopy became an acknowledged diagnostic tool as well as an established approach for limited range of treatment objectives such as pleurodesis, and or the treatment of empyema thoracis.

In the 1990s availability of a range of equipment and instruments to be used in the chest cavity for thoracoscopy procedures allowed Thoracoscopy to become an approach for surgery of the chest and to emerge, with its new cloak as Video-Assisted Thoracoscopic Surgery -VATS.

The reduced post-operative pain, the increased post procedural mobility of patients and the shorter duration of hospitalization (with its attached cost) were appealing factors for VATS to flourish in last two decades.

VATS INCISIONS AND PORTS

From the beginning of VATS, the camera and instruments were introduced into the chest via an incision or through a cannula inserted to the chest by a trocar. Either way, the channels are referred to as 'ports'. The Trocar and canula Port could be made of either metallic or plastic.

Port(s) placement has to be considered carefully to get an optimal view of the target area and instrumentations in use within thoracic cavity. It may vary in position in order to achieve the objective of the operative procedure in relation to the topography of the target lesion within the chest. Also, to some extent, port placement should fit in with the preference of the surgeon.

However, in the "classical" VATS the principle of triangulation with the optic and instruments entering the chest at the corner of the notional triangle is usually observed (Fig. **10**).

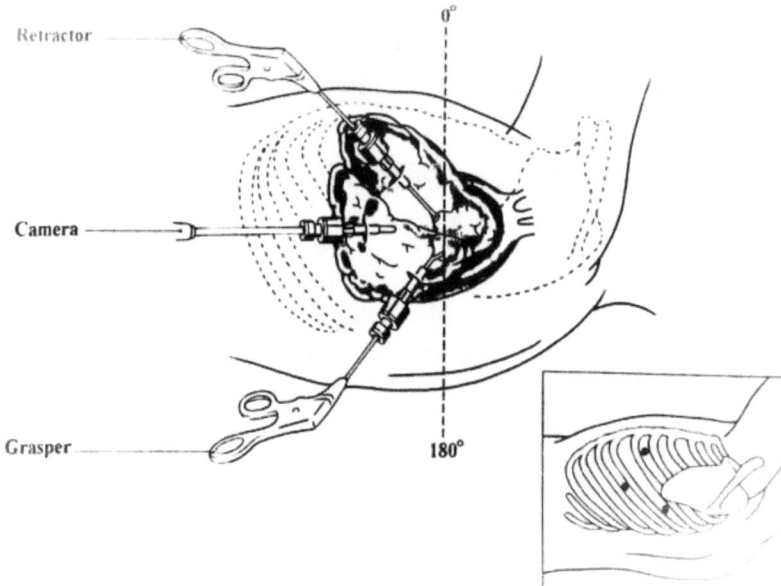

Fig. (10). The use of a three port approach to achieve "trianglulation". The ports are positioned so as to allow the operator to place the operative area of the apex of a notional pyramid defined by the optic and operating instruments the relative positions of which can be rotated as required.

This design which has been followed, by and large, until the present time, provides a clear view of the operative field and the various instruments which would be entering the field without clashing and obstructing the view on the screen.

There have been in the course of time variations in the number of Ports as well as their positions, matching on the one hand the advances in optics and instrumentation, and also as a continuing drive to minimisation.

One of the early variations came about with the necessity of finding a way of retrieval of the resected specimen safely and cleanly (a kind of the "kamel through the eye of a needle"). This was going to be either: a totally new short incision appropriately placed in a position near to the location of the resected specimen to be retrieved and called "the utility " incision. Or, alternatively the utility incision could be part of an existing Port, which has to be slightly larger than otherwise would be required for instrumentation (Fig. **11**).

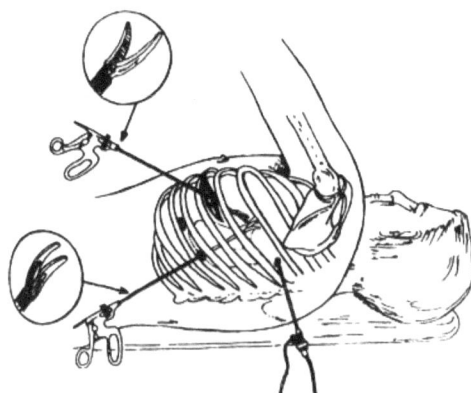

Fig. (11). Classical port arrangement for pulmonary surgery. Note the enlarged anterior port used as "utility" incision/port.

MINIMIZATION OF MINIMAL ACCESS INCISIONS AND PORTS

For the past 2 decades there has been a trend to further minimize the mini access /VATS by reducing the number of Ports and/or the size of the incision.

The idea of reducing the number of Ports goes back to the very beginning of VATS when some simple procedures including lung biopsy and pleurodesis could be carried out under vision using two Ports. More formally the application of 2 Ports-VATS also known as "Single utility Port" coincided with growing confidence and an ever expansion of range in instrumentations allowing pulmonary resection.

A number of studies which followed the trend, showed that the results of two Port VATS were in all measured parameters similar to those of three Ports-VATS.

Many practitioners used a 1.5 incision made at the level of 8 intercostal space along the posterior axillary line for the 30-degree Thoracoscope. According to the position of the lesion another 3-4 cm incision is also made over the 4th or 5th intercostal space along the anterior axillary line.

Basically, the position of the two incisions can be variable depending on the topography of the lesion in a segment or lobe of the lung.

Moghissi *et al* used the two Ports VATS initially in order in order to be able to use NdYAG laser within the pleural cavity. Subsequently they used two Ports VATS as a method of illumination (exposure to laser light) for Photodynamic Therapy (PDT), in a pre-sensitized cancer in the peripheral lung (See Chapter of Lasers in Lung Cancer.

- Uni-portal VATS: The feasibility of Uniportal VATS was first demonstrated by Meglire and colleagues in 2000.

At the "Thoracic surgery and interdisciplinary symposium" on the threshold of the third millennium. An international continuing medical education programme. Naples, Italy 2000:29-30.", Migliore and colleagues. presented a series of 58 different procedures performed through a single port. On this occasion these authors described a handcrafted 20 mm flexible circular trocar, rigid enough to avoid its collapse For anatomical lung resection 3-5 cm incision is regarded by many to be adequate. However, one has to take into account the physical build of the patients and a other factors. Therefore rational planning than rigid attitude needs to be applied.

Dr. Migliore who is the real unsung hero of the uniportal VATS discusses this issue more adequately in a separate chapter in this book (see chapter 10 on Uniportal VATS).

There is also the issue of the retrieval of the resected specimen. Placement of the incision should match the design of the operation and fit the topography of the pathology. The 4th and sixth intercostal spaces in the midaxillary line appears to be the site suitable for most procedures.

Uni-VATS has also been described for subxiphoid, trans axillary, transsternal and transcervical approaches.

CONCLUSION

In this Chapter the common incisions to accesses the Thoracic Cavity and its structures, are described. The trends to minimisation of incision and expansion of "key hole" access to thoracic structures, with all their well documented metabolic and other advantages, should be regarded as a mean to achieve a planed objectives of an operation and not because of simplicity and advantages . Minimal Access, Video Assisted Thoracoscopic Surgery (VATS) and its variants have still limitation for a number of operations despite most sophisticated instrumentation and advanced optics technology. There also is an important issue concerned with availability of required equipment in a number of countries in the world.

For now and for foreseeable future the surgeon should have the basic practical knowledge of approaches to thoracic cavity through various "classical" incisions, in addition to methods of minimal access surgery.

NOTES

Some of the illustrations in this chapter are taken from Moghissi's Essentials of

Thoracic & Cardiac Surgery. Second Edition. Edited by K Moghissi, J A C Thorpe, F Cuilli 2003 Elsevier Science. The copy right was relinquished by the publishers to the principal Editor on 7th November 2007.

CONSENT FOR PUBLICATION

Not applicable.

CONFLICT OF INTEREST

The author declares that there is no conflict of interest in this chapter.

ACKNOWLEDGEMENTS

Kate Dixon & Janet Melvin.

FURTHER READING

[1]   Socci L, Martin-Ucar AE. Access to the Chest Cavity: Safeguards and Pitfalls in Core Topics in Thoracic Surgery. Cambridge University Press 2016; pp. 25-37.
       [http://dx.doi.org/10.1017/CBO9781139565905.004]

[2]   Moghissi K. Thoracic incisions – surgical access to thoracic operations.Moghissi's Essentials of Thoracic and Cardiac Surgery. 2nd ed. Elsevier Science 2003; pp. 47-59.

[3]   Baeza OR, Foster ED. Vertical axillary thoracotomy: a functional and cosmetically appealing incision. Ann Thorac Surg 1976; 22(3): 287-8.
       [http://dx.doi.org/10.1016/S0003-4975(10)64918-1] [PMID: 962416]

[4]   Bethencourt DM, Holmes EC. Muscle-sparing posterolateral thoracotomy. Ann Thorac Surg 1988; 45(3): 337-9.
       [http://dx.doi.org/10.1016/S0003-4975(10)62479-4] [PMID: 3348708]

[5]   Dartvelle PG, Chapelier AR, Machiarini P. Anterior trans thoracic approach for radical resection of lung tumours invading the thoracic inlet. J Thorac Cardiovasc Surg 1994; 108: 389-92.

[6]   Ginsberg RJ. Alternative (muscle-sparing) incisions in thoracic surgery. Ann Thorac Surg 1993; 56(3): 752-4.
       [http://dx.doi.org/10.1016/0003-4975(93)90972-K] [PMID: 8379788]

[7]   Kittle CF. Which way in?--The thoracotomy incision. Ann Thorac Surg 1988; 45(3): 234.
       [http://dx.doi.org/10.1016/S0003-4975(10)62454-X] [PMID: 3348693]

[8]   Kraus D h, Huo J, Burt M. Surgical access to tumours of the cervicothoracic junction. Head Neck 1995; 17: 131-6.
       [http://dx.doi.org/10.1002/hed.2880170210] [PMID: 7558810]

[9]   Lardinois D, Sippel M, Gugger M, Dusmet M, Ris HB. Morbidity and validity of the hemiclamshell approach for thoracic surgery. Eur J Cardiothorac Surg 1999; 16(2): 194-9.
       [http://dx.doi.org/10.1016/S1010-7940(99)00156-6] [PMID: 10485420]

[10]   Mitchell RL. The lateral limited thoracotomy incision: standard for pulmonary operations. J Thorac Cardiovasc Surg 1990; 99(4): 590-5.
       [http://dx.doi.org/10.1016/S0022-5223(19)36930-2] [PMID: 2319778]

[11]   Moghissi K. Median sternotomy wound disruption: A surgical technique of repair. J R Coll Surg Edinb 1977; 22(2): 156-7.

[PMID: 323478]

[12]   Rothenberg SS, Pokorny WJ. Experience with a total muscle-sparing approach for thoracotomies in neonates, infants, and children. J Pediatr Surg 1992; 27(8): 1157-9.
[http://dx.doi.org/10.1016/0022-3468(92)90579-V] [PMID: 1403554]

[13]   Lewis RJ, Caccavale RJ, Sisler GE. Special report: video-endoscopic thoracic surgery. N J Med 1991; 88(7): 473-5.
[PMID: 1891124]

[14]   Jacobaelis H C. The Cauterization of adhesions in artificial pneumothorax treatment of pulmonary tuberculosis under thoracoscopic control. Proc Roy Soc Med 16 (Jul) Parts 1 & 2 Section of electrotherapeutics 1922; 1922-9123. 45 - 60

[15]   Jacobaeus HC. Uber Die, Moglichkeit Die Zystoskopie Bei Untersuchung Seroser Hohllungen Anzuwenden. Munch Med Wochenschr 1910; 57: 2090-2.

[16]   Richards JM, Dunning J, Oparka J, Carnochan FM, Walker WS. Video-assisted thoracoscopic lobectomy: the Edinburgh posterior approach. Ann Cardiothorac Surg 2012; 1(1): 61-9.
[PMID: 23977469]

[17]   Landreneau RJ, Mack MJ, Keenan RJ, Hazelrigg SR, Dowling RD, Ferson PF. Strategic planning for video-assisted thoracic surgery. Ann Thorac Surg 1993; 56(3): 615-9.
[http://dx.doi.org/10.1016/0003-4975(93)90930-G] [PMID: 8379753]

[18]   Landreneau RJ, Mack MJ, Hazelrigg SR, *et al.* Video-assisted thoracic surgery: basic technical concepts and intercostal approach strategies. Ann Thorac Surg 1992; 54(4): 800-7.
[http://dx.doi.org/10.1016/0003-4975(92)91040-G] [PMID: 1417251]

[19]   Hansen HJ, Petersen RH. Video-assisted thoracoscopic lobectomy using a standardized three-port anterior approach - The Copenhagen experience. Ann Cardiothorac Surg 2012; 1(1): 70-6.
[PMID: 23977470]

[20]   Moghissi K. (Taken from Walker W S, Video assisted thoracic surgery (VATS). Thoracic incisions – surgical access to thoracic operations.Moghissi's Essentials of Thoracic and Cardiac Surgery. 2nd ed. Elsevier Science 2003; pp. 47-59.

[21]   Mineo TC, Ambrogi V. Erratum to a glance at the history of uniportal video-assisted thoracic surgery. J Vis Surg 2018; 4: 112.
[http://dx.doi.org/10.21037/jovs.2018.05.21] [PMID: 29963401]

[22]   Reinersman JM, Passera E, Rocco G. Overview of uniportal video-assisted thoracic surgery (VATS): past and present. Ann Cardiothorac Surg 2016; 5(2): 112-7.
[http://dx.doi.org/10.21037/acs.2016.03.08] [PMID: 27134837]

[23]   Kim HK, Sung HK, Lee HJ, Choi YH. The feasibility of a Two-incision video-assisted thoracoscopic lobectomy. J Cardiothorac Surg 2013; 8: 88-95.
[http://dx.doi.org/10.1186/1749-8090-8-88] [PMID: 23587171]

[24]   Migliore M, Giuliano R, Deodato G. Video-assisted thoracic surgery through a single port. Thoracic surgery and interdisciplinary symposium on the threshold of the third millennium an international continuing medical education programme 2000; 29-30.http://xoomer.virgilio.it/naples2000/index.html Naples, Italy

[25]   Migliore M, Deodato G. A single-trocar technique for minimally-invasive surgery of the chest. Surg Endosc 2001; 15(8): 899-901.
[http://dx.doi.org/10.1007/s004640090033] [PMID: 11443464]

[26]   Migliore M. Initial History of Uniportal Video-Assisted Thoracoscopic Surgery. Ann Thorac Surg 2016; 101(1): 412-3.
[http://dx.doi.org/10.1016/j.athoracsur.2015.07.053] [PMID: 26694295]

[27]   Rocco G. History and indications of uniportal pulmonary wedge resections. J Thorac Dis 2013; 5

(Suppl. 3): S212-3.
[PMID: 24040526]

[28]   Sharpe DA, Dixon C, Moghissi K. Thoracoscopic use of laser in intractable pneumothorax. Eur J Cardiothorac Surg 1994; 8(1): 34-6.
[http://dx.doi.org/10.1016/1010-7940(94)90130-9] [PMID: 8136167]

[29]   Moghissi K, Dixon K, Thorpe JA. A method for video-assisted thoracoscopic photodynamic therapy (VAT-PDT). Interact Cardiovasc Thorac Surg 2003; 2(3): 373-5.
[http://dx.doi.org/10.1016/S1569-9293(03)00073-2] [PMID: 17670074]

Principle of Standard (Conventional) Pulmonary Resection for Lung Cancer

Keyvan Moghissi[*]

The Yorkshire Laser Centre, Goole & District Hospital, Goole, UK

Abstract: In this chapter, the principles of standard techniques of pulmonary resection are described. The chapter comprises of a number of sections:

In the first section, the focus of attention has been the issues related to the pulmonary arteries and veins and their safe and secure handling.

1. In the second, reference is made to some aspects of bronchoplastic operation.

2. Surgery for lung cancer affecting the lower tracheal bifurcation (carina and main stem bronchi) is dealt with in a separate section.

3. A separate section is devoted to lung cancer involving the lung, carina and also portion of the lateral wall of the trachea, which needs carinal resection or tracheal Sleeve Pneumonectomy (TSP).

4. Pancoast tumour/Superior Sulcus tumour is also a separate section.

5. Finally, lung cancer invading the chest wall is dealt with separately.

6. The reason for targeting the above topics in lung cancer surgery in separate sections is that each of these requires separate expertise and their surgical treatment needs special consideration and expertise.

Keywords: Bronchoplastic/parenchyma conservative of lung cancer surgery, General Principles of standard/conventional surgery for lung cancer, Surgery for superior sulcus/Pancoast Tumour, Surgery for lung cancer invading the chest wall, Tracheal bifurcation surgery, Tracheal Sleeve Pneumonectomy/Carinal Pneumonectomy.

[*] **Corresponding author Keyvan Moghissi:** The Yorkshire Laser Centre, Goole & District Hospital, Goole, UK; Tel: 01724 290456; E-mail: kmoghissi@yorkshirelasercentre.org

Keyvan Moghissi, Jack Kastelik, Philip Barber & Peyman Sardari Nia (Eds.)

INTRODUCTION

In whatever way the thoracic cavity is approached, the aim is to first visually explore and then expose the target organ prior to carrying out surgical procedure.

Also, irrespective of access, the principle of cancer surgery, which is complete removal of cancer and precancerous lesion together with all relevant and potentially relevant nodes, will have to be applied.

In standard methods of access to the chest cavity, the lung parenchyma is examined from the apex down to the base visually and by palpation. This is followed by the examination of the root and fissures. Particular attention is paid to the anterior aspect of the hilum and freedom of the major vessels from invasion by the pathological process as well as lymphadenopathies.

After the introduction of Video-Assisted- Thoracoscopic- Surgery (VATS) and its routine usage towards the close of the 20th Century, there has been a gradual decrease in standard (conventional) approach to the chest cavity and with it, an inevitable change in pulmonary resection methods and to some extent its indications.

Staplers in thoracic and pulmonary operation made their debuts in the 1980s, at the time only for pulmonary wedge resection and for the closure of the bronchial stump.

Expansion of VATS necessitated the development of a whole range of novel surgical instruments and devices. Amongst these, vascular staplers were of particular importance. Despite accelerated advances of VATS, in the opinion of this author and many others, a thoracic surgeon must be able and should be trained to use either the standard/conventional approach or VATS according to the requirement of the case. This in practicc means for now and in the near foreseeable further that a pulmonary surgeon should master both methods of "conventional", VATS and yet more Avant-guard surgery.

Relevant to this chapter are:

• Pulmonary vessels of the part of the lung to be excised need to be secured as per conventional methods, between ligatures and divided, or alternatively be secured and divided by stapler's automated action applied by the operator, who is able and knowledgeable to its use.
• In general: Staplers are convenient and safe to be used to close and divide the bronchial branch.
• It is important for a pulmonary surgeon to realise that in principle, suturing a

bronchus implies that the surgeon can put an individual stitch in an area when it calls for insertion of a stitch, whereas stapler is applied by the operator who has no choice in inserting a single stitch where needed.

Except for biopsy or wedge excision, all pulmonary resections are based first on the dissection of the corresponding bronchovascular structures. In practice, this means that the pulmonary vascular branches are divided between ligatures individually and the bronchi are closed separately. In pneumonectomy, the main pulmonary artery, the two main pulmonary veins (superior and inferior), and the main bronchus at, or just below, the division of the trachea have to be dealt with.

In lobectomy, the branches of the pulmonary artery and vein to the lobe concerned are to be divided between ligatures. With minor anatomical variations on each side, the number of pulmonary arterial branches to a lobe is equal to the number of its constituent segments.

In lobar resection, the artery to the lobe can be dealt with before it gives off segmental branches. In segmental resection, arteries to the segment have to be dealt with individually because they are given off separately from the trunk of the main lobar artery. The vein to a lobe is a single one which then divides. Therefore, the lobar vein can be divided between ligatures, as a single structure, before its division. Likewise, the bronchial branch to a lobe is given off as a single trunk, which then divides and, therefore, the lobar bronchus can be dealt with separately.

The segments are the smallest pulmonary anatomical unit, which can be excised. They receive a single arterial branch, one or two veins and a single bronchial branch. In segmentectomies, these are dealt with individually.

DISSECTION AND LIGATION OF VESSELS

With minor variations, the anatomical arrangement of the pulmonary arterial and venous systems are similar for the right and left lung. There is a superior and an inferior pulmonary vein on each side. On the right side, the superior vein is concerned with the upper and the middle lobe. On the left, it gives off branches to the upper lobe proper and the lingula. The inferior pulmonary vein on either side is concerned with the lower lobe. The veins are anterior structures of the hilum and are surrounded by a pericardial cuff. The inferior vein can be easily identified in the anteroinferior aspect of the lung within the inferior pulmonary ligament on each side. The superior pulmonary vein is adjacent and inferior to the pulmonary artery.

Like veins, the main pulmonary artery is an anterior structure on both sides. After giving off segmental branches to the anterior and apical segments of the upper lobe, the main artery passes posteriorly and turns into the oblique fissure to run along its axis. Therefore, the segmental arterial branches, except for the upper lobe, are given off from the pulmonary arterial trunk in the oblique fissure.

As a general rule, the arterial trunk in the fissure is overlaid by the pleura and lymph nodes. The latter are a good landmark. The branches of the pulmonary artery are ligated and divided. The veins are dealt with in a similar fashion. It is a wise precaution to suture the main pulmonary artery and the main trunks of the pulmonary veins in addition or as an alternative to ligating them.

In certain circumstances, intrapericardial division of pulmonary vessels is mandatory as there may not be an uninvolved length outside the pericardium to allow extra-pericardial ligation and division as described above. It is imperative to suture vessels when they are to be divided intrapericardially. Simply tying them off is a recipe for disaster which happens only once to a patient and should never happen to a surgeon. In recent years stapling devices have been used by many to deal with pulmonary vessels safely and efficiently.

BRONCHIAL CLOSURE

Staplers are now safe and efficient instruments for bronchial closures; however stitches still present an opportunity to place individual sutures exactly in the place that the surgeon desires it to be. In such cases, it is best to clamp the bronchus distal to the line of incision. The alternative of dividing the bronchus between two clamps will produce crushing of the tissues at the site of the closure and unnecessary tissue injuries. The two edges of the bronchial cut are stitched together, and the bronchus opening is closed. Vascular staplers are used by many surgeons and have been shown to be safe and easy to apply. To categorically state, which is the best method of bronchial closure and what suture material is the most appropriate is neither scientific nor particularly useful. The reason being that during long training, surgeons have come to select their preference as to whether to use hand suturing or staplers, and maybe, in some cases both.

Each surgeon has been trained to use a particular method and will continue to practice it unless it proves unsatisfactory. A trainee surgeon should be 'au fait' with hand sewing as well as stapling. Many surgeons have a method of covering the bronchial stump with living tissues in cases of pneumonectomy, with the aim of reducing the risk of broncho-pleural fistula formation. Pedicle intercostal graft, pleura, pericardium and pedicle omental graft have been extensively used for this purpose. The author has used the pedicle graft of the pericardium for many years and has, as a result, had no cases of bronchopleural fistula following pneumonectomies' in a 10-year period (over 140 consecutive cases).

Additional Tips on Pulmonary Resection

- It is easier to divide pulmonary and pleural adhesions when the lung is ventilated rather than the alternative of collapsing the lung. Therefore, at the start of the operation with the lung expanded adhesions are divided and exploration (both visual and by palpation) is done. The lung is then collapsed for further exploration.
- It is easier to separate and dissect the lobes of the lung by incising the adhesion and the pleura in the fissures when the lung is expanded and ventilated.
- The way to mobilise a very adherent lung which is attached to the chest wall, is to strip the parietal pleura with the lung (*i.e.* extrapleural mobilisation) from the chest wall and then enter the pleural space in a convenient place where the lung is free, usually on the mediastinal aspect of the lungs.
- Following the bronchial closure, it is a wise precaution to test the closure against a ventilation pressure of 30-40 cm water generated by the anaesthetic machine through the endotracheal tube, whilst 500 ml of warm (body temperature) saline is poured into the pleural space to submerge the stump and thus demonstrate any air leak.
- It is important to handle the lung with extreme gentleness since trauma or rough manipulation will result in air leak and/or pulmonary contusion, either/both of which will prolong recovery.
- Electro-diathermy and coagulation should not be used near the bronchial stump; bleeding vessels should be ligated or sutured.

BRONCHO PLASTIC PROCEDURES

These operations are designed to offer an economic resection of the lung by preserving the healthy pulmonary parenchyma whilst allowing the surgical excision of a diseased bronchus. In physiological terms, the tissues which are responsible for effective ventilation (*i.e.* parenchyma) are conserved, whereas a part of the dead space is excised. In practice, this is achieved by excision of a bronchus without resection of its distal lung tissue. In some cases, the bronchial excision is undertaken, and the remnant bronchus is attached to nearby lobar or segmental bronchial branches.

There are a number of issues that Surgeons need to address before undertaking any bronchoplastic operations:

- There should be adequate, viable un-involved length of distal and proximal site

of the proposed residual bronchi allowing infiltrated bronchial mucosa and its external wall by cancer.
- White Light Bronchoscopy (WLB) and Auto Fluorescence Bronchoscopy (AFB) should be a mandatory pre-operative undertaking in cases submitted for bronchoplastic lung resection in order to assure lack of neoplastic infiltration of the mucosa.

Peri bronchial lymphatic infiltration can also easily be missed and cause an early recurrence of the tumour. Studies that observed at bronchial margin infiltration after pulmonary resection for lung cancer suggest that the rate of bronchial margin infiltration in all resection is in the order of 4-6%. This rate could be a staggering 30% in central lung cancer. In the absence of AFB facilities, some surgeons recommend resorting to frozen section biopsies from the bronchial margin before proceeding to anastomosis.

The common varieties of bronchoplastic procedures are:

Main Stem Bronchial Excision without Pulmonary Resection

Based on anatomical consideration, in practice, a malignant tumour which could involve either of the main stem bronchi that could allow bronchoplastic operation without added pulmonary resection (i. e; excision of short segment of bronchus and plastic reconstruction) will have to be:

- Either, a short-localised carcinoma in situ, which in the opinion of this author should be treated by Photodynamic therapy (PDT) and not surgical methods.
- Or, a cancer of the main bronchus which extends to and involves also the lower trachea. Such a tumour requires bifurcation resection (lower trachea and both bronchi) resection followed by reconstruction.

In practical term the anatomical features of main stem bronchi are not compatible for excision of left main stem and/or even shorter right main bronchus.

Bronchoplastic Procedures with Conservation Lung Resection

Right Upper Lobectomy with Sleeve Bronchial Resection (Fig. 1)

The principle of sleeve resection is to excise the upper lobe of the lung together with the sleeve of the main bronchus and then to reconstruct the bronchial tree by joining the trunk of the lower lobe bronchus to the trachea. On the right side this is easily achieved because the upper lobe bronchus branch is given off very near the horizontal plane of the carina. Therefore, after ligation and division of the Azygos vein, the carina, the intermedius and right upper lobe bronchi are individually encircled and whilst the lung is collapsed (contralateral ventilation) division and anastomosis (reconstruction) are done.

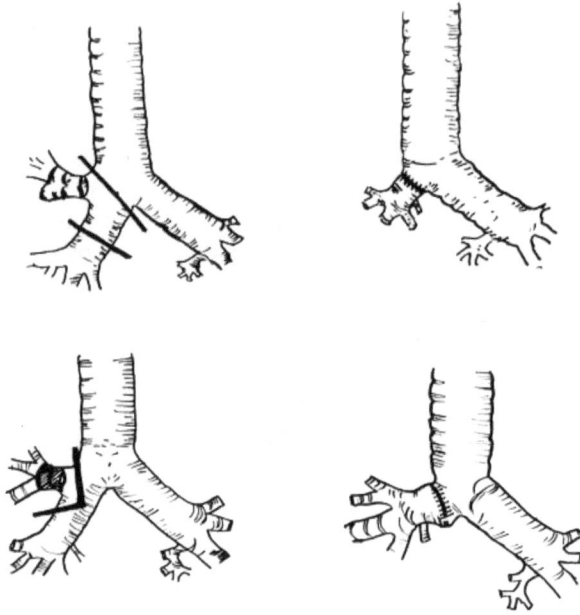

Fig. (1). Above lobectomy with sleeve resection of the main bronchus (left) and reconstruction (right). Below lobectomy with wedge excision of the main bronchus (left) and reconstruction (right).

The variant of classical sleeve lobectomy is the right upper lobectomy together with a wedge excision of the lateral wall of the right main bronchus. This is then followed by anastomosis of the lateral wall of the intermedius bronchus to the remnant of the lower trachea (Fig. **1**).

It is mandatory to have a clear evidence that all the remnant bronchial margins are un-involved.

Left Upper Lobectomy Sleeve Resection

The sleeve resection on the left upper lobe is rather more complicated than the right because of the anatomical position of the pulmonary artery, its branches to the left lung and their relationship with the left main bronchus.

Nevertheless, the method is similar to that of the right upper lobectomy sleeve resection. Basically, in a classical sleeve; resection whilst the upper lobe arteries and veins are secured and divided, the left main bronchus is severed above and below the left upper lobe bronchus branch, which in this case has the left upper lobe proper and lingula segments. The left upper lobe remnant below the carina is then anastomosed with the left lower lobe bronchus division. It is, at times, possible to save the lingula. In this scenario, the plastic repair requires some "tailoring".

In the case of wedge excision of the left main bronchus together with the left upper lobe and its bronchus, only the partial circumference of the left main bronchus is removed together with the left upper lobe bronchus and the lower lobe bronchial division is connected to the left main bronchus remnants. (Fig. **2**).

Because of the topography of the pulmonary artery in relation to the bronchus, the main left pulmonary artery may have to be divided and reconstructed in all bronchoplastic procedures on the left side. Homologous pericardial patch for the left pulmonary artery reconstruction is a useful tissue to be used, should patch grafting of the pulmonary artery become necessary.

Other Broncho Plastic Procedures

There are numerous possibilities of broncho plastic procedures in which a portion of the main bronchus, with a lobe of the lung, is excised and the reconstruction is carried out by swinging the remaining lobar bronchus to join with the trachea or available healthy bronchi. In some, the whole circumference of the bronchus is excised, and re-implantation of the residual bronchi is undertaken. In others, partial circumferential excision of the main bronchus (wedge excision) is performed with standard lobectomy followed by reconstruction as required, similar to the diagram shown in Figs. (**1** and **2**).

In all plastic procedures, it is wise to provide a protective cover to the anastomosis by pericardium or pleura. In some cases, pedicle intercostal graft can be provided for covering.

Excision of the Carina, Right and Left Main-Stem Bronchi (Bifurcation Resection) - Followed by Reconstruction of the Air Way

In this operation, the two main bronchi and carina involved by the tumour are excised together with a total circumference of a small portion of the lower trachea. The remnant of the right main and left main bronchi are then connected to the lower tracheal remain.

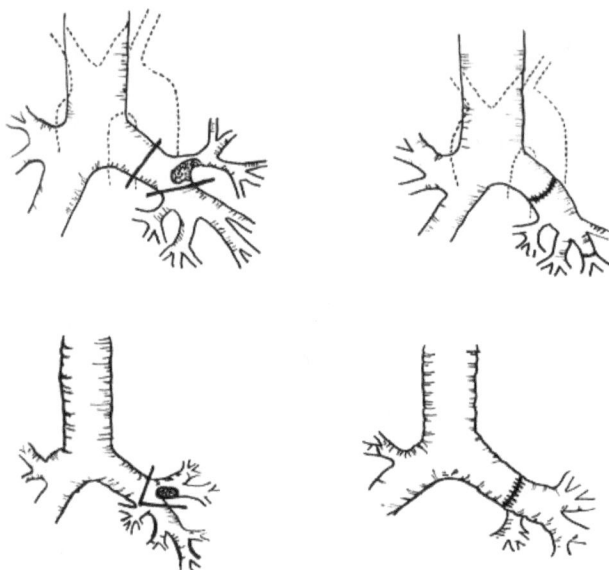

Fig. (2). Above upper lobectomy and sleeve resection of the main bronchus (left) and reconstruction (right). Below upper lobectomy with wedge resection of left main bronchus (left) and reconstruction (right).

Pre-operative workup should be thorough in order to allow the surgical team to have the virtual model of the operative field and involvement of various components of airway and the extent of the lesion within and without the lumen of each component of the lower trachea and main bronchi.

- In addition to the standard preoperative workup and staging procedures, it is crucial to know the extent of the tumour involvement of the lower trachea, the right and the left main stem bronchi as well as the expanse of the precancerous lesion which could be invisible by a naked eye using the ordinary "white light". This assessment needs to be within the 3D diagrammatic model, which includes:
  ○ Posterior, anterior and the lateral walls of the lower trachea right and left main bronchi.
  ○ Taking the account of a relative shortness of the right main bronchus before it gives off the right upper lobe bronchus, that for all practical purpose is level with the carina.

When measuring the length of the lower tracheal involvement by the tumour, it is mandatory to measure the total length of the trachea. In the experience of this author with over 150 cases of the trachea and tracheobronchial resection and reconstruction, there is a variation in the order 1.5-2cm of the length of the trachea (from Larynx/ which is about 2 cm below the cords at endoscopy to carina.

Besides the total length of the trachea in a patient who is undergoing surgery, the surgeon needs to have a clear measurement of:

a. The total length of the tumour free trachea (length of the trachea from the larynx to the upper limit of the tumour).
b. The total length of the tumour from its upper edge to its lower limit in the right main bronchus.
c. The length of the tumour from its upper edge in the trachea to its lower limit in the left main bronchus.

Imaging plays an important role in the design of the bifurcation resection and reconstruction, however, the rigid and flexible bronchoscopies are important from the decision-making point of view.

The rigid bronchoscope (RB) is important in the measurement of the extent of the tumour and tumour free airway. Also, its rigid consistency allows appreciation of the suppleness of the tissues as an index of their infiltration by the tumour and or its lack of elasticity which is important to prevent tension on the suture lines which join the lower trachea to the right and left bronchi reconstruction.

The role of Flexible Fibreoptic Bronchoscope (FFB) is to determine the limits of the margin of the tumour by white light (WL) and Auto Fluorescence bronchoscopy (AFB).

Provided that the pre-operative work up is meticulous and extensive, and the model of the airway and the extent of the pathology can be made with precise measurements, the gap between the trachea and two bronchi should not present any surprises and real problems at operation either in its excision or the reconstruction phases of the operation.

The simple operative access is basically *via* an extended right postero-lateral thoracotomy through the 4th intercostal space. This approach affords suitable access to mobilisation of good portion of the trachea and carina as well a good length of the main bronchi. Alternative approach of extended median sternotomy, bilateral thoracotomies have been used in cases which cannot be managed with a right thoracotomy.

There are various possibilities of reconstruction. The basic and easiest would be to join right and left bronchial remnants to make a "neo carina" which can be attached to the lower tracheal tail end. Variation to this simple method is to carry out and end (bronchus) to side (tracheal) anastomosis.

Anaesthesia and ventilation during such an operation which needs to have part of the main airway exposed and "open", need a close cooperation with the anaesthetic team. This should consider the basic facts that ventilation (oxygenation) is life support and yet the anaesthetic method or its devices should not hinder clear view and free surgical maneuvers.

It is tempting for those trained in the use of Cardio-Pulmonary Bypass (CPBP) with the use of "pump-oxygenator" to consider the method which obviates manipulation of endo-airway tubes. However, based on personal experience (3 cases) we find the method adds to the total operating time and anticoagulation can still be an added hazard. Nevertheless, in cases requiring a more extensive mobilization and more complicated anastomosis, it is reasonably simple to carry out all parts of the operation without CPBP and to start the bypass only for the phases of excision of the "bifurcation" and anastomosis reconstruction suturing of the operation.

Our method of "double circuit" ventilation is quite simple and seems to work well. The method consists of having two anaesthetic and ventilator systems and circuits to use at different phases of the operation.

Circuit A

This consists of standard (single lumen) endotracheal tube which is placed at the start of the operation. The lower tip of this tube should sit above the upper part of the tumour in the trachea (Fig. **3**, Top-left).

Circuit B

A shorter and narrower endo tracheal tube is connected to a separate sterile airway tubing ready at hand on the instrument trolley wrapped in a sterile towel to be used later on during the operation.

At the start of surgery, Circuit A is used entirely for anaesthetic and ventilation.

When all mobilisation and accessory parts of the operation are completed the surgeon incises the trachea and excises the lower trachea and the bronchi. During this time the endo tracheal tube of Circuit B is introduced in the top of right (and in some cases the left) main bronchial opening through the operative field by the surgical team and one lung ventilation is continued (Fig. **3**, Top-right).

The edges of the right and left main bronchi are sewn together posteriorly to create a new carina. The posterior layer of anastomosis is carried out and completed easily with the endo bronchia (Circuit B) in place and is looked after by an assistant.

Once the posterior layer of the anastomosis is completed the anaesthesia and ventilation are taken over by the Circuit A. This is done by pushing the endotracheal tube which has remained in the upper part of the trachea to enter the right or left main bronchus passing over the posterior anastomosis suture line (Fig. 3, Bottom-left).

The anterior layer of anastomosis is now easily undertaken with the ventilation continuing through the endo bronchial tube of the Circuit A (Fig. 3, Bottom-right).

After the completion of the anterior suture line the whole of the anastomosis is wrapped with a pedicle graft of the pericardium for security.

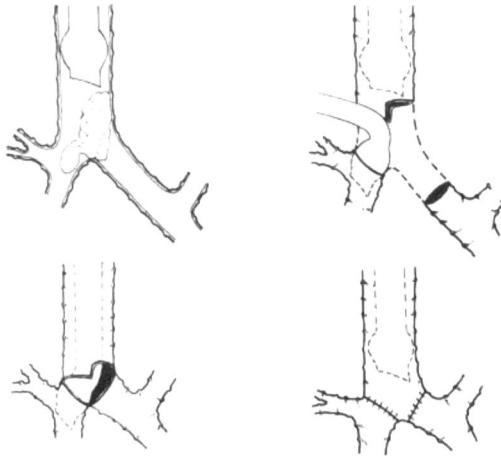

Fig. (3). Illustration ventilation management during the excision of the lower trachea and main branchial tumours. Top-left, Endotracheal tube. Top-right, Excision of the tumour. Bottom-left, The suturing of the posterior wall. Bottom-right, Anterior wall anastomosis.

Tracheal Sleeve Pneumonectomy (Synonym Carinal Pneumonectomy) for Lung Cancer Extending to the Latera Wall of the Trachea

Tracheal Sleeve pneumonectomy is an extensive operation which is designed to surgically treat a complex type of lung cancer that involves a great part of the lung with extension to the lateral wall of the trachea and often the carina may be of no exaggeration to suggest that the new generation of Thoracic Surgeons rarely and exceptionally have the opportunity to handle such cases. This is because the current trend in triage of lung cancer cases for surgery, at least in developed countries, tends to label such extensive tumours as unsuitable for surgery at presentation. This, coupled with a tendency in the training of Thoracic Surgeons towards "minimalization", shunts the management of this complex tumour (and similar complex types of lung cancer) to the path of unsuitability for surgery and on to the chemo-radiation track. This is an issue of concern and has been referred to by a number of senior Thoracic Surgeons in Europe and beyond.

It needs also to be noted that the cherished and "*sine qua non*" idea of controlled clinical trials to show the validity of surgery in these rare types of lung cancer is unrealistic because of variabilities in the components of this complex cancer and by its sheer paucity in number.

For now, it is important to keep the flame of interest alive and accept that in the hands of an experienced team, this type of surgery can provide a worthwhile long-term survival with an acceptable quality of life in a selected cohort of patients.

Selection of patients for TSP is rigorous and can only be made following full imaging and endoscopic examination with precise mapping of the extent of the tumour and its ramifications.

The local extent must consider that the limiting factors in classical reconstruction of the air way, after excision of the tumour with safety margin, is the length of the lower tracheal involvement. A figure of 2-3 cm has been advocated by a number of experts as the limit of lower tracheal extent of the tumour, after excision of which anastomosis between the remnants of air way structures can be made without tension [1].

Study of surgical anatomical pathology of this complex tumour appears to indicate that in the majority of cases, the involvement of the lateral wall of the trachea is an expansion from the main stem bronchus and is not a total circumferential but partial, thus leading this author in the early and mid 1970s, to introduce a "Bio-Prosthesis" for patch partial circumflex grafting the lower trachea.

The Bio-Prosthesis was made by heavy Marlex mesh and pedicle graft of the pericardium. Marlex mesh (Mm) is a polypropylene and high-density polyethylene (HDPE). It was introduced in early the 1960s and used experimentally and clinically by Beal et al (1963) [2] for tracheal reconstruction.

The addition of the pedicle graft of the Pericardium to Mm prevented air leak through the mesh and allowed incorporation within the host tissues (Moghissi 1975, Moghissi 1979 and Sharpe et al 1996) [3-5]. It proved invaluable for patching partial circumferential tracheal defects after excision. The use of prosthesis of Mm-Pericardium allowed simplification of the technique of operation for TSP in some cases. Standard operation consists of a pneumonectomy, complete circumferential excision of the lower trachea followed by reconstruction by direct anastomosis of residual airway.

In 101 tracheo-bronchoplastic operations where the Mm-Pericardium had been used in 20 patients, there was no graft failure for a period up to 5 years (Moghissi 1979) [6].

In the 1970's there were also other prothesis for tracheal substitution, but they were essentially made of plastic and intended for total circumferential replacement of the trachea [7]. Our bio prothesis is basically for patch grafting.

We believe it is always preferable not to resort to prosthesis. However, if a choice has to be made between inoperability and the use of patch graft of Mm-Pericardium, based on limited experience of some 40 cases, we will have no hesitation to use the prosthesis as shown on Fig. (**4**) and Fig. (**5**).

Rigorous pre-operative work up with evaluation of cardio-pulmonary functions and preparation of patients for such an operation is of prime importance.

Selection of patients for TSP is partially governed by the experience of the surgical team, the stage of the disease, together with the attitude towards the use of Chemo-radiation as induction therapy.

Using TNM stage classification, M+ cases are excluded from selection by all.

Attitudes towards T factor is reasonably clear: Those surgeons who are not prepared to delve into the use of prosthesis of any kind (such as many authors of the most recent publications on the subject) generally consider 2-3 cm of the lower tracheal involvement as a limit beyond which the case would be unsuitable for TSP. We do subscribe to this view.

Nevertheless if 3-4 cm of the lateral wall of the trachea needs to be excised, we believe patch grafting (covering the defect) will provide another 1.5 to 2.5 cm extra length which makes a difference between operability and inoperability. In all cases pre surgical random biopsy or Auto Fluorescence Endoscopy with targeted biopsy is mandatory. Also, it is a good precaution to carry out Frozen Section biopsy at operation.

The N factor and inclusion /exclusion based on it, is also the matter of surgical experience and attitude.

High para-tracheal nodal involvement and even lower N-2 cases pose a problem for investigation of these patients. Clearly it is necessary, or at least desirable, to have information on N factor of TNM before embarking or even selecting a patient for TSP to add mediastinoscopy and Endobronchial Ultra Sound (EBUS) to the list of investigations for more accurate staging of the N factor. However, both these procedures have the disadvantage of creating scar and fibrous tissue in the area of the lower trachea and bifurcation which adversely affects the surgery and pollutes the surgical field. This issue has been raised by authors of recent publications (Weder et al 2016) [1].

We believe each centre should have a protocol based on their experience and use the inclusion/exclusion criteria which best suits their particular setting.

There is evidence that Induction Therapy in selected centres is not attended by a higher overall operative mortality or survival. However, the tangible benefit of such an undertaking is debatable.

The T factor has not been an issue for this author in the complex of TSP as in these cases, the tumour usually expands within 2-3 cm from the bifurcation of the trachea.

Even in limited lower tracheal involvement, we would willingly use our patch graft, if we found it difficult anastomosis between trachea and the top of the residual main stem bronchus after carinal resection en block with the resected lung.

The literature review on TSP confirms our attitude that operative treatment should be considered in centres which can devote time and effort to patients with such complex lung cancer scenarios. This is not the kind of operation which should be undertaken by every Thoracic Surgery Centre.

Post-operative radiotherapy is a worthwhile undertaking, but this is based on observational studies rather than controlled studies for the very reasons given before about the rarity of such cases to provide statistically meaningful information.

It is important to note that: Firstly, the technical and oncological operability is greater for the right compared with left lung [8]. Secondly some of the cases in which the Bio-prosthesis were used in our initial studies [3,4] would have been considered as inoperable without the uses of the prosthesis.

Anaesthesia and ventilation during the operation is a matter of experience of the Surgeon's and anaesthetic teams. We prefer a single lung (the un-affected lung by the cancer) intubation and manipulate the position of the tube with a pre-operative planned protocol with the anaesthetic team.

Alternatively, the double intubation system as used for bifurcation resection as described above. We could rarely select patients who could benefit from TSP when the culprit lung was a "left lung". Basic operative procedure and exposure is an extended postero-lateral thoracotomy through the 4th interspace.

All centres concerned with TSP agree that the selection of patients for the right is easier and commoner than that for the left lung.

We have had no 5 years survival for patients with left TSP. The cases are usually more advanced at presentation and also technically they are more difficult to master. Furthermore, the standard postero-lateral thoracotomy appears not to be the most suitable approach for the left side. "Clamshell" or an antero-lateral thoracotomy with median sternotomy allows better access.

For the commoner right pneumonectomy TSP, the lung is removed *en block* with sleeve of the trachea (full circle) and carina. The remnant airway; that is the left main stem bronchus is then anastomosed with trachea.

Sometimes adjustment should be added if tracheal diameter is too wide to match comfortably the left main bronchus. This can be done by various manoeuvres such as elliptical incision of the bronchus and the tracheal ends. Posterior membranous layer is best anastomosed using a running stitch. The anterior layer is best to be carried out by series of interrupted stitches. We have always wrapped the anastomosis with pedicle graft of pericardium. Small drains on each side of the neck should be soft; silicon and be underwater /sealed and not open to air.

When Mm-pericardial graft patch is to be used to cover the tracheobronchial defect resulted from the excision of the tumour, the lung en block with the bronchus, the carina and the lower trachea is excised. The latter only in its partial circumferential leaving 50% of the opposite lateral and the posterior wall of the trachea in situ. The defect is carefully measured and an appropriately sized Marlex mesh is tailored as a patch to cover the gap. The patch is sewn to the tracheal edges above and to the medial wall of the left main stem bronchus below (Fig. **4** and **5**). Once this is done a graft of the pericardium with its vascular pedicle intact is prepared and sewn over the Marlex mesh. Sometimes an additional intercostals muscle is faced over the pericardium.

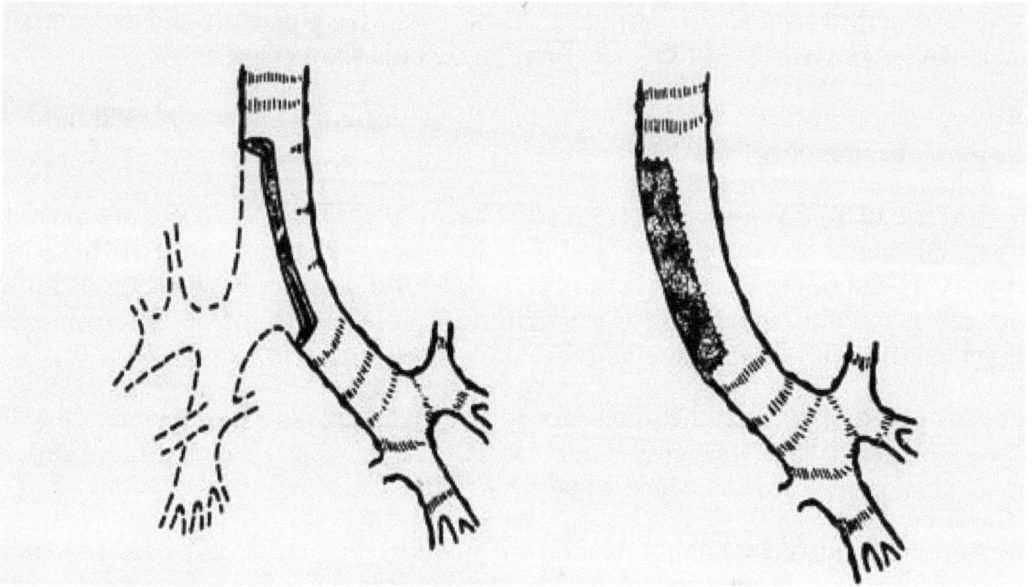

Fig. (4). Use of Marlex mesh prosthesis in excision and reconstruction of limited (2-3 cm lateral wall of the trachea in STP. On the left-hand side is the sketch showing the extent of airway excision (the whole of the right lung, carina and 2 – 3 cm of partial circumferential excision of the lower trachea. On the right-hand side, the sketch shows the coverage of the defect with prothesis of Marlex mesh.

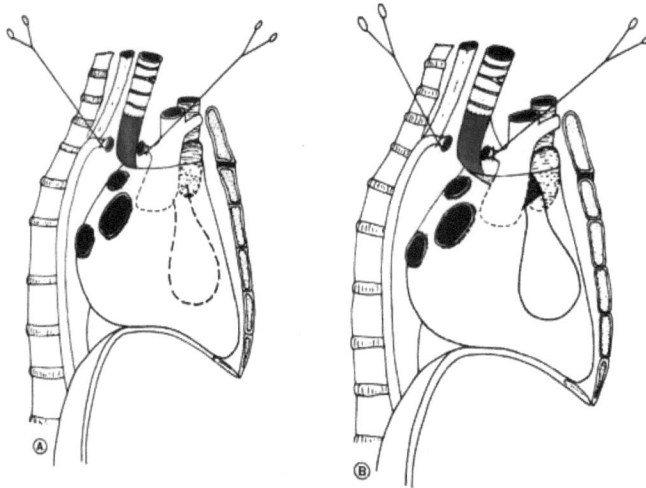

Fig. (5). Use of pedicle graft of pericardium covering (added to) the Marlex mesh as per Fig. (4) (A) A lateral view of the right hemithorax shows the tracheal defect covered over with Marlex mesh. The heavy interrupted line indicates the outline of the pedicle graft of pericardium to be prepared. The azygos vein is ligated and divided. (B) The pericardial patch attached to its pedicule is passed beneath the superior vena cava. It is sutured to the trachea over the Marlex mesh. Taken from Moghissi K, The trachea in Moghissi's Essentials of Thoracic and Cardiac Surgery, Second Edition. Published by Elsevier 2003 page 220.

The role of chemo radiation in TSP is governed by the histology of the tumour and the N status, similar to any lung cancer and the attitude of a particular lung cancer team [9].

At the present time with the advances in laser surgery and Photodynamic Therapy (PDT), we believe:

• Nd YAG laser is a very good tool to debulk the tumour particularly if needed in the lower trachea.
• Post-operative recurrence at the site of the anastomosis can be successfully treated with or without additional external beam radiotherapy by PDT.
• PDT can also be used as an induction therapy to convert an inoperable tumour by reason of its involvement of the carina and the opposite main bronchus (T factor) to operable one by destroying the local extent of the cancer allowing less extensive surgery to be undertaken.

All follow up of such patients should have a defined protocol which uses clinical examination, chest radiography and trachea bronchoscopy using White Light and AFB.

Results of TSP in the world literature varies between 19 and 50, this is entirely a matter of mix of cases primarily N factor. Whilst the N0 in the hands of an experienced centre can be expected to have >40% 5 years survival, N2 cases have generally 0% 5 years expectation of survival. Some histologies such as adenoid cystic carcinomas have far better results. Our current attitude on such tumours, particularly in the case of node involvement is to offer alternative treatment such as PDT. In a small number of 4 cases with the condition and N+ PDT provided over 5 years (actual) survival for all.

Pancoast Tumours (Synonym Superior Sulcus Tumour)

In 1932 Dr Henry Pancoast a radiologist described a cancer located in the apex of the lung with affinity to grow through the chest wall, the neuro-vascular structures of the thoracic inlet, the root of the neck and the brachial plexus. Apart from the general symptoms and signs of lung cancer which may or not be present, the tumour involves upper ribs and the thoracic vertebral column sooner or later causing pain and a complex set of distressing symptoms [1].

In advanced cases the stellate ganglion become affected and patients develop Horner's syndrome consisting of: miosis, anhidrosis, ptosis and enophthalmos.

Many cases are diagnosed in an advanced stage of the disease and the radical operation which is an extensive surgery, needs to be considered. Such an operation requires thorough investigations and definite histological diagnosis.

In the early 1950s the condition was almost always fatal despite efforts at heroic and adventurous surgery [2].

At that time Shaw and Paulson [3, 4] introduced combined radiotherapy and surgery with a 5-year survival of approximately 30%.

Since mid-1990s the tri-modality treatment has been the byword with induction Chemo-radiation followed by extensive surgery. The Paulson's approach, through an elongated postero-lateral thoracotomy, extended to the neck posteriorly, despite its extensive skin incision and soft tissues surgical cutting, provides somewhat restricted exposure, even after excision of the first or more ribs. Alternative anteriorly placed incision affords a better exposure in an overall majority of cases. This incision is basically an L shaped cervicothoracic incision which was proposed by Dartevell in the 1990s [5, 6]. It or its variant is used by many, including this author and provides a less hazardous "en block" excision of all component of the tumour under vision.

The pulmonary upper lobe tumour per se could only be a small component of the totality of the cancer mass. Therefore, the anterior approach is more in line with exposing the most component of the tumour which ideally should be excised "en block" and in total. In practice this means all or part of the following structures:

- Excision of the 1st or any other ribs, with contained and intervening soft tissues.
- Part of the body of the upper thoracic vertebrae often attached or involved to the main body of the cancer.
- Involved nerve roots, lower trunk of the brachial plexus.
- The upper lobe of the lung and mediastinal node clearance.
- Involved parts subclavian vessels with immediate reconstruction.

Plans for reconstruction of the chest wall have to be made pre-operatively in conjunction with plastic and reconstructive surgical team. When a number of ribs are excised the reconstruction requires more than soft tissue remodelling and the use of materials such as Marlex mesh with/or without Methyl methacrylate "stiffeners" will be required.

In terms of indications and contraindications, experience of the surgical team does matter. Nevertheless, there is a general consensus that tumours with distant metastases and those with N3 are not candidates for extensive resection. The vertebral body involvement of >50% is also regarded by many as a major contra indication.

The role of induction therapy and/or addition of chemo-radiation to surgery is also not clear [7-10].

It is the opinion of this author that whilst trimodality treatment for Pancoast tumours is the best which can be offered to patients, it is nevertheless mandatory that, one should as a surgeon use all possible methods of investigation to be able to prognosticate on length of survival as well as the quality of survival of the patient before delving into an extensive surgery.

The copious literature on the Pancoast is not clear about the many aspects of prognostication. This is partly due to the fact that Pancoast is a relatively rare tumour and making relevance purely on statistical evidence with so many variable factors from case to case make the reliance to statistic much harder.

The 5 years survival using trimodality treatment is reported to be between 40-50% of operated cases (N0- N1) [11, 12].

Clearly Pancoast tumours should not be dealt with by every Thoracic Surgical Centre but by designated centres with a multi-disciplinary team dedicated to treating such complex cancers and operations which enable availability of resources and continuing experience (See Chapter 16 Lung Cancer Centre)

Lung Cancer Invading the Chest Wall

It is a general agreement that survival of patients with lung cancer, with involvement of the chest wall after resection, is essentially dependent on two principal factors, namely; the nodal status and the completeness of the resection. This has been observed by many groups since the late 1960s and 1970s. It then became a fact and "cast in iron" since the 1990's. Nevertheless, firstly on critical analysis, and a personal study of this author, it has become clear that, chest wall involvement in terms of ribs, intercostals muscles and other soft tissues outside the ribs is almost always a local extension and invasion by the cancer, whereas involvement of the parietal pleura and endo-thoracic fascia are often an expression of a wider spread infiltration. Secondly, and more importantly from the surgical/ technical stand point, the chest wall involvement by the cancer should be thought as two entities:

1. Ribs, intercostal muscles and the related soft tissue external to the ribs.
2. Parietal pleura and endothoracic fascia, internal to ribs

This is because, purely from the technical aspect, surgery for lung cancer invading the chest wall should take account of the architecture of the thorax and the functional anatomy of bones; in this case, the ribs.

Ribs not only maintain the integrity of the chest morphology but are also responsible for harmonious breathing in which there is symmetry between the two sides of the chest in the two phases of ventilation (inspiration and expiration). Surgical removal of segments of a number of ribs, which can be the case in chest wall excision on one side, will disturb symmetrical movements of the chest (inflation and deflation) and will create paradoxical movement of the chest in inspiratory and expiratory phases of ventilation and disturb gas exchange as its consequence.

Clearly therefore, whilst oncologically the chest wall invasion by cancer, irrespective of its depth, is classified as T3, surgically speaking the group with ribs and more outward invasion require a totally different surgical tactic.

Chest wall invasion by lung cancer is uncommon, with a prevalence of less than 10% of cases, of which about 60% (6% overall) have rib and extra-costal soft tissue involvement.

The surgical management of local neoplastic involvement of the non-bony chest wall is simple and no different than any other resectional surgery for lung cancer, the extent of which is governed by oncological requirements.

Stripping or excising the parietal pleura and the layer of endothoracic fascia do not pose any technical challenges.

Since 1986 we, and those trained in laser surgery, use the laser (Nd YAG) as a surgical cutting and coagulating device which offers added safety in destroying malignant cells at the margin of excision.

The decision regarding Induction Therapy (IT) in these cases is also similar to other lung cancer with N+ management.

Cases in which the bony chest wall is involved by cancer deserve specific description in this chapter, as almost 50% of such patients require excision of 3-4 (on average) ribs (Fig. **6**). All of these patients require reconstruction of the chest wall and around 60% require a prosthetic device.

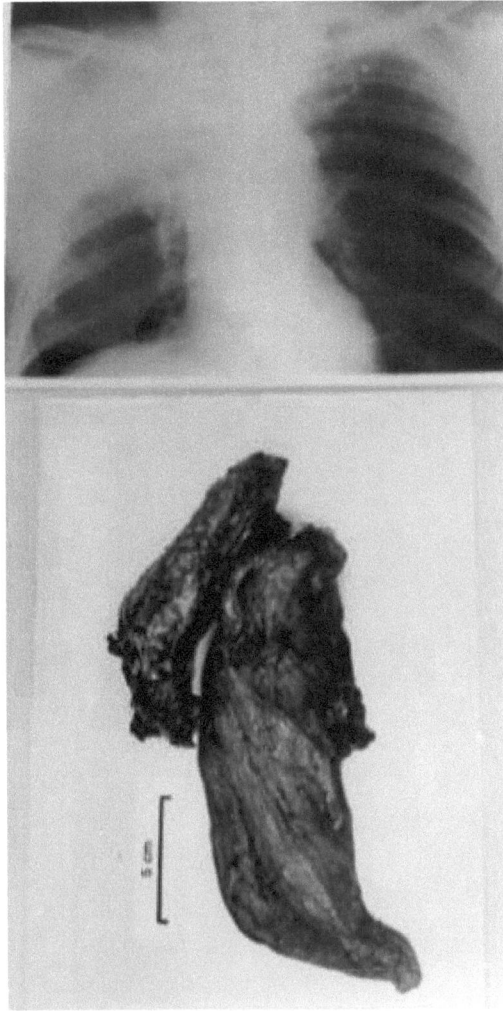

Fig. (6). Above chest radiograph of a patient with right lung cancer and involvement of chest wall. Below a pneumonectomy together with the portion of 3 ribs, in this case there was no necessity to reconstruct the chest wall with the use of prosthesis.

This seems to accord with the data of 58 patients treated by Shah *et al.*, (1999), in which near 50% had a different length of between 3-5 ribs excision (together with their soft tissues). Interestingly 50% (29 amongst 58 patients) required reconstruction with Marlex mesh or composite prosthesis of Marlex –methyl methacrylate.

Our prosthesis has been Marlex mesh covered muscles and soft tissue imported from the extra thoracic component. In some such cases, we have planned the operation in cooperation with a plastic and reconstructive surgeon's team. Wide margin is the rule of this type of cancer surgery as infiltration in the muscular tissue is difficult to evaluate without a frozen section, which in these cases can be so tedious as to become impractical.

We do not subscribe to the view of routine post-operative radiotherapy. A recent Editorial by Suzuki and colleagues seems to use of Post-operative Radio Therapy (PORT).

A multidisciplinary team approach is an important consideration and in the era of trends in shortening the duration of postgraduate training, early involvement of oncologists and plastic and reconstructive surgeons is imperative.

The 5-year survival of patients undergoing lung cancer with chest wall resection operation is recorded to be between 25-40% for N0 cases. In many series, there is no 5 years' survival for the T3-N2 cases.

CONCLUSION

Chapter 9 is a compound collection of a variety of complicated types of operations with a defined indication within the repartee of thoracic surgery. It describes broncho plastic operations, tracheal plastic after extensive pulmonary resection/(STP), Pancoast tumour and invasion of chest wall locally by lung cancer.

There has been little variation in the methods used in these operations and because of the relative rarity of each component of the chapter (operations), most of the recent publications are of retrospective nature.

Whilst VAT is used routinely in a range of relatively simple lung cancer operations, its role in complicated operations can only be supportive and subsidiary for the procedures described in this chapter.

Also, the principle of conventional operations should and is the way of teaching to those who aspire to become a Thoracic Surgeon. In 21st Century VATS and Classical Conventional Surgery must be within the repertoire of Thoracic Surgeons; they are not competitive but complementary.

FURTHER READING

Further Reading for Bronchoplastic Operation

Kara M, Dizbay Sak S, Orhan D *et al.* Proximal bronchial extension with special reference to tumor localization in non-small cell lung cancer. Eur J Cardiothorac Surg 2001;**20**:350–355.

"Tumors often have extensive microscopic proximal extension in excess of the apparent gross tumor. This is more common for central tumors (30.3% of the central tumors had microscopic tumor extending past the grossly visible tumor in one study."

Moghissi K. Les procedes broncho plastiques; A propos de 101 casconsecutifs Chirurgie 1979;105:460-467

Maygarden Susan J, Detterbeck F C &Funkhouse W K

Bronchial Margin in Lung Cancer Specimens: Utility of Frozen Section and cross evaluation Modern Pathology 2004; 17:1080–1086

"Pathology reports for all lobectomy and pneumonectomy specimens at UNC Hospitals between 1991 and 2000 (n=405) were reviewed for correlation between frozen section and final bronchial margin, gross distance between tumor and margin and tumor type. Frozen section was performed in 268 cases (66%). A total of 243 were true negatives (90.6%), 16 (6.0%) were true positives, four (1.5%) were false positives and five (1.9%) were false negatives. The site of tumor in true-positive cases was mucosal (11), submucosal (three), lymphatics (one)"

Yildizeli B, Fadel E, Mussot S, Fabre Dm Chaaigner O and

Dartevelle P. Morbidity, Mortality and long term survival after sleeve lobectomy for non-small cell lung cancer. **EJCTS**, 2007; 31: 95–102, https://doi.org/10.1016/j.ejcts.2006.10.031

"The presence of microscopic deposits of tumour cells at the bronchial resection margin (BRM) may adversely affect the prognosis of patients. Residual tumour cells were identified at the BRM in 40 (5.4%) of 735patients who had been operated on for non-small cell lung carcinoma (NSCLC)."

Further Reading for Tracheal Sleeve Pneumonectomy

de Perrot M, Shields TW, LoCicero J, *et al.* Tracheal Sleeve Pneumonectomy. In: Shields TW, LoCicero J, Reed CE, *et al.* editors. General Thoracic Surgery. 7th Edition. Ambler: Lippincott Williams & Wilkins, 2009.

Dartevelle P, Macchiarini P. Techniques of pneumonectomy. Sleeve pneumonectomy. Chest Surg Clin N Am 1999;9:407-17.

Dartevelle PG, Macchiarini P, Chapelier AR. 1986: Tracheal sleeve pneumonectomy for bronchogenic carcinoma: report of 55 cases. Updated in 1995. Ann Thorac Surg 1995;60:1854-5] doi: 10.21037/shc.2017.08.11.

Grillo HC. Surgery of the trachea and bronchi. London: BC Decker Inc., 2004

Grillo HC. Carinal reconstruction. Ann Thorac Surg 1982;34:356-73. Weder W, Inci I. Carinal resection and sleeve pneumonectomy. J Thorac Dis 2016;8:S882-S888.

Perelman MI, Koroleva NS. Primary tumors of the trachea. In: Grillo HC, Eschapasse H. editors. Major challenges. Philadelphia, PA: Saunders, 1987:91-106.]

Porhanov VA, Poliakov IS, Selvaschuk AP, *et al.* Indications and results of sleeve carinal resection. Eur J Cardiothorac Surg 2002;22:685-94. 10.1016/S1010-7940(02)00523-7.

Further Reading for Lung Cancer Invading the Chest Wall

Downey RJ, Martini N, Rusch VW, Bains MS, Korst RJ, Ginsberg RJ.

Extent of chest wall invasion and survival in patients with lung cancer. Ann Thorac Surg. 1999;68:188-93.

"Survival of patients with lung cancer invading the chest wall after resection with curative intent is highly dependent on the extent of nodal involvement and the completeness of resection, and much less so on the depth of chest wall invasion ...."

Lanuti M. Surgical Management of Lung Cancer involving the Chest Wall

Thorac Surg Clin. 2017; 2:195-199. doi: 10.1016/j.thorsurg.2017.01.013.

Suzuki M, Mori T, Shiraishi K, Ikeda K, Masuda Y, Matsubara E, Shirakami C, Hinokuma H. What is the optimal adjuvant therapy for T3N0 lung cancer invading the chest wall? Editorial J Thoracic Disease, 2017; 9: 4233-4235

CONSENT FOR PUBLICATION

Not applicable.

CONFLICT OF INTEREST

The author declares that there is no conflict of interest in this chapter.

ACKNOWLEDGEMENTS

The author would like thank Kate Dixon, Janet Melvin, and Sally Gibbins.

REFERENCES FOR TSP

[1]   Weder W, Inci I. Carinal resection and sleeve pneumonectomy. J Thorac Dis 2016; 8: S882-8.

[2]   Beall AC, Harrington OB, Greenberg SD, *et al.* Circumferential replacement of thoracic trachea with marlex mesh. JAMA 1963; 183: 1082-4.
[http://dx.doi.org/10.1001/jama.1963.63700130001011]

[3]   Moghissi K. Tracheal reconstruction with a prosthesis of marlex mesh and pericardium. J Thorac Cardiovasc Surg 1975; 69: 499-506.

[4]   Moghissi K. Reconstruction of trachea with Marlex mesh pericardium following circumferential excision. J R Coll Surg Edinb 1975 ; 20(5): 327-1.

[5]   Sharpe DA, Moghissi K. Tracheal resection and reconstruction: A repot of 82 patients. Eur J Cardiothorac Surg 1996; 10(12): 1040-5.

[6]   Moghissi K. Les procedes broncho plastiques; A propos de 101 casconsecutifs. Chirurgie 1979; 105: 460-7.

[7]   Neville WE, Bolanowski PJ, Soltanzadeh H. Prosthetic reconstruction of the trachea and carina. J Thorac Cardiovasc Surg 1976; 72: 525-38.

[8]   Galetta D, Spaggiarri L. Early and long-term results of tracheal sleeve pneumonectomy for lung cancer after induction therapy. Ann Thoracic Surgery 2018; 105: 1017-23.

[9]   Banki F, Wood DE. Techniques of performing left carinal pneumonectomy. Oper Tech Thorac Cardiovasc Surg 2007; 12: 194-209.

REFERENCES FOR PANCOAST TUMOUR

[1]   Pancoast HK, Inci I. Superior pulmonary sulcus tumor. Tumor characterized by pain, Horner's syndrome, destruction of bone and atrophy of hand muscles. JAMA 1932; 99: 1391-96.

[2]   Chardack WM, Maccallum JD, *et al.* Pancoast syndrome due to bronchiogenic carcinoma: successful surgical removal and postoperative irradiation; a case report. J Thorac Surg 1953; 25: 402-12.

[3]   Shaw RR, Paulson DL, Kee JL. Treatment of superior sulcus tumor by irradiation followed by resection. Ann Surg 1961; 154: 29-40.

[4]   Paulson DL. Carcinomas in the superior pulmonary sulcus. J Thorac Cardiovasc Surg 1975; 70: 1095-104.

[5]   Dartevelle PG, Chapelier AR, Macchiarini P, *et al.* Anterior transcervical-thoracic approach for radical resection of lung tumors invading the thoracic inlet. J Thorac Cardiovasc Surg 1993; 105: 1025-34.

[6]   Dartevelle PG. Herbert Sloan Lecture. Extended operations for the treatment of lung cancer. Ann ThoracSurg 1997; 63: 12-9.

[7]   Shahian DM, Neptune WB, Ellis FH. Pancoast tumors: improved survival with preoperative and postoperative radiotherapy. Ann Thorac Surg 1987; 43: 32-8.

[8]   Gandhi S, Walsh GL, Komaki R, *et al.* A multidisciplinary surgical approach to superior sulcus tumors with vertebral invasion. Ann Thorac Surg 1999; 68: 1778-84; discussion 1784 Rusch VW. Management of Pancoast tumours. Lancet Oncol 2006;7:997-1005.

[9]   Rusch VW, Giroux DJ, Kraut MJ, *et al.* Induction chemoradiation and surgical resection for superior sulcus non-small-cell lung carcinomas: long-term results of Southwest Oncology Group Trial 9416 (Intergroup Trial 0160). J Clin Oncol 2007; 25: 313-8.

[10]   Kwong KF, Edelman MJ, Suntharalingam M, *et al.* High-dose radiotherapy in trimodality treatment of Pancoast tumors results in high pathologic complete response rates and excellent long-term survival. J Thorac Cardiovasc Surg 2005; 129: 1250-7.

[11]   Collaud S, Waddell TK, Yasufuku K, *et al.* Long-term outcome after en bloc resection of non-smal--cell lung cancer invading the pulmonary sulcus and spine. J Thorac Oncol 2013; 8: 1538-44.

[12]   Marulli G, Battistella L. Mammana, Calabrese F and Rea F.Superior sulcus tumors (Pancoast tumors).Ann Transl Med. 2016 Jun; 4(12): 239.
        [http://dx.doi.org/10.21037/atm.2016.06.16]

CHAPTER 10

Video-Assisted Thoracoscopic Surgery

Mahmoud Loubani[1,*] and **Marcello Migliore**[2,*]

[1] *Hull University Teaching Hospitals NHS Trust, Hull, UK*

[2] *Thoracic Surgery, Department of Surgery and Medical Specialties, Policlinico University Hospital, University of Catania, Catania, Italy*

Abstract: (Section 1) Video-Assisted Thoracoscopic Surgery has evolved significantly over the last twenty years and is increasingly becoming the preferred method for lung resection. It has and continues to be refined and improved with an increasing body of evidence to support it over open surgery.

(Section 2) In this chapter, the author defines and briefly describes Mini-Uniportal VATS (Uni-VATS).

The introduction of Video-assisted thoracic surgery (VATS) *via* a short (Mini) Single skin incision and a port (trocar) provides an alternative to already established access to the thoracic cavity and a novel surgical approach to pulmonary operations.

There has been a debate about the definition of "Uni- VATS" and how short in extent characterizes the adjective "mini"? Many surgeons define "uniportal" as a VATS operation performed through an incision of 4-8 cm, others believe that when the skin exceeds 2 cm the name should be mini-thoracotomy. We define Uni-VATS an operation in which the operation in the chest is performed when a port (trocar) is introduced *via* a minimal skin incision of 2-3 cm, whereas when a larger incision is made, the operation should be called single–incision-video assisted-mini thoracotomy.

Uni- VATS for lung cancer has been successfully used to perform a range of pulmonary operations from wedge excision to pneumonectomy and more sophisticated procedures. Double lumen tube and controlled ventilation is the preferred method to carry out Uni-VATS, but more recently, the feasibility of non-intubated normal breathing method has also been explored in selected patients undergoing major lung resection. Although the first uniportal lobectomy was performed almost 10 years ago, there have only been a few retrospective comparative studies and only one prospective randomized trial between single-port and multi-port lobectomy.

[*] **Corresponding authors Mahmoud Loubani and Marcello Migliore:** Hull University Teaching Hospitals NHS Trust, UK and Thoracic Surgery, Department of surgery and medical specialties, Policlinico University Hospital, University of Catania, Catania, Italy;
E-mails: Mahmoud.loubani@hey.nhs.uk and mmiglior@hotmail.com

Keyvan Moghissi, Jack Kastelik, Philip Barber & Peyman Sardari Nia (Eds.)

With the advance in technology and imaging devices matched by experience and surgical expertise, one may speculate that within a decade uniportal computer-assisted, instrument-controlled surgery will open up a new horizon, allowing Uni- VATS to become a routine practice for surgical treatment of lung cancer.

Keywords: Lung cancer, Minimally invasive thoracic surgery, Minimal incision, NSCLC, Single port, Single trocar, Uniportal, VATS, Video-Assisted Thoracoscopic Surgery.

SECTION 1

VIDEO-ASSISTED THORACOSCOPIC SURGERY (BY MAHMOUD LOUBANI)

INTRODUCTION

Video-Assisted Thoracoscopic Surgery (VATS) was first introduced in the early twentieth century and has since become the main access for Thoracic Surgeons. The first clinical application of VATS was reported in 1910 when a cystoscope was introduced into the chest for examination of the pleural cavity [1]. The equipment and technical ability has since become more specific for Thoracic Surgery especially with the introduction of the video and now more recently 3-dimensional video capabilities. Surgery rates in England and Wales continue to increase for Non-small Cell Lung Cancer (NSCLC) with a further increase from 17.5% in 2016 to 18.4% in 2017 as seen in the National Lung Cancer Outcomes [2]. This has been accompanied by an increase in the uptake of the VATS approach for the treatment of lung cancer and reported in the UK to account for over 30% in 2015 [3]. There is however variability between different hospitals and this is also reflected in results for the United States. Of 55,972 cancer lobectomies performed at 905 hospitals, 17,072 (30.5%) were VATS. Crude hospital VATS use varied widely between 4.4% to 42.3% even after case-mix adjustment [4]. This is multifactorial relating to the availability of expertise and suitability of patients but also due to the lack of Level 1 evidence which might be provided by the multicenter randomized Violet Trial [5] comparing one-year outcomes of VATS versus Open Surgery. Patients must have disease suitable for resection by both VATS and open surgery, to be considered eligible. It excludes patients who have a previous malignancy that influences life expectancy, in whom robotic surgery is planned or those having pneumonectomy or non-anatomic resection.

THE VATS INCISIONS

Three Ports VATS

This is the first described and most popular access for lobectomy and has been in practice for more than 20 years [6]. It involves the triangulation of a camera port at the apex of an inverted triangle in the 7th or 8th intercostal space at the anterior axillary line. The posterior port is placed near the position of the end of a thoracotomy incision anterior to the scapula and an anterior utility port in the 4th or 5th intercostal space just lateral to the pectoralis muscle, 4th for an upper lobe and 5th for a lower lobe. The utility port normally measures 3-5 cms and serves to allow the delivery of the lobe following completion of the resection and takes advantage of the wider intercostal space anteriorly. This approach is technically easy to learn and allows excellent exposure and access to all the hilar vessels and to complete lymph node dissection. This approach doesn't involve rib spreading, reducing the pain involved in a full thoracotomy, but still has the drawback of three separate incisions in three different intercostal spaces with potential acute or chronic pain in any of these spaces.

The order of the incisions is somewhat debatable with proponents of the utility port first suggesting that performing this first allows the accurate placement of the other two ports especially the camera port which could make a significant difference to the conduct of the operation. On the other hand, performing the utility port first could commit the surgeon to an anterior thoracotomy should the case be unsuitable for a thoracoscopic approach. Inserting the Camera port first allows inspection of the pleural space for significant adhesions or unexpected tumors which will have an impact on the conduct of the operation. This still allows a posterolateral thoracotomy to be performed if required which is the normal open approach for a lobectomy. However, as surgeons become more experienced with the anterior VATS approach an anterior thoracotomy becomes the incision of choice to approach hilar structures in the same manner and order.

Two Port VATS

In this approach, a utility incision is used accompanied by a lower camera port but no posterior incision is performed. Two-port VATS has shown to reduce operative and postoperative pleural drainage as well as extubation time and postoperative hospitalization compared with three-port VATS. This has been shown to be safe and feasible [7]. However, this study and others have not demonstrated a significant reduction of the trauma to the chest wall and potential acute and chronic pain. The two-port approach has formed the base for further evolution into a uniportal incision.

Uniportal VATS

The evolution of thoracoscopic surgery resulted in the advent of a uniportal approach for lobectomy and lung resections. The concept of Uniportal VATS was first described for simpler procedures over a decade ago [8, 9] before being used to perform lobectomies for lung cancer with a good early result [10, 11]. This although technically more challenging potentially reduces the problem encountered with the three ports by reducing the trauma to the chest wall and the pain from three different incisions although the evidence is not fully elucidated. The normal approach is to use the utility incision of the three-port approach as the only incision and use it for the thoracoscopic video camera as well as all the instrumentation and ultimately retrieval of the resected lung. A 30 degrees camera is essential for this approach to allow visualization of hilar structures during the dissection.

ROBOTIC ASSISTED SURGERY

This is the latest technological advance in lung resection surgery which was first reported in 2002 [12] and is continuously evolving. Affordability of robots in different hospitals and sharing this resource with other surgical specialties has contributed to its availability allowing for widening popularity for the treatment of early-stage non-small cell lung cancer (NSCLC) [12]. The advantages of this approach include a magnified three-dimensional (3D) view and the endo-wrist technology that reproduce the natural movements of a surgeon's hand [14 - 16]. The robotic approach requires 4 incisions which might be seen as a step backward from the previous advances reducing the number of incisions required to perform the resection. However, proponents counteract this argument by the fact that the fulcrum of the instruments is not at the chest wall resulting in a reduction of the pain caused by pressure on intercostal nerves. Nonetheless, with robotic surgery, the tactile sensation is lost as the surgeon operates from the console and is not touching the patient or the instruments.

CONVERSION TO THORACOTOMY

Intraoperative conversion from VATS to an open approach can be prohibitive to take up VATS procedures in borderline cases and is reported to range from 5% to 23% with almost 50% of the conversions performed as an emergency [17 - 19]. Most of the evidence comes from retrospective series describing the outcomes related to conversions having greater perioperative morbidity compared to successful VATS completion [17] while others show similar outcomes [20]. A study examining 1227 lobectomy patients [21] reported that 42% were completed by VATS with a 7% conversion rate, while 51% were performed *via* planned thoracotomy. Complications in the postoperative period were significantly more frequent in the conversion group 46% versus 23% in the VATS group (p<0.001), but similar to the open group (42%, p=0.56). The causes of conversion were due to vascular causes in 25% of the cases and 9% for lymph nodes and the major cause accounting for 64% of the cases was for anatomical reasons such as adhesions and tumor size. The conversion rate for VATS lobectomy dropped from 28% to 11% over the study period which is a natural reduction with increasing experience.

SECTION 2

MINI SINGLE SKIN INCISION VIDEO-ASSISTED THORACIC SURGERY (UNIPORTAL –VATS) FOR LUNG CANCER OPERATIONS (BY MARCELLO MIGLIORE)

INTRODUCTION

Since the emergence of VATS 30 years ago and its universal expansion, there has been a dramatic change in thoracic surgical practice in general and in pulmonary resection more specifically. Several advantages of VATS compared with standard access to the chest have been amply documented in the literature. Reduced pain postoperatively, minimal scar and shorter postoperative recovery in VATS compared with the traditional have been highlighted in all studies. Nevertheless, a further step has been the introduction 20 years ago of VATS performed through a port (trocar) inserted *via* a minimal skin incision [1 - 3].

Definition

There appears to be no universally accepted definition for Uni-VATS. This is illustrated in Table **1**. Basically, all these names describe the same method to operate the chest where the surgeon works *via* a minimal skin incision and through a very small trocar/port using instruments that are separated from the optic. The length and the extent of the skin incision have been the subject of discussions and debates.

Table 1. Different names for the same mini single skin incision VATS technique.

Single access
Single trocar
Single port
One port
Uniportal

Some surgeons call uniportal an operation performed through an incision of 4-8 cm (Fig. **1**), others believe that when a skin incision is larger than 2 cm, the procedure should be called VATS mini-thoracotomy. In the year 2000, a careful clarification about the various types of VATS techniques has been published [4], and in 2016, there was another endeavor to define uniportal VATS [5]. Although many surgeons believe that the rib retractor should not be used when uniportal VATS is used, in daily practice, it is sometimes necessary to enlarge the space in order to retrieve the resected specimen to avoid the increase in the size of the skin incision.

Unfortunately, the recently published "European Society of Thoracic Surgeons Consensus Report on uniportal video-assisted thoracic surgery lobectomy" provides no real clarification and adds confusion to already confused terminology [6]. It follows that, the term uniportal VATS is still imprecise and subject to variation and that in essence there is no consensus regarding the definition, but the ambiguous word "uniportal" is arousing enthusiasm within the population of thoracic surgeons, and many journals are happy to publish papers with the word uniportal in the title.

Short History

On the 20th of June 2019, the author searched the Google Scholar database, the word uniportal appears in 598 papers. According to the Scopus database, the increase of papers with the word uniportal in the title is evident. For the first time the word uniportal appeared in the medical literature in 1991 for a "uniportal arthroscopic microdiscectomy and decompression" [7]. In thoracic surgery, the first experience on video-assisted thoracic surgery through a single port was presented in abstract form in 2000 at the annual congress of the SAGES in Atlanta- USA and at the VIII Congress of the European Society of thoracic surgery in London. Then full-length papers were published in 2000, 2001, 2002 and 2003 (1-4). At that time, the technique had been used for: lung biopsy and decortications, haemothorax, pneumothorax, sympathectomy, empyema, as well s staging lung cancer, biopsy of the lung and mediastinal nodes and treatment of pleural effusion. But the technique became known worldwide only when an inferior lobectomy has been performed through a 5 cm skin incision [8]. Currently, many centres are adopting the method. It is also of note that Respiratory Physicians are adopting Thoracoscopy/and Video thoracoscopy to become interventionists in line with their colleagues in cardiology to become Interventional Respiratory Physicians.

Instrumentations

When the skin incision is 2 cm the trocar to be used must be flexible and have a diameter of 15–20 mm to allow the simultaneous introduction of the optic and endoscopic dedicated devices including a light source, an optic, an endocamera, two monitors, and an electrosurgical unit. The optic, which has a diameter ranging from 5 to 10 mm, is chosen based on the surgeon's preference. We prefer the 0° or 30° angle scope. Endoscopic instruments are available from several manufacturers and should be no longer than 20 cm. Atraumatic graspers, dissecting tampon, suction and irrigating system, 5-mm endoscopic clip appliers, and the 5-mm ultracision are useful for simultaneous coagulation and cutting of vessels smaller than 7 mm. In some circumstances, standard open instruments can be used. The instrumentation for a thoracotomy in an emergency setting must always be ready at hand.

Anesthesia for Uniportal VATS

Double lumen tube is the preferred method to perform uniportal VATS, and clearly intubated thoracic surgery offers many advantages to the patient. Zhao *et al.* [9] have shown that one-lung ventilation (OLV) technique is fundamental in minimally invasive thoracic surgery. This can be achieved *via* a double-lumen endotracheal tube or placing a bronchial blocker through a single-lumen endotracheal tube [9]. More recently, non-intubated thoracic surgery has been also used in selected patients for major lung resection [10]. The so-called "Awake Surgery" has been described for patients not suitable for general anesthetic [9]. Moreover, patients have a significantly reduced incidence of postoperative respiratory complications, such as pneumonia and ARDS. Awake thoracic surgery may also reduce stress hormone response, attenuate the impact on the immune system, and lower the effects of postoperative lymphocyte response [11].

Indications for Uniportal VATS in NSCLC

Notwithstanding the lack of universal agreement on the definition of Uniportal - VATS, we believe a range of pulmonary operation can safely be performed using single skin incision ranging from 2 or 8 cm without a need for an additional one. This however relies largely on the availability and usage of appropriate" tools" such as the harmonic scalpel which permits to safely secure blood vessels of all calibers (*e.g* large pulmonary vessels) without the need for additional "tie". Currently, the indications for uniportal VATS for NSCLC are shown in Table **2**.

Table 2. Reported Uniportal VATS procedure for SNCLC.

| Pleural biopsy |
| Pleurectomy |
| Lymphadenectomy |

(Table 2) cont.....

Wedge resection
Segmentectomy
Lobectomy
Pneumonectomy
Sleeve resection

UNIPORTAL VATS FOR LUNG CANCER

Initially, uniportal VATS for lung cancer was performed mainly for staging lung cancer and to treat malignant pleural effusion. For staging procedure, a 2 cm skin incision and a flexible trocar (port) were used to obtain mediastinal node and lung biopsy samples [1 - 3,]. After the introduction of sophisticated coagulation device and dedicated staplers, it was possible to perform major lung resection through a small port. Although the first lobectomy through a small (5cm skin incision) VATS was performed (8), there have been few retrospective comparative studies between single-port and multi-port lobectomy and only one prospective randomized trial (Table **3**).

Table 3. (Evidence table) Uniportal VATS for lung cancer. * the only prospective study.

Author /year	Reference number	Type of operation	N° patients	Size of skin incision	Main message
Zhu *et al.* 2015	13	lobectomy	33 *vs* 49	3.5-4.5	No significant difference
Gonzales rivas /2011	8	Lobectomy	1	5	feasible
Ersen /2018	14	Lobectomy	21 *vs* 81	3.5–4.5	Longer operative time
Hirai/2016	18	Lobectomy	84	4.2 mean	Longer operative time
Ugalde/2019	15	Lobectomy	274 *vs* 448	3-8	No difference
Perna / 2016 *	16	Lobectomy	51 *vs* 55	4-5	No advantages

Zhu *et al.* [13] have shown, in a retrospective comparative study between single-port and triple-port lobectomy, that no significant differences in total mediastinal lymph node harvest intraoperative blood loss, chest drainage duration, postoperative hospital stay, and complications between the two groups ($P>0.05$). In that study, operative time of single-port group was significantly longer than that of the triple-port group (181.3 ± 27.5 *vs*. 149.5 ± 30.9 min, $P<0.05$), but the postoperative pain was less in the single-port group (3.6 ± 0.7 *vs*. 5.5 ± 1.0, $P<0.05$).

Ersen *et al.* [14] performed a comparative study between uniportal and multi portal VATS on 102 patients. A significant difference was found in the duration of chest tube drainage, pain visual analog scale score, length of hospital stay, perioperative blood loss, amount of postoperative drainage, number of harvested lymph nodes or complication rate. However, operative time was shorter (189 min *vs.* 256 min, p < 0.005) in the multiport group than in the uniportal group.

Bourdages-Pageau *et al.* [15] in a comparative study between two groups of 274 Uni-VATS and 448 multi-VATS showed that Uni-VATS group was associated with fewer pneumonia (P= 0.012), as well as decreased intraoperative bleeding (P< 0.001), faster surgery (P< 0.001), shorter duration of chest tube drainage (P= 0.001), and shorter hospital stay (P< 0.001).

The only one randomized trial [16] comparing 51 patients undergoing Uni-VATS with 55 patients who had M-VATS showed no superiority of the Uni-VATS group over-M-VATS in respect of postoperative pain, length of hospital stay, duration of chest tube drainage, or postoperative complications.

Moreover, a systematic review [17] and meta-analysis showed no benefits of U-VATS with regards to the duration of surgery, intraoperative bleeding, and conversion to thoracotomy. In the propensity-matched data, no benefit associated with U-VATS lobectomy was identified.

In the first Japanese experience, Hirai *et al.* [18] have shown in 84 stage I lung cancer patients, undergoing Uni-VATS lobectomy, a mean operative time of 175 ± 21 min, operative blood loss of 92 ± 18 mL, and duration of drain placement 1.9 ± 0.6 days. The duration of the postoperative hospital stay was 7.1 ± 1.7 days. Only 2 patients (2.4%) were converted into open thoracotomy.

Although it is unclear as to how the entire lung can be withdrawn through a single 4 cm skin incision of Uni- VATS, this appears to be feasible provided that skin incision can be extended to 6-7 cm, as reported by Halazeroglu [19]. Uniportal VATS can also be used to treat complications after major lung resection such as empyema post pneumonectomy [20, 21]. There are very few publications concerned with the use of 5cm uniportal VATS to perform more sophisticated operations such as sleeve arterial and bronchial resection [22].

Modification of the Uniportal VATS

Modification of uniportal technique has also been recently reported. Wang *et al.* [23] have shown a thoracic needled suspending device which was useful to reduce operation time 120.2 ± 40.32 min versus the control group (P<0.05). Moreover, new devices, such as an articulated arm to hold the camera, have been introduced to increase ergonomics and optimization of surgical resources [24].

Uniportal VATS lobectomy has been also performed *via* the subxiphoid approach [25, 26]. Song *et al.* [26] showed that the average pain scores 8 hours, day 1, 2 and 3 after surgery, as well as the day before discharge, were 2.39±0.99, 2.06±0.85, 1.68±0.87, 1.29±0.78, and 0.48±0.51, respectively, which were significantly lower than those in the control group (standard intercostal uniportal VATS).

Uniportal robotic surgery is now a reality as it has been described its use for mediastinal masses in 14 patients as a safe and feasible procedure, and an uniportal subxiphoid port has been applied to robotic pulmonary lobectomies with success [27, 28]. The authors concluded that more complex procedures could be done with the advent of new uniportal technology in the near future.

A WORD OF CAUTION

One of the problems with VATS and uniportal VATS is the intraoperative localization of small pulmonary nodules or ground-glass opacity [29 - 32]. Ujiie *et al.* [33] showed that computed tomography-guided percutaneous indocyanine green injection and intraoperative near-infrared localization of small nodules are safe and feasible with 90% success rate (18 of 20 patients).

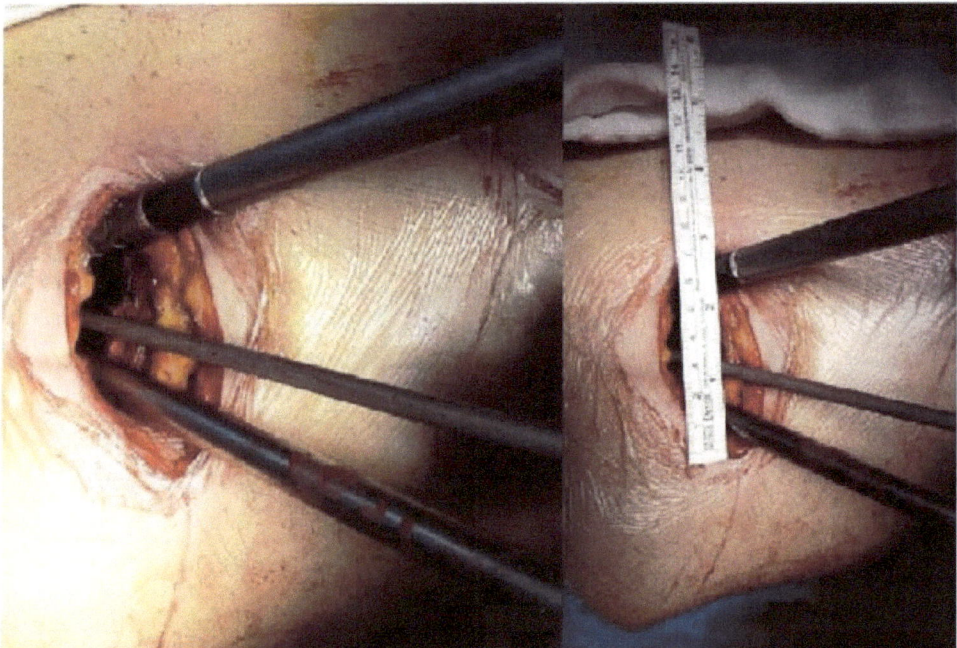

Fig (1). Single skin incision of 7 cm in a 195 cm height patient. Should this incision be considered uniportal or it is a single incision video-assisted mini-thoracotomy?

Nevertheless, Augustin and Smith [34] affirm the lack of scientific evidence for the superiority of one minimally invasive approach over the other and these situations reflect a gut feeling rather than solid arguments in favor of uniportal VATS. Furthermore, Hirai *et al.* [35] report that uniportal VATS involves a restricted ability to manipulate surgical instruments and therefore careful consideration of the surgical indications for U-VATS should depend on the tumor characteristics and patient's physical condition. Nevertheless, although the short-term outcomes of U-VATS are good, the oncological validity of U-VATS remains unclear, even for early-stage lung cancer. Nowadays, it is hard to suggest one VATS technique as the preferred method to perform major lung resection for lung cancer. For the same reasons, the surgeon should choose the VATS method that suits best [36, 37].

THE FUTURE

It is important to emphasize the primary purpose and the principle of lung cancer surgery demand: complete removal of cancer and precancerous component, clearance of relevant lymph nodes and cancer-free bronchial section. The thoracotomy method is a secondary consideration.

At the end of the story, the goal is the same irrespective as to whether the operation is performed through VATS or Uni-VATS, and for as long as it is achieved safely to operate lung cancer and not inferior to other approaches, but the need for randomized controlled trials is compulsory to confirm its strengths.

In the next decade, we may witness an increase in computer-assisted, instrument-controlled surgery [38]. Hopefully, uniportal VATS robotics will make surgery far simpler for all users and will open up a new horizon for precise and safer surgery. However, the enthusiasm for getting a new technology should match with patient safety. In the face of all technology, one needs to consider safety [39, 40].

CONCLUSION

This chapter is comprised of 2 sections.

In the first section, the author describes what is the standard method of VATS in the context of standard pulmonary resection. Nevertheless, additional issues related to standard VATS are also briefly discussed.

In the second section, Mini-VATS and Uni-Portal VATS are discussed and their perspectives are debated.

This chapter must be read with part of chapter 1 concerned with the Thoracoscopic Anatomy of the Thorax (chapter 1) and VAT Incision in chapter 8

(Thoracic incision).

CONSENT FOR PUBLICATION

Not applicable.

CONFLICT OF INTEREST

The author declares that there is no conflict of interest in this chapter.

ACKNOWLEDGEMENTS

Declared none.

REFERENCES (SECTION 1)

[1]   Jacobaeus HC. Über die Möglichkeit, die Zystoskopie bei Untersuchung seröser Höhlungen anzuwenden. Munch Med Wochenschr 1910; 57: 2090-2.

[2]   National Lung Cancer Audit Annual report 2018 (for the audit period 2017) Published May 2019.https://www.rcplondon.ac.uk/projects/outputs/nlca-annual-report-2018

[3]   SCTS 2014-15 Thoracic Registry Data.   https://scts.org/_userfiles/pages/file/Audit%20and%20 Outcomes/3_year_data_summary_2015.pdf

[4]   Abdelsattar ZM, Allen MS, Shen KR, *et al.* Variation in hospital adoption rates of video-assisted thoracoscopic lobectomy for lung cancer and the effect on outcomes. Ann Thorac Surg 2017; 103(2): 454-60.
       [http://dx.doi.org/10.1016/j.athoracsur.2016.08.091] [PMID: 27825690]

[5]   VIdeo assisted thoracoscopic lobectomy versus conventional Open Lobectomy for lung cancer, a multi-centre randomised controlled trial with an internal pilot. The VIOLET Study https://www.journalslibrary.nihr.ac.uk/programmes/hta/130403#/

[6]   Landreneau RJ, Mack MJ, Hazelrigg SR, *et al.* Video-assisted thoracic surgery: basic technical concepts and intercostal approach strategies. Ann Thorac Surg 1992; 54(4): 800-7.
       [http://dx.doi.org/10.1016/0003-4975(92)91040-G] [PMID: 1417251]

[7]   Yan X, Chen X, Li G, Chen S. Two-portal versus three-port video-assist thoracoscopic surgery for early stage nonsmall cell lung cancer: A retrospective study. Medicine (Baltimore) 2017; 96(33)e7796
       [http://dx.doi.org/10.1097/MD.0000000000007796] [PMID: 28816968]

[8]   Rocco G, Khalil M, Jutley R. Uniportal video-assisted thoracoscopic surgery wedge lung biopsy in the diagnosis of interstitial lung diseases. J Thorac Cardiovasc Surg 2005; 129(4): 947-8.
       [http://dx.doi.org/10.1016/j.jtcvs.2004.08.027] [PMID: 15821673]

[9]   Jutley RS, Khalil MW, Rocco G. Uniportal vs standard three-port VATS technique for spontaneous pneumothorax: comparison of post-operative pain and residual paraesthesia. Eur J Cardiothorac Surg 2005; 28(1): 43-6.
       [http://dx.doi.org/10.1016/j.ejcts.2005.02.039] [PMID: 15927479]

[10]   Gonzalez D, Paradela M, Garcia J, Dela Torre M. Single-port video-assisted thoracoscopic lobectomy. Interact Cardiovasc Thorac Surg 2011; 12(3): 514-5.
       [http://dx.doi.org/10.1510/icvts.2010.256222] [PMID: 21131682]

[11]   Gonzalez-Rivas D, Paradela M, Fernandez R, *et al.* Uniportal video-assisted thoracoscopic lobectomy: two years of experience 2013; 95(2): 426-32.
       [http://dx.doi.org/10.1016/j.athoracsur.2012.10.070]

[12] Melfi FM, Menconi GF, Mariani AM, Angeletti CA. Early experience with robotic technology for thoracoscopic surgery. Eur J Cardiothorac Surg 2002; 21(5): 864-8.
[http://dx.doi.org/10.1016/S1010-7940(02)00102-1] [PMID: 12062276]

[13] Veronesi G, Novellis P, Voulaz E, Alloisio M. Robot-assisted surgery for lung cancer: State of the art and perspectives. Lung Cancer 2016; 101: 28-34.
[http://dx.doi.org/10.1016/j.lungcan.2016.09.004] [PMID: 27794405]

[14] Park BJ, Flores RM, Rusch VW. Robotic assistance for video-assisted thoracic surgical lobectomy: technique and initial results. J Thorac Cardiovasc Surg 2006; 131(1): 54-9.
[http://dx.doi.org/10.1016/j.jtcvs.2005.07.031] [PMID: 16399294]

[15] Dylewski MR, Ohaeto AC, Pereira JF. Pulmonary resection using a total endoscopic robotic video-assisted approach. Semin Thorac Cardiovasc Surg 2011; 23(1): 36-42.
[http://dx.doi.org/10.1053/j.semtcvs.2011.01.005] [PMID: 21807297]

[16] Cerfolio RJ, Bryant AS, Skylizard L, Minnich DJ. Initial consecutive experience of completely portal robotic pulmonary resection with 4 arms. J Thorac Cardiovasc Surg 2011; 142(4): 740-6.
[http://dx.doi.org/10.1016/j.jtcvs.2011.07.022] [PMID: 21840547]

[17] Samson P, Guitron J, Reed MF, Hanseman DJ, Starnes SL. Predictors of conversion to thoracotomy for video-assisted thoracoscopic lobectomy: a retrospective analysis and the influence of computed tomography-based calcification assessment. J Thorac Cardiovasc Surg 2013; 145(6): 1512-8.
[http://dx.doi.org/10.1016/j.jtcvs.2012.05.028] [PMID: 22698554]

[18] Sawada S, Komori E, Yamashita M. Evaluation of video-assisted thoracoscopic surgery lobectomy requiring emergency conversion to thoracotomy. Eur J Cardiothorac Surg 2009; 36(3): 487-90.
[http://dx.doi.org/10.1016/j.ejcts.2009.04.004] [PMID: 19502073]

[19] Gazala S, Hunt I, Valji A, Stewart K, Bédard ER. A method of assessing reasons for conversion during video-assisted thoracoscopic lobectomy. Interact Cardiovasc Thorac Surg 2011; 12(6): 962-4.
[http://dx.doi.org/10.1510/icvts.2010.259663] [PMID: 21388988]

[20] Jones RO, Casali G, Walker WS. Does failed video-assisted lobectomy for lung cancer prejudice immediate and long-term outcomes? Ann Thorac Surg 2008; 86(1): 235-9.
[http://dx.doi.org/10.1016/j.athoracsur.2008.03.080] [PMID: 18573430]

[21] Puri V, Patel A, Majumder K, *et al.* Studying Intraoperative Conversions from Video-Assisted Thoracoscopic Surgery (VATS) Lobectomy to Open Thoracotomy. J Thorac Cardiovasc Surg 2015; 149(1): 55-62.
[http://dx.doi.org/10.1016/j.jtcvs.2014.08.074] [PMID: 25439768]

REFERENCES (SECTION 2)

[1]   Migliore M, Giuliano R, Deodato G. Video assisted thoracic surgery through a single port 2000.http://xoomer.virgilio.it/naples2000/index1.html

[2]   Migliore M, Deodato G. A single-trocar technique for minimally-invasive surgery of the chest. Surg Endosc 2001; 15(8): 899-901.
        [http://dx.doi.org/10.1007/s004640090033] [PMID: 11443464]

[3]   Migliore M. Efficacy and safety of single-trocar technique for minimally invasive surgery of the chest in the treatment of noncomplex pleural disease. J Thorac Cardiovasc Surg 2003; 126(5): 1618-23.
        [http://dx.doi.org/10.1016/S0022-5223(03)00592-0] [PMID: 14666042]

[4]   Migliore M, Deodato G. Thoracoscopic surgery, video-thoracoscopic surgery, or VATS: a confusion in definition. Ann Thorac Surg 2000; 69(6): 1990-1.
        [http://dx.doi.org/10.1016/S0003-4975(00)01302-3] [PMID: 10892980]

[5]   Migliore M, Halezeroglu S, Molins L, *et al.* Uniportal video-assisted thoracic surgery or single-incision video-assisted thoracic surgery for lung resection: clarifying definitions. Future Oncol 2016; 12(23s): 5-7.
        [http://dx.doi.org/10.2217/fon-2016-0370] [PMID: 27712092]

[6]   Bertolaccini L, Batirel H, Brunelli A, Gonzalez-Rivas D, Ismail M, Ucar AM, *et al.* Uniportal video-assisted thoracic surgery lobectomy: a consensus report from the Uniportal VATS Interest Group (UVIG) of the European Society of Thoracic Surgeons (ESTS). European journal of cardio-thoracic surgery: official journal of the European Association for Cardio-thoracic Surgery 2019 May 5;

[7]   Schaffer JL, Kambin P. Patient selection and indications for uniportal arthroscopic microdiskectomy and decompression. Semin Orthod 1991; 6(2): 109-12.

[8]   Gonzalez-Rivas D, de la Torre M, Fernandez R, Mosquera VX. Single-port video-assisted thoracoscopic left upper lobectomy. Interact Cardiovasc Thorac Surg 2011; 13(5): 539-41.
        [http://dx.doi.org/10.1510/icvts.2011.274746] [PMID: 21828107]

[9]   Zhao ZR, Lau RWH, Ng CSH. Anaesthesiology for uniportal VATS: double lumen, single lumen and tubeless. J Vis Surg 2017; 3: 108.
        [http://dx.doi.org/10.21037/jovs.2017.07.05] [PMID: 29078668]

[10]   Gonzalez-Rivas D, Aymerich H, Bonome C, Fieira E. From open operations to nonintubated uniportal video-assisted thoracoscopic lobectomy: minimizing the trauma to the patient. Ann Thorac Surg 2015; 100(6): 2003-5.
        [http://dx.doi.org/10.1016/j.athoracsur.2015.07.092] [PMID: 26652512]

[11]   Mineo TC, Sellitri F, Vanni G, Gallina FT, Ambrogi V. Immunological and Inflammatory Impact of Non-Intubated Lung Metastasectomy. Int J Mol Sci 2017; 18(7): 1466.
        [http://dx.doi.org/10.3390/ijms18071466] [PMID: 28686211]

[12]   Cajozzo M, Lo Iacono G, Raffaele F, *et al.* Thoracoscopy in pleural effusion--two techniques: awake single-access video-assisted thoracic surgery versus 2-ports video-assisted thoracic surgery under general anesthesia. Future Oncol 2015; 11(24) (Suppl.): 39-41.
        [http://dx.doi.org/10.2217/fon.15.288] [PMID: 26638922]

[13]   Zhu Y, Liang M, Wu W, *et al.* Preliminary results of single-port versus triple-port complete thoracoscopic lobectomy for non-small cell lung cancer. Ann Transl Med 2015; 3(7): 92.
        [PMID: 26015934]

[14]   Erşen E, Kılıç B, Kara HV, *et al.* Uniportal versus multiport video-assisted thoracoscopic surgery for anatomical lung resections: a glance at a dilemma. Wideochir Inne Tech Malo Inwazyjne 2018; 13(2): 215-20.
        [http://dx.doi.org/10.5114/wiitm.2018.75897] [PMID: 30002754]

[15]   Bourdages-pageau E, Vieira A. outcomes of uniportal vs multiportal video-assisted thoracoscopic lobectomy. Seminars in thoracic and cardiovascular surgery 2019 may 29; wb saunders.

[16]   Perna V, Carvajal AF, Torrecilla JA, Gigirey O. Uniportal video-assisted thoracoscopic lobectomy versus other video-assisted thoracoscopic lobectomy techniques: a randomized study. Eur J Cardiothorac Surg 2016; 50(3): 411-5.
[http://dx.doi.org/10.1093/ejcts/ezw161] [PMID: 27174549]

[17]   Harris CG, James RS, Tian DH, *et al*. Systematic review and meta-analysis of uniportal versus multiportal video-assisted thoracoscopic lobectomy for lung cancer. Ann Cardiothorac Surg 2016; 5(2): 76-84.
[http://dx.doi.org/10.21037/acs.2016.03.17] [PMID: 27134832]

[18]   Hirai K, Takeuchi S, Usuda J. Single-port video-assisted thoracic surgery for early lung cancer: initial experience in Japan. J Thorac Dis 2016; 8 (Suppl. 3): S344-50.
[PMID: 27014483]

[19]   Halezeroğlu S. Single incision video-assisted thoracic surgery pneumonectomy for centrally located lung cancer. Future Oncol 2018; 14(6s): 41-5.
[http://dx.doi.org/10.2217/fon-2017-0422] [PMID: 29664351]

[20]   Migliore M, Borrata F, Nardini M, *et al*. Awake uniportal video-assisted thoracic surgery for complications after pneumonectomy. Future Oncol 2016; 12(23s): 51-4.
[http://dx.doi.org/10.2217/fon-2016-0362] [PMID: 27744718]

[21]   Migliore M, Calvo D, Criscione A, Borrata F. Uniportal video assisted thoracic surgery: summary of experience, mini-review and perspectives. J Thorac Dis 2015; 7(9): E378-80.
[PMID: 26543631]

[22]   Gonzalez-Rivas D, Fernandez R, Fieira E, Rellan L. Uniportal video-assisted thoracoscopic bronchial sleeve lobectomy: first report. J Thorac Cardiovasc Surg 2013; 145(6): 1676-7.
[http://dx.doi.org/10.1016/j.jtcvs.2013.02.052] [PMID: 23507125]

[23]   Wang S, Meng C, Jiang Z, *et al*. Self-made thoracic needled suspending device with a snare: An excellent aid for uniportal video-assisted thoracic lobectomy and segmentectomy for lung cancer. Oncol Lett 2019; 17(4): 3671-6.
[http://dx.doi.org/10.3892/ol.2019.10030] [PMID: 30881492]

[24]   Sesma J, Bolufer S, Gálvez C, *et al*. Video-assisted thoracic surgery assisted by articulated arm (AVATS): a new way towards ergonomics and optimization of surgical resources. Shanghai Chest 2019; 4.

[25]   Liu CC, Wang BY, Shih CS, Liu YH. Subxiphoid single-incision thoracoscopic left upper lobectomy. J Thorac Cardiovasc Surg 2014; 148(6): 3250-1.
[http://dx.doi.org/10.1016/j.jtcvs.2014.08.033] [PMID: 25240526]

[26]   Song N, Zhao DP, Jiang L, *et al*. Subxiphoid uniportal video-assisted thoracoscopic surgery (VATS) for lobectomy: a report of 105 cases. J Thorac Dis 2016; 8 (Suppl. 3): S251-7.
[PMID: 27014471]

[27]   Park SY, Kim HK, Jang DS, Han KN, Kim DJ. Initial Experiences With Robotic Single-Site Thoracic Surgery for Mediastinal Masses. Ann Thorac Surg 2019; 107(1): 242-7.
[http://dx.doi.org/10.1016/j.athoracsur.2018.08.016] [PMID: 30296424]

[28]   Nardini M, Migliore M, Jayakumar S, ElSaegh M, Mydin IM, Dunning J. Subxiphoid port applied to robotic pulmonary lobectomies. J Vis Surg 2017; 3: 35.
[http://dx.doi.org/10.21037/jovs.2017.03.01] [PMID: 29078598]

[29]   Migliore M, Fornito M, Palazzolo M, *et al*. Ground glass opacities management in the lung cancer screening era. Ann Transl Med 2018; 6(5): 90-0.
[http://dx.doi.org/10.21037/atm.2017.07.28] [PMID: 29666813]

[30]   Nardini M, Bilancia R, Paul I, *et al*. ^{99m}Technetium and methylene blue guided pulmonary nodules resections: preliminary British experience. J Thorac Dis 2018; 10(2): 1015-21.
[http://dx.doi.org/10.21037/jtd.2018.01.143] [PMID: 29607175]

[31]   Santambrogio R, Montorsi M, Bianchi P, Mantovani A, Ghelma F, Mezzetti M. Intraoperative ultrasound during thoracoscopic procedures for solitary pulmonary nodules. Ann Thorac Surg 1999; 68(1): 218-22.
[http://dx.doi.org/10.1016/S0003-4975(99)00459-2] [PMID: 10421144]

[32]   Ambrogi MC, Melfi F, Zirafa C, *et al.* Radio-guided thoracoscopic surgery (RGTS) of small pulmonary nodules. Surg Endosc 2012; 26(4): 914-9.
[http://dx.doi.org/10.1007/s00464-011-1967-8] [PMID: 22011947]

[33]   Ujiie H, Kato T, Hu HP, *et al.* A novel minimally invasive near-infrared thoracoscopic localization technique of small pulmonary nodules: A phase I feasibility trial. J Thorac Cardiovasc Surg 2017; 154(2): 702-11.
[http://dx.doi.org/10.1016/j.jtcvs.2017.03.140] [PMID: 28495056]

[34]   Augustin F, Schmid T. A word of caution-when uniportal VATS should not be done. J Vis Surg 2018; 4: 29.
[http://dx.doi.org/10.21037/jovs.2018.01.06] [PMID: 29552511]

[35]   Hirai K, Enomoto Y, Usuda J. For which thoracic operation is U-VATS superior? J Vis Surg 2017; 3: 103.
[http://dx.doi.org/10.21037/jovs.2017.07.06] [PMID: 29078664]

[36]   Migliore M. Video-assisted thoracic surgery techniques for lung cancer: which is better? Future Oncol 2016; 12(23s): 1-4.
[http://dx.doi.org/10.2217/fon-2016-0465] [PMID: 27885852]

[37]   Migliore M, Criscione A, Calvo D, *et al.* Safety of video-assisted thoracic surgery lobectomy for non-small-cell lung cancer in a low-volume unit. Future Oncol 2016; 12(23s): 47-50.
[http://dx.doi.org/10.2217/fon-2016-0367] [PMID: 27764965]

[38]   Dunning J. Disruptive technology will transform what we think of as robotic surgery in under ten years. Ann Cardiothorac Surg 2019; 8(2): 274-8.
[http://dx.doi.org/10.21037/acs.2019.03.02] [PMID: 31032213]

[39]   Migliore M. Uniportal video-assisted thoracic surgery, and the uni-surgeon: new words for the contemporary world. J Vis Surg 2018; 4: 45.
[http://dx.doi.org/10.21037/jovs.2018.02.11] [PMID: 29682455]

[40]   Migliore M. How surgical care is changing in the technological era. Future Science 2016; 2(no. 2)
[http://dx.doi.org/10.4155/fsoa-2016-0010]

CHAPTER 11

The Role of Radiotherapy in the Management of Lung Carcinoma

Andrzej Wieczorek[1,*] and Nilesh S. Tambe[2]

[1] *Consultant Clinical Oncologist, Queens Centre for Oncology & Haematology, Castle Hill Hospital, Hull University Teaching Hospitals NHS Trust, Castle Road, Cottingham, UK*

[2] *Radiotherapy Clinical Scientist, Radiation Physics Department, Queens Centre for Oncology & Haematology, Castle Hill Hospital, Hull University Teaching Hospitals NHS Trust, Castle Road, Cottingham, UK*

Abstract: The aim of this chapter is to describe the role of radiotherapy in the management of lung carcinoma. The introduction covers general information about radiotherapy followed by a more detailed description of the basic principles of nuclear physics and radiotherapy treatment planning and delivery showing the influence of recent rapid progress in technology on the efficacy of this treatment modality. Following the introduction of technical aspects of radiation oncology, the role of radiotherapy, emphasising novel techniques of stereotactic ablative body radiotherapy, is described as the definitive treatment in early non-small cell lung carcinoma. The next part of the chapter presents the current role of radiotherapy with curative intent in locally advanced inoperable non-small cell lung cancer in combination with chemotherapy and immunotherapy. The use of radiotherapy in operable locally advanced lung carcinoma is also analysed to complete all clinical indications for this clinical entity. The role of radiotherapy in the management of small cell lung carcinoma is subsequently presented where consolidation chest radiotherapy and prophylactic cranial irradiation in combination with standard chemotherapy and its input to overall outcome are analysed for both limited and extensive disease. The basic principles of standard palliative radiotherapy are then presented with its input in the management of incurable stage of lung carcinoma in addition to palliative systemic treatment and the best supportive care. A brief description of new stereotactic techniques in the palliative setting is also presented. The chapter concludes with the management of radiotherapy related toxicity presenting most frequently observed side effects and their treatment.

* **Corresponding author Andrzej Wieczorek:** Consultant Clinical Oncologist, Queens Centre for Oncology & Haematology, Castle Hill Hospital, Hull University Teaching Hospitals NHS Trust, Castle Road, Cottingham, UK; Tel: 01482 461310; Fax: 01482 607739; E-mail: Andrzej.Wieczorek@hey.nhs.uk

Keywords: 3D-conformal radiotherapy, 4D-computer tomography, Adjuvant immunotherapy, Adjuvant radiotherapy, Chemo-radiotherapy, Consolidation chest radiotherapy, Intensity modulated radiotherapy, Non-small cell lung carcinoma, Palliative radiotherapy, Prophylactic cranial irradiation, Radiotherapy principles, Radiotherapy toxicity, Radiation oesophagitis, Radiation pneumonitis, Small cell lung carcinoma, Standard radiotherapy, Stereotactic radiotherapy, Volumetric modulated arc therapy.

INTRODUCTION

Radiotherapy has a very important role in the management of lung carcinoma and is one of the main therapeutic modalities used in the treatment of lower respiratory tract malignancies. Nowadays, the gold standard in oncology is combined treatment, therefore radiotherapy is mainly used together with systemic treatment and/or less frequently with surgery in various therapeutic sequences. In the early stages of the non-small cell lung carcinoma, radiotherapy could be however used as monotherapy with curative intent. The megavoltage photon external beam radiotherapy is the main treatment modality used for the treatment of lung carcinomas since the late fifties. Over the last three decades, an unprecedented improvement in the quality of external beam radiation delivery was observed due to progress in the technology of treatment machines. The radiotherapy technique evolved from a simple combination of the two opposed fields initially followed by oblique 3-4 field techniques used in the eighties and the beginning of the nineties where the dose was calculated just in one central plane (so-called 2D technique) to conformal radiotherapy in the nineties where the dose was calculated in all planes across the target volume in three-dimensions (3D) based on CT scans obtained during the treatment planning session. At the beginning of the current millennium, further development of radiotherapy was observed as intensity modulated radiotherapy (IMRT) equipped treatment machines became widely available and this technique was introduced to the majority of radiotherapy departments worldwide. The use of IMRT in thoracic malignancies is based on a much higher conformality of dose distribution than those achievable with conventional 3D conformal radiotherapy and based on better normal organ sparing. Currently, lung IMRT is mainly delivered with volumetric arc therapy (VMAT) either on standard linear accelerators or helical therapy on tomotherapy machines and this technique has replaced the first generation of IMRT techniques with fixed fields.

Radical radiotherapy total dose is delivered with several smaller doses called fraction dose over the period of time. The most frequently used regimen is called standard fractionation and uses 1.8-2Gy per fraction five days a week. The total radiotherapy dose varies between 60 to 70Gy in 30 to 35 fractions. Another form of the dose delivery is hypo-fractionated radiotherapy with doses of 50-55Gy in 20 fractions and is considered to be an alternative to standard fractionation especially for elderly patients with significant comorbidities when shortening the overall time of the treatment is essential. It is offered in the minority of radiotherapy departments mainly in the UK.

Stereotactic ablative body radiotherapy (SABR) is the special form of radical radiotherapy developed recently which delivers very precisely focused radiation to treat mainly peripheral early lung non-small lung carcinoma. It uses high fractionation doses every 2-3 days with the total doses 50-60Gy in 3-8 fractions. In advanced cases of lung carcinoma when curative intent is no longer possible, radiotherapy can be used with palliative intent mainly aiming to improve the quality of patient life and symptom control. Lower doses compare to radical intent are used with a smaller number of fractions.

Nuclear physics is the basic science to support clinical use and development of radiation oncology and general principles of it will be presented in the next paragraphs of this chapter. Radiobiology and molecular biology are also basic sciences to give support and development of radiotherapy but the presentation of general principles is beyond the scope of this textbook and can be found in other publications.

BASIC PRINCIPLES OF RADIOTHERAPY NUCLEAR PHYSICS

X-rays are a very commonly used type of radiation for treating cancer patients.

Production of Kilo-voltage (kV) X-ray

kV photons are produced by abruptly stopping electrons accelerated across the potential difference between a cathode and an anode within a vacuumed X-ray tube (Fig. **1A**). In this process, a part or the entirety of the kinetic energy of the electrons is transformed into electromagnetic energy. The energy and the quality of the X-ray beam are dependent on the potential applied across the cathode and the anode. A spectrum of X-rays is produced with the higher energy being equal to the energy of the most energetic incident electron. The electrons produced *via* thermionic emission in the cathode are accelerated and strike the high atomic number target material/anode (*e.g.* tungsten) producing X-rays mainly *via* the following three interactions.

1. When relatively low energy electrons (energy lower than the binding energy of the orbital electrons) are incident on the electron cloud of the target material, a small deflection is caused resulting in loss of energy causing excitation and heat production. These regard the majority of interactions.
2. The incident electrons with energy higher than the binding energy of the orbital

electrons of the target may eject electrons from the inner orbit and the vacancies created are filled by electrons from the outer shell emitting photons of the energy equal to the difference in energy between two shells. These are called characteristic X-rays. The energy of these X-rays depends on the energy difference between orbital shells which, in turn, depends on the atomic number of the target material.

3. Braking or the bremsstrahlung X-rays are produced as a result of the deceleration of the highspeed incoming electrons when passing close to a positively charged target nucleus. This type of interaction produces the majority of X-ray photons.

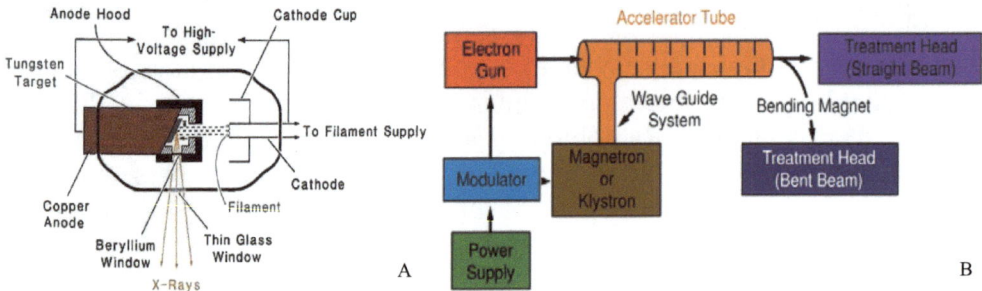

Fig. (1). A: Schematic of the x-ray tube on left and B: a block diagram of the medical linear accelerator (right) [1].

Megavoltage (MV) X-ray

Megavoltage photons are generated in a linear accelerator. Instead of using potential difference, electrons are accelerated towards a target material by interacting with a synchronised radio-frequency electromagnetic field (Fig. **1B**). A spectrum of bremsstrahlung X-rays is produced by hitting the target material with the maximum energy being equal to the energy of the most energetic incident electron. In order to be used for treatment, the low energy X-rays are eliminated from the treatment beam by adding a filter that absorbs these low energy X-rays (Fig. **2A**). This increases skin sparing whilst treating deep seated tumours. Electron beams produced within linear accelerators can be used for treating superficial lesions. In this case, the X-ray target is retracted from the beam path and replaced by a scattering foil which spreads the incident electron beam making it uniform for treatment (Fig. **2B**). The secondary collimator consists of movable multi leaf collimators (MLCs: thickness between 0.25cm to 1cm) and jaws these are used for defining radiotherapy treatment field [1].

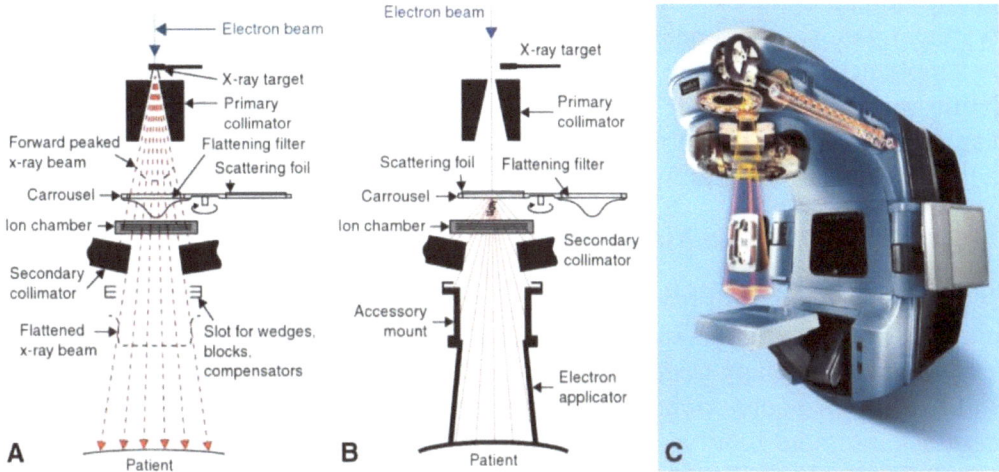

Fig. (2). Schematic of a linear accelerator head. X-ray mode (A), electron mode (B) and linear accelerator with accelerating waveguide (C) [1].

BASIC PRINCIPLES OF RADIOTHERAPY TREATMENT PLANNING AND DELIVERY

Lung radiotherapy treatment planning is nowadays a very complex and technology-driven treatment process requiring teamwork to assure proper and safe delivery. Radiotherapy delivery is preceded by a treatment planning session. A very important part of it is the immobilisation of the patient to assure good accuracy and reproducibility of planned radiation.

CT Simulation

Lung cancer patients are positioned supine with the arms above the head using a wing board with hand poles (to avoid treating though the arms) and a knee rest for comfort and stability. If both arms cannot be raised above the head, then an attempt should be made to raise one arm above the head if possible. Both the wing board and knee rest are fixed to the treatment couch using locking bars. The position of locking bars, arm poles and head position is recorded on the patient's setup sheet so that the patient can be reproducibly set-up in the same position as at the CT simulation during the entire course of radiotherapy treatment which is delivered in several fractions. Any deviation from the planned/simulated treatment position could introduce errors in treatment delivery (especially if pre-treatment imaging is not performed). Immobilisation devices limit patient motion during treatment so that the treatment can be accurately delivered as planned.

Performing a planning CT scan in the treatment position constitutes a standard localisation procedure for subsequent radiotherapy and also enables the computer treatment planning systems to calculate the prescribed dose. CT localisation could be supplemented by image fusion with MRI or PET CT for better accuracy in delineating head and neck tumour. 4D CT (four-dimensional) to track tumour respiratory motion is currently considered as the gold standard in radical radiotherapy for lung carcinoma.

Internal Target Motion Management

One of the challenges of treating lung cancer patients with radiotherapy is tumour motion due to breathing. It is essential to account for the tumour motion in the process of radiotherapy treatment planning, as, if unaccounted for; tumour motion could lead to be geometric miss (not treating the entire tumour due to motion). To account for tumour motion, lung cancer patients with regular breathing undergo a four-dimensional (4D) CT scan; patients with irregular breathing may not be suitable for 4DCT as it could cause significant motion artefacts in the resultant scans and could affect target delineation. Patients with irregular breathing undergo a 3D-CT scan (this is a fast scan which only represents the tumour position at the time of the scan). A patient's breathing trace is acquired during a 4DCT scan (Fig. 3) using external surrogates such as an infrared reflective marker block positioned on the patient's chest/abdomen. The signal from the reflective markers is captured by a camera and stored in the database. Following the completion, the scan, the acquired CT data is binned into different bins (6 to 12 bins are possible; 10 bins are commonly used); binning of CT data is done based on phase/time or amplitude of the acquired trace. In phase/time binning, each breathing cycle is divided into 10 equal time points and each time point forms a scan. Subsequent breathing cycles are then binned in the corresponding bin. In amplitude binning, the data are binned based on the amplitude within each breathing cycle. 4D-CT scanning enables the capture of tumour motion associated with the respiratory breathing cycle.

Target Volume Delineation

Target volume and organs at risk delineation is a very important task for radiation oncologists as it has a big influence on the overall outcome of the treatment and its toxicity. The principles involved in lung cancer are no different from those that apply elsewhere in the body. The target volumes typically consist of GTV (gross tumour volume) and CTV (clinical target volume). The GTV is the primary tumour and thoracic lymph nodes metastases visualised on cross-sectional radiology images. The CTV is a tissue volume that contains a demonstrable GTV and/or is considered to contain microscopic, subclinical extensions at a certain probability level. In thoracic radiotherapy, a subclinical extension of the primary tumour and thoracic lymph nodes metastases together with thoracic lymph nodes groups harboring occult metastases is included in the CTV. The principle rules of GTV and CTV delineation in radical lung radiotherapy [2] have been agreed among the radiation oncologist community. A detailed discussion of principles of target volume and organ at risk delineation for lung cancer is beyond the scope of this chapter and is covered in other textbooks. The PTV-planning target volume is the margin that needs to be added to CTV to compensate for uncertainties in planning and delivery. When 3D CT is used for treatment planning, the PTV is additionally expanded by a standard margin to compensate for respiratory tumour motion, in addition to the margin applied to account for uncertainties in treatment setup. In 4D CT planned radiotherapy, respiratory motion is individually assessed for the patients and an ITV (internal target volume) is created. It consists of an internal margin added to the CTV and/or GTV to compensate for internal physiologic movement (*e.g.* breathing) (Figs. **4** and **5**). This ITV is then expanded by a margin accounting for set up uncertainties to create the final 4D PTV.

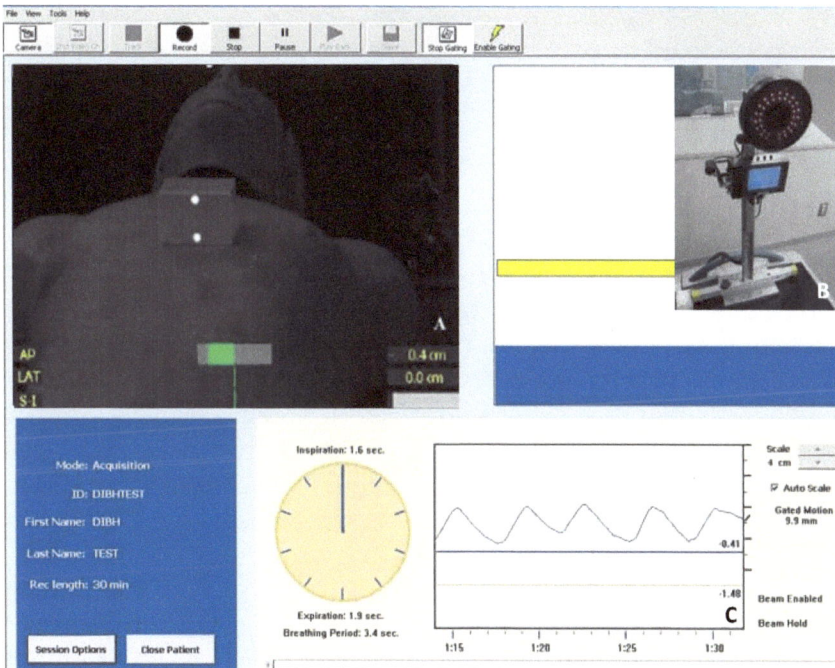

Fig. (3). Showing Varian's real time positioning management (RPM) system, image A showing infrared marker block placed on patient's chest and the infrared camera in image B. The real time breathing trace acquired by the RPM system is shown in image C. The acquired breathing trace is saved on a local RPM database and used to segregate the acquired CT data into the required number of bines.

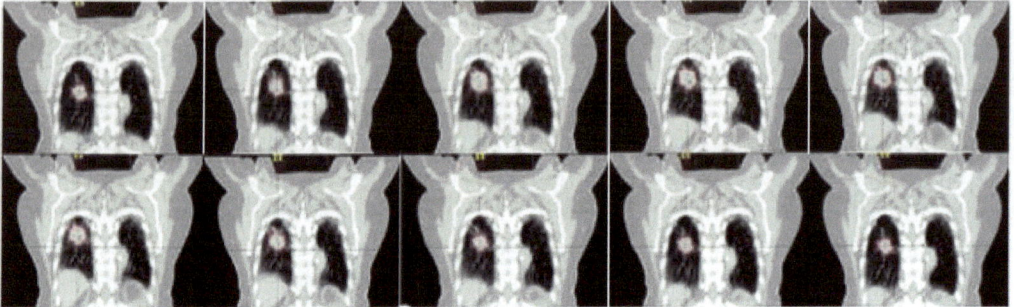

Fig. (4). Showing tumour motion (mainly in the superior and inferior direction around cross-hair) on a ten-phase 4DCT scan.

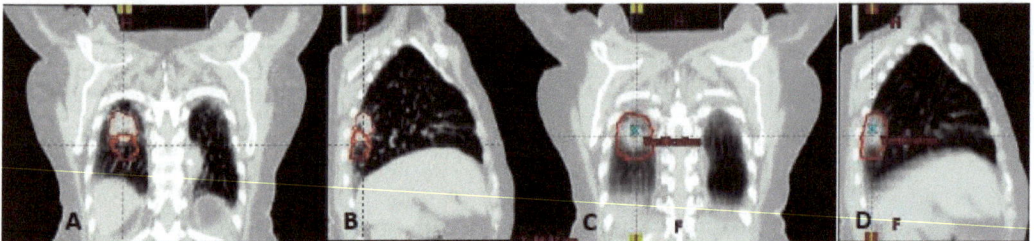

Fig. (5). Displaying the maximum motion of gross tumour volume (GTV) in A and B. On C and D images, the volume in orange showing a reduction in internal target volume (ITV) when gated on phase 20 to 60 were selected for treatment delivery compared to the total ITV (red).

Treatment Planning

Radiotherapy treatment planning for the management of cancer patients can be considered as a two-part process: The first part includes the clinical treatment planning, where the treatment intent, modality, radiation dose prescription, target volumes and clinical structures are decided. The second part regards the technical aspect of treatment planning where information about a patient's position and immobilisation, are used to drive decision around treatment beam geometry, aperture and energy are decided to produce individualised optimal treatment plans for a certain patient [3]. The aim is to deliver the prescription dose to the target volume whilst minimising the dose to healthy tissues (OARs), following guidance published by the ICRU. Achieving the desired target coverage whilst minimising OAR dose can be challenging, especially when the target volume is in close proximity with the dose-limiting structures (*e.g.* spinal cord), which, if over irradiated, could severely impact on a patient's quality-of-life, producing effects such as paralysis. Treatment planning is performed on high speed computer software either in the forward planning 3D conformal technique, where staff choose from which angles the radiation beams are incident on the patient and adjust the relative contribution of these beams manually, or inverse planning IMRT where the computer treatment planning system intelligently selects the most appropriate way to deliver radiation, based upon a series of constraints fed into the system by staff. The latter radiation technique is used with increasing frequency due to its advantages over 3D conformal radiotherapy.

Different radiotherapy treatment planning and delivery techniques have been developed over the years. In the early days of radiotherapy, patients were planned using two-dimensional (2D) images acquired on a conventional simulator. Treatment fields were defined based on poorly differentiated anatomical and tumour boundaries and dose distribution and treatment time were calculated manually using 2D dosimetry data [3, 4]. Following the development of the CT scanner in 1979 [5], there has been a significant improvement in the radiotherapy planning process; three-dimensional (3D) CT images are currently being used for delineating target volumes and establishing a true 3D target volume. After 1999, the development of 3D treatment planning systems (TPS) and the multi-leaf collimator (MLC) allowed the shaping of the aperture of treatment beams to the target volume using the beam's eye view (BEV) mode resulting in the superior conformation of isodoses to the target volume whilst minimising dose to OARs. Multiple static fields are placed around the target volume using the beam's eye view (BEV) visualisation tool; BEV helps to avoid or minimise beam incidence through critical structures. Plans are optimised by changing the weighting (contribution) from different beams and by using wedges to compensate for body obliquity. Although target conformity improved with 3DCRT planning as compared with 2D planning, the delivery of the prescription dose to the entire target volume is often limited due to the proximity of OAR. Furthermore, the dose to OAR structures located in the groove region of a concave target volume cannot be reduced below the prescription dose unless target coverage is compromised [6].

Advanced Radiotherapy Techniques

In 1982, the intensity modulated radiotherapy (IMRT) planning technique was first proposed by Brahme *et al.* [6]. Since then, the use of IMRT in clinical practice has increased significantly and has currently become the standard of care for radiotherapy treatment of different sites. IMRT is a more complex form of conformal radiation therapy where conformity is achieved by modulating the intensity of beams. Each IMRT field consists of multiple segments/beamlets formed using MLCs and their intensities within the field are defined using monitor units (MUs).

IMRT can be used to produce significantly superior conformity of the dose distribution as compared with 3D-CRT. In addition, it can produce a more homogeneous dose distribution across the PTV and achieve a sharper dose fall-off at the PTV edge. A sharper dose fall-off from the PTV boundary may allow a significant reduction of the OAR volume receiving higher doses. These features allow dose escalation to target volumes - whilst keeping OAR doses within clinical tolerance - thus improving treatment outcome. Reduction in OAR doses reduces the complication rate and improves patients' quality of life.

IMRT plans can be delivered using step and shoot or dynamic techniques. In step and shoot treatments, the radiation beam is turned off whilst MLC are moving to the next segment as well as between gantry rotation. In dynamic delivery, the radiation beam is switched off only during gantry motion to the next planned position.

The VMAT technique is even more complex to deliver as gantry speed, dose rate and MLC aperture change continuously during treatment delivery. VMAT plans produce more conformal dose distributions than IMRT plans as there are more degrees of freedom which also result in the total number of monitor units in VMAT plans to be significantly lower as compared to IMRT plans. However, a larger volume of normal tissues is usually exposed to low radiation doses in VMAT plans as compared to IMRT and 3D-CRT plans due to the nature of delivery (*i.e.* arc delivery) (Fig. **6A**). VMAT plans usually consist of one or two full (360°) or partial (180°) arc(s).

Treatment Delivery

Treatment is delivered by computer driven linear accelerators using 4-15MV photons with sub millimetre accuracy allowing radiation to be focussed on the tumourous tissues and minimising radiation to normal tissue structures. Image-guided radiotherapy (IGRT) and dosimetry play a very important role in quality assurance of external beam radiation delivery. The whole process of radiation treatment planning and delivery is based on the International Commission on Radiation Units & Measurements ICRU62 report for 3D conformal techniques and ICRU83 report for IMRT [7].

Radiotherapy treatments are delivered in fractionated schedules; mainly five-times a week (typically on weekdays) for 4 to 7 weeks depending on the dose and fractionation regime chosen for an individual patient. This approach ensures normal tissues are given time to recover from the sub-lethal damage caused by radiation. The time between different fractions also allows redistribution of tumour cells from the resistant phase of the cell division cycle (*i.e.* S phase) to more sensitive phases (*i.e.* late G2 and M). Furthermore, it allows the re-oxygenation of hypoxic tumour cells improving tumour cell killing. Repair and repopulation of the normal cell during breaks between fractions improve tolerance to treatment [8].

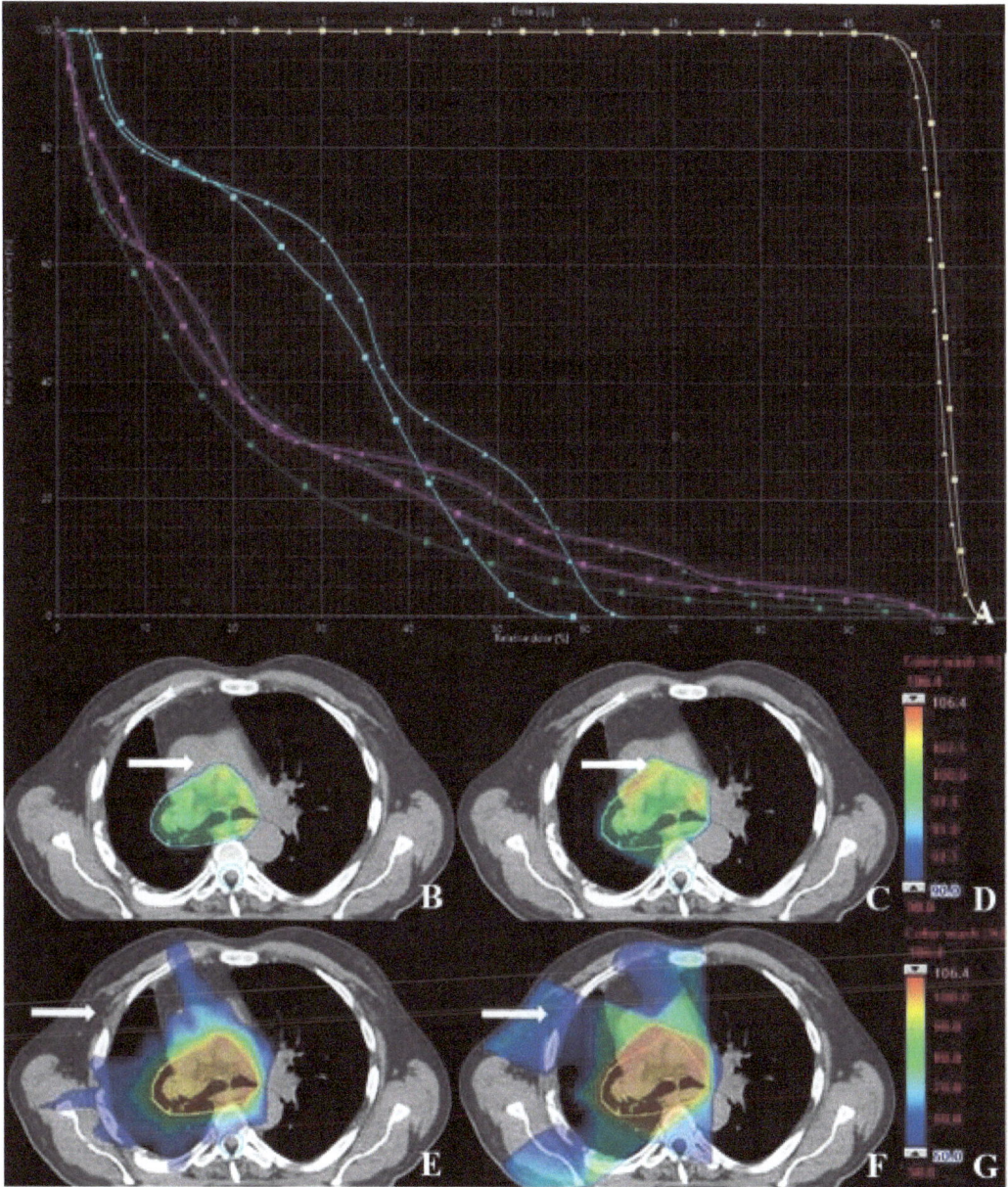

Fig. (6). A: Dose volume histogram (DVH) displaying lung (pink), spinal cord PRV (cyan), heart (green) and PTV (orange) curves for both 3DCRT (in triangle) and VMAT (in square) plans. It can be seen from the DVH plot that VMAT increases the volume receiving lower doses and reduces the volume receiving higher doses compared to the 3DCRT plan. The axial slices show dose distribution in colour wash, B and C: colour wash with 90 % dose threshold and E and F: with 50 % dose threshold. It can be seen from these images (B, C, E and F) that dose conformity is significantly higher in VMAT plan compared to the 3DCRT plan. D and G: showing dose legend.

Pre-treatment Imaging

Patients are positioned on the treatment couch of the linear accelerator in the same position as during the treatment planning simulation. 2D (planar kV or MV images) (Fig. **7A**) or 3D [cone beam computerised tomography (CBCT)] (Fig. **7B**) imaging is performed immediately prior to treatment delivery to confirm treatment position; these images are compared with planning CT images (2D images are compared with digitally reconstructed radiographs (DRR)) and any setup differences are corrected by shifting the couch accordingly prior to treatment delivery. Volumetric (CBCT) imaging is preferred for lung patients as it allows visualisation of internal anatomical changes during treatment. Recent further technological development in on-board imaging technology allows the performance of a 4D-CBCT enabling accurate visualisation of tumour motion and tumour matching prior to treatment delivery.

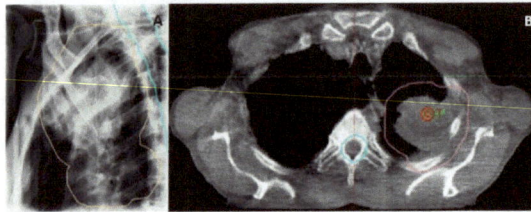

Fig. (7). Showing 2D planar image (A) and 3D CBCT slice (B) planar image with planning target volume (PTV) and spinal cord PRV (planning at risk volume) contours displayed. The CBCT images on the right display internal anatomy and tumour more clearly compared to the 2D image.

3D imaging provides information about soft tissues changes as compared with 2D images which mostly display bony anatomy. Potential anatomical changes (of internal or external anatomy) can be seen on CBCT images and can help to assess if a patient requires adaptive radiotherapy planning (ART: the treatment plan is adjusted to anatomical changes seen on images).

THE ROLE OF RADIOTHERAPY IN EARLY STAGE NON-SMALL LUNG CARCINOMA

Surgery remains the standard treatment for early stage I-II non-small lung carcinoma; however, a substantial proportion of patients are medically inoperable or refuse surgery. The number of such patients has been increasing over the last decades due to ageing population. Patients are medically inoperable mainly due to poor respiratory function or serious comorbidities, such as cardiovascular disease. Quite a substantial proportion of these patients can still be offered alternative treatment in the form of radical external beam radiotherapy. For small, less than 5 cm in maximum diameter peripheral lung tumours with no hilar lymph adenopathy, stereotactic ablative body radiotherapy (SABR) became standard of care over the last decade and gives a very valuable option for medically inoperable patients with early stage non-small lung carcinoma. A method for stereotactic body radiotherapy for extracranial targets was developed at the Karolinska University Hospital in Stockholm in the early nineties [9] and since then, the interest in this treatment technique has grown exponentially leading to further development and research which became the foundation to recognise this treatment modality as the standard of care nowadays. There is an extensive amount of literature confirming excellent results in terms of local control, overall survival (Table 1) and low toxicity profile [10 - 23] with the suggestion that the results of SABR can be either slightly inferior or similar to the results reported for segmentectomy or lobectomy [24, 25].

Table 1. Lung SABR reported survival outcome and local control in 35 studies [26].

	Studies with Mean ± SD Median (range)	Mean ± SD	Median (range)
Overall survival (%)			
12 months	15	82.8 ± 11.4	83.0 (52 – 100)
24 months	21	64.5 ± 15.5	65.4 (32 – 91)
36 months	18	57.7 ± 16.0	55.9 (32 – 91)
60 months	9	45.3 ± 20.1	47.0 (18 – 77.5)
Cause-specific survival (%)			
12 months	7	93.7 ± 2.7	94.0 (88 – 96)
24 months	15	77.3 ± 9.9	82.0 (53.5–88)
36 months	14	72.0 ± 11.9	70.0 (53 - 90.5)
60 months	7	56.9 ± 16.2	50.0 (40 –78)
Local control (%)			
12 months	8	91.8 ± 3.5	92.0 (85.3 – 96)
24 months	11	86.9 ± 9.7	88.0 (67.9 – 96)
36 months	11	80.6 ± 13.6	84.0 (57 – 95)
48 months	1	89.0 ± 0.0	89.0 (n/a)
60 months	1	86.0 ± 0.0	86.0 (n/a)

SABR has a very well-established role for the peripheral lung tumours; however, the use of SABR for centrally located lesions remains controversial because of concerns about the potential for very severe or even lethal toxic effects when ablative doses of radiation are delivered to critical structures such as bronchial tree, oesophagus, major vessels, heart, and the brachial plexus/phrenic nerve [27]. The IASLC has defined 'central tumours' as tumours located within 2 cm in all directions of any mediastinal critical structure, including the bronchial tree and other organs listed above [28]. For tumours located in the hilar region or so-called moderately central tumours, SABR seems to be feasible option to achieve high local control rates with limited toxicity [29]. In many centres, less intense dose fractionation with 60Gy in 8 fractions is used but has not been fully accepted worldwide as the gold standard and currently there is plenty of research likely to identify the dose regimens, planning optimization, and normal tissue dose-volume constraints for using SABR to treat moderately central NSCLC. However, care should be taken to distinguish moderately central tumours as described before from so-called 'ultra-central' lesions where radiotherapy high dose volume overlaps the trachea or main bronchi. In the latter anatomical localisation, SABR proved to cause an unacceptable risk of severe toxicity and therefore cannot be recommended in clinical practise [30]. When SABR cannot be offered to medically inoperable early stage NSCLC due to unacceptable risk of the severe toxicity, standard radical radiotherapy remains an alternative option still offering curative intent; however, reported results remained significantly inferior to surgery or SABR [31].

THE ROLE OF RADIOTHERAPY IN LOCALLY ADVANCED NON-SMALL LUNG CARCINOMA

Locally advanced non-small lung carcinoma patients consist of a very heterogenous group mainly in the unresectable stage of the disease. The prognosis is poor and significantly worse compared to the early stage. Single modality treatment either surgical or radiotherapy results in very poor outcomes, therefore, combination treatment for this clinical entity remains standard of care for patients with good performance status and respiratory function where radical intent therapy can be offered. For those patients who have poor performance status, poor respiratory function or big volume disease, treatment with palliative intent remains the only available option. Until recently concurrent chemo-radiotherapy remained the standard of care for the locally advanced non-small cell lung cancer patients treated with radical intent showing its superiority over other sequential chemo-radiotherapy However, outcomes remained disappointing in the past because most patients have had disease progression following completion of treatment, with approximately 15 to 30% of patients remaining alive at 5 years [32]. The long-term results of the RTOG 0617 trial reporting 32.1% 5-year overall survival rate in the standard arm set a new 5-year landmark for the patients with unresectable stage III non-small lung carcinoma since it is higher to any previously published prospective data [33]. The toxicity of concurrent chemo-radiotherapy although reversible and manageable remained very substantial [34 - 36]. Concurrent chemo-radiotherapy typically uses standard fractionation regimen with the total doses of 60-66Gy in 30/33 fractions together with concurrent chemotherapy using cisplatin+ etoposide or cisplatin+ vinorelbine, or paclitaxel+ carboplatin, or cisplatin+ pemetrexed if non-squamous histology for two to six cycles administered concomitantly to radiation. Numerous attempts to improve the poor outcome of concurrent chemo-radiotherapy by intensifying chemotherapy in form of either adding additional induction [37] or adjuvant [35, 38 - 40] cycles of a cytotoxic treatment or increasing total dose of radiotherapy [34] failed to show the better outcome.

The recent publication of the results of the PACIFIC trial showed significant improvement in overall survival for patients who had adjuvant immunotherapy durvalumab intravenously at a dose of 10 mg per kilogram of body weight every 2 weeks for up to 12 months in addition to concurrent chemo-radiotherapy [41, 42]. This publication has opened a new chapter for combining immunotherapy with standard chemo-radiotherapy and is considered to be the long-awaited breakthrough to improve treatment results for the locally advanced good performance inoperable non-small lung carcinoma. The 24-month overall survival rate was 66.3% (95% confidence interval [CI], 61.7 to 70.4) in the durvalumab group, as compared with 55.6% (95% CI, 48.9 to 61.8) in the placebo group (two-sided P = 0.005) [42]. Updated analyses regarding progression-free survival were similar to those previously reported, with a median duration of 17.2 months in the durvalumab group and 5.6 months in the placebo group (stratified hazard ratio for disease progression or death, 0.51; 95% CI, 0.41 to 0.63) [41, 42]. Following the publication of the PACIFIC trial, adjuvant immunotherapy became recently the standard of care for this group of patients.

For elderly and/or less fit patients with clinically relevant comorbidities when concurrent chemo-radiotherapy is deemed to be too toxic, the sequential approach can be a good choice [43]. The accelerated RT schedules which are delivered in a shorter overall treatment time showed a small absolute benefit of 2.5% in 5-year OS over standard fractionation [44].

The treatment of the small group of patients presented with resectable locally advanced non-small cell lung carcinoma remains a matter of controversy and is not very well defined. The postoperative adjuvant radiotherapy failed to show survival benefit and is not routinely recommended [45]. For N0 and N1 disease postoperative radiotherapy was found to be detrimental in the outcome. An unexpected N2 disease discovered at surgery was showing no overall survival differences but was found to produce better local control therefore in some centres postoperative radiotherapy to mediastinum is used sequentially in addition to adjuvant chemotherapy. The use of postoperative radiotherapy after positive surgical resection appears empirically reasonable to prevent local relapse and is accepted indication worldwide, but it is not supported by high-quality evidence

[45]. The very aggressive approach to the management of resectable locally advanced non-small cell lung carcinoma with induction chemo-radiotherapy failed to show an overall survival benefit for the trimodality treatment but showed significant improvement in disease-free survival [46 - 48]. The use of trimodality treatment remains therefore controversial owing to the lack of survival benefit; however, in many countries is considered to be an acceptable choice for the very selected group of resectable locally advanced non-small cell lung carcinoma [43].

THE ROLE OF RADIOTHERAPY IN SMALL LUNG CARCINOMA.

Cisplatin or Carboplatin in combination with Etoposide remains the main treatment modality for all stages of small cell lung carcinoma. The role of radiotherapy for this clinical entity is limited and complementary to systemic treatment aiming to improve overall and disease progression-free survival. About one-third of patients will present with a locally advanced disease which can be safely encompassed with high dose radiotherapy volume and is commonly described as a limited disease (LD) but the remaining two-thirds will present with either stage IV disease or locally advanced with big volume disease where delivery of high dose radiotherapy is unsafe due to anticipated high rate of severe, unaccepted toxicity and is commonly called extensive disease (ED). Although TNM staging remains the gold standard, the above terminology is very useful to understand the role of radiotherapy in the management of small cell lung carcinoma and is still used by many oncologists in addition to recommended TNM assessment.

In LD, consolidation chest radiotherapy and prophylactic cranial irradiation are routinely used in addition to chemotherapy. Prophylactic cranial radiotherapy is added sequentially following good response to systemic treatment whereas consolidation chest radiotherapy can be used either concurrently or sequentially to chemotherapy. Consolidation chest radiotherapy improves survival over chemotherapy alone with a median survival of 15–20 months and 2-year survival rates reported to be 20%–40%. The proportion of patients who survive for 5 years has been reported to be 20%–25% [49 - 51]. Concurrent chemo-radiotherapy is the most effective combination and should be used in LD patients if the irradiated volume assures safe delivery precluding severe toxicity and patients are of good performance status and respiratory function. The timing of radiotherapy seems to be very essential with an early start during the first or second cycle of cisplatin-based chemotherapy proved to lead to improved overall survival compared with delayed radiotherapy [52 - 55]. Twice daily radiotherapy with a total dose of 45Gy in 30 fractions delivered over 3 weeks remains the most effective regimen [56]; however, 66Gy in 33 fractions over 6.5 weeks gives the same results with similar toxicity and can be alternatively used depending on patient's preference and service availabilities of a radiotherapy department [57]. The majority of LD patients cannot be treated with concurrent chemoradiotherapy due to tumour size or comorbidities. The sequential chemoradiotherapy is the best alternative for them; however, with an inferior outcome to concurrent treatment. There is no definitive evidence to indicate the optimal radiotherapy dose in this patient group. 50-60Gy in 20-30 fractions over 4-6 weeks or 40Gy/15 over 3 weeks are usually delivered after completion of chemotherapy to patients with a good response to systemic treatment.

Patients with ED have a poor prognosis with a median overall survival of 8–13 months and palliative chemotherapy with Cisplatin/Carboplatin and Etoposide for four to six cycles is the standard of care. Sequential consolidation chest radiotherapy improves overall survival and progression-free survival for the patients who responded to initial palliative systemic treatment [58, 59]. The CREST study using radiotherapy with 30 Gy in 10 fractions in patients with any response after 4–6 cycles of chemotherapy led to a 2-year survival rate of 13% compared with 3% without chest irradiation [58]. Following this publication in 2015 sequential chemo-radiotherapy was accepted as the gold standard for this patient group.

The propensity of small-cell lung cancer (SCLC) to seed in the brain is well known. Autopsy studies have shown brain metastases in 50–65% of patients with SCLC with a cumulative probability of brain metastases reaching 80% for patients who live 2 or more years [60, 61]. The prophylactic cranial irradiation (PCI) in LD can reduce the risk of brain metastases from 59% to 33% at 3 years and is accompanied by a survival benefit (21% *versus* 15%) [62 - 64]. Based on this data PCI is now recognised as the part of the standard of care in patients with LD-SCLC with partial or complete response to initial treatment. The standard dose for PCI is 25 Gy in 10 fractions. Higher doses do not improve outcomes but increase mortality [65] and chronic neurotoxicity [63]. The role of PCI in ED remains controversial. The EORTC trial published in 2007 reported that PCI had signi-ficantly reduced symptomatic brain metastases in ED (14.6% *versus* 40.4%) and had increased overall survival at 1 year (27.1% *versus* 13.3%) [66]. It led the PCI to be considered a standard treatment for these patients similarly to LD. A limitation of this study was that no brain imaging was required before PCI. Recently, a Japanese randomised phase III trial showed in the same setting which required that all patients underwent brain magnetic resonance imaging (MRI) after completing chemotherapy and during follow-up that PCI reduced the incidence of brain metastasis (48% vs.69%, P < 0.001) with overall survival being marginally shorter in PCI group than in the observation (control) group [67]. Since that no universally accepted guidelines are available regarding the use of PCI for patients with ES and both therapeutic options are acceptable subject of clinician and patient preference [68].

PALLIATIVE RADIOTHERAPY IN LUNG CARCINOMA

Palliative radiotherapy offers a quick, inexpensive, and effective way of reducing many of the focal symptoms and improves the quality of life in patients suffering from locally advanced or metastatic lung cancer in the incurable stage of the disease when radical treatment cannot be offered. It can be used together with the best supportive care and palliative systemic treatment. Palliative treatments are delivered at the same treatment machines as radical radiotherapy; linear accelerators and utilises lower total doses using much shorter courses of larger fraction size (hypo-fractionation) with the focus shifting to symptom control while minimising treatment burden and toxicity. It can be used to treat symptomatic locally advanced lung tumours or distant metastases. It uses simple radiotherapy techniques like one direct or two parallel opposed fields with short and uncomplicated treatment planning. The most frequently used palliative regimens are: 8-10Gy in a single fraction, 20Gy in 5 fractions and 30 Gy in 10 fractions. The most widely accepted indications related to locally advanced lung carcinoma are: airway obstruction, chest wall pain, cough control and haemoptysis. Painful bone metastases or metastatic spinal cord compression are frequent indications for palliative radiotherapy either. Symptomatic brain, soft tissue or lymph node metastases can be also treated with palliative radiotherapy but its role is uncertain and more controversial than previously listed indications. The basic principles and indications to standard palliative radiotherapy were developed 5-6 decades ago and were modified over this time but not fundamentally changed and are very well covered on international or national guidelines [69, 70]. Recent progress in technology permitted to use more intense, in terms, of total dose delivered palliative irradiation with stereotactic techniques in selected cases of incurable lung carcinoma patients with better local control and overall survival compare to standard palliative radiotherapy outcome. The oldest and most commonly accepted therapy with this technique is stereotactic radiosurgery for solitary or oligo brain metastases. This treatment can be only offered to patients with low volume brain metastases with good performance status and when the extracranial disease is already controlled or can be potentially treated with the life expectancy over 6 months. Total dose 15-24 Gy in the single fraction is used and results in better local control and overall survival compare to standard palliative whole-brain radiotherapy [71, 72]. The hippocampal-sparing during cranial irradiation is the approach that can potentially delay or reduce the severity of the neurocognitive decline. A phase II clinical trial (RTOG0933) showed that conformal avoidance of the hippocampus during whole-brain radiation therapy for brain metastases was associated with preservation of memory and quality of life relative to a historical control group [73]. Recently presented early results NRG Oncology CC001 [NCT02360215] phase III trial showed better preservation of neurocognitive function with hippocampal avoidance with memantine [74] The hippocampal sparing whole brain radiotherapy although promising is not accepted worldwide as the standard of care and further clinical data with long term observation is awaited. Stereotactic ablative body radiotherapy (SABR) can be offered to patients with solitary, unresectable and less than 6 cm non-small lung cancer adrenal metastasis where the extra-adrenal disease is either absent or limited and potentially treatable with life expectancy over 6 months. The total doses of 30-36Gy in 3 fractions over 6-7 days or 45Gy in 5 fractions over 10 days results in a local control rate over 90% at 2 years and a median survival range 8 to 22 months with acceptable toxicity [75 - 77]. Spinal oligometastatic disease in non-small cell lung cancer patients who have or have not received prior external beam radiotherapy can be offered SABR with good local and pain controls and acceptable toxicity. 24-27Gy in 2-3 fractions are most frequently used with a less intense dose of 30Gy in 5 fractions recommended when re-irradiation [78]. There is no good enough evidence to support the routine use of SABR to other localisations of metastatic disease in non-small cell lung carcinoma [78].

THE FUTURE DIRECTIONS OF DEVELOPMENT OF RADIOTHERAPY FOR LUNG CANCER

Radiotherapy has been recently transformed by the rapid development of technology mainly driven by progress in computer sciences and this trend is due to continue in the future. The new generation of computer programs so-called artificial intelligence will change the entire field in medicine in general with radiotherapy being subjected to it in particular. The whole chain of processes leading to the delivery of radiotherapy to the patients is very likely to be automatized in the future to transform this service with significantly less workforce needed to produce a better outcome. It will almost certainly cause significant repercussions for the patients, providers and healthcare as a whole compared by some authors to changes imposed by the industrial revolution on the society in the past [79]. The other direction of travel in near future would be combining radiotherapy with immunotherapy or other novel anticancer therapies to improve the outcome in more advanced cases as it was successfully initiated already based the results of Pacific trial [42] with the increased use of stereotactic techniques to deliver ultra hypofractionated radiotherapy both in radical or palliative settings. Finally, particle beam therapies although currently showed no statistically proven advantages over standard photon beam radiotherapy in lung cancer [80], will almost certainly have its role in anticancer treatment in the distant future once technology related to its delivery improves with simultaneous decrease of the cost of this therapy.

MANAGEMENT OF RADIOTHERAPY RELATED TOXICITY

Radiation-induced toxicities are divided into acute (early) toxicities with radiation-induced oesophagitis or radiation-induced pneumonitis (RP) being the most frequently observed which generally occur either during treatment or within first six months of the radiotherapy and chronic (late) toxicities (*e.g.* lung fibrosis) which usually develop between six months to several years after treatment. There is no causative treatment for radiation-induced toxicity and symptomatic management is the only therapeutic option available for the patients experiencing side effects of radiotherapy. Common Terminology Criteria for Adverse Events (CTCAE v4.0) [81] is used for scoring acute and late toxicity caused by radiotherapy. The current progress in technology with IMRT being widely used in radical lung radiotherapy affected in a significant decrease in the occurrence and severity of treatment-related toxicity. Radiotherapy toxicities are predicted based on the dose received by a certain volume of normal tissues and can be significantly reduced during the treatment planning process simultaneously maintaining good coverage of high dose for target volumes containing cancer. Radiation-induced oesophagitis is frequently observed acute toxicity during radical radiotherapy to centrally located lung cancers with onset in the second half of the radiation course with the maximum at the completion. Increasing dysphagia and pain on swallowing are the symptoms of this toxicity. It is mostly managed by adequate, very often opioid, analgesia and appropriate calorie daily intake and hydration with routine use of supplements. When the severe grade of radiation-related oesophagitis tube feeding and intravenous hydration may be required. This is nowadays seldom necessary as the current state of technology usually prevents severe oesophageal toxicity. Oesophageal stricture is rarely observed late toxicity and is treated with endoscopic dilatation [82]. Radiation-induced pneumonitis (RP) is another common toxicity occurring as an aftereffect of delivering radical doses to the lung parenchyma. It usually starts 6-12 weeks following completion of radiation and causes shortness of breath on exertion, persistent non-productive cough, chest pain especially that which worsens with breathing and low-grade fever. The duration of RP is usually 1-4 weeks. The treatment consists of a high dose of corticosteroids; 60 mg/day of prednisolone orally in 1-4 divided doses, cough suppressants, pain killers and apyrexials. Severe RP could cause respiratory distress which may require hospitalisation for respiratory failure management. The incidence of RP is between 15-40% and is usually of mild or moderate severity. The incidence and severity of RP are dose-dependent. The V20 (the percentage of lung receiving more than 20Gy) is the most frequently used dose constrain in radiotherapy treatment planning. The current standard of radiotherapy treatment planning is to keep V20< 30-35% which makes the incidence of moderate RP less than 20% [82]. Radiotherapy induced pulmonary fibrosis is the most common and irreversible late side effects and can lead to severe alteration of respiratory function. Treatment for this toxicity is similar to the treatment of lung fibrosis other than radiation-related etiologies.

Chest wall pain and osteoporotic rib fracture is the specific toxicity related to SABR delivered to very peripheral lung tumours with close location to ribs. Chest wall pain is reported in approximately 10% of patients with severe grade 3 toxicity in about 2.0% [83] and a median time to onset of more than 6 months following treatment end. The risk of symptomatic rib fracture is less than 5% with the median time of onset at 22 months when dose tolerances for chest wall are kept below recommended constrains [84]. The other toxicities are either mild or moderate like skin reaction or rare like cardiac toxicity or very rare like spinal cord radiation induced myelopathy or brachial plexopathy and are treated similarly to the same conditions caused by other clinical entities [82].

CONCLUSIONS/KEY LEARNING POINTS

1. Due to the recent progress of technology, radiotherapy became a very precise and effective treatment modality maintaining good efficacy with fairly low toxicity profile and have a very important role in the management of lung carcinoma.
2. Stereotactic ablative body radiotherapy (SABR) is a very valuable option for medically inoperable patients with early stage non-small lung carcinoma.
3. Concurrent chemo-radiotherapy followed by adjuvant immunotherapy gives the best results in the treatment of locally advanced non-small lung carcinoma with low volume disease and good performance status.
4. Prophylactic cranial irradiation and chest consolidation radiotherapy for patients responding to chemotherapy is the only recent significant advance in the management of small cell lung carcinoma.
5. Palliative radiotherapy especially delivered with stereotactic techniques is a very valuable therapeutic modality in the management in patients with the incurable stage of lung carcinoma.
6. Symptomatic management is the only therapeutic option available for the patients experiencing side effects of radiotherapy.

CONSENT FOR PUBLICATION

Not applicable.

CONFLICT OF INTEREST

The author declares that there is no conflict of interest in this chapter.

ACKNOWLEDGEMENTS

Declared none.

REFERENCES

[1]   Khan FM. The physics of radiation therapy. 5th ed., Baltimore: Williams & Wilkins 2010.

[2]   De Ruysscher D, Faivre-Finn C, Moeller D, *et al.* European Organization for Research and Treatment of Cancer (EORTC) recommendations for planning and delivery of high-dose, high precision radiotherapy for lung cancer. Radiother Oncol 2017; 124(1): 1-10.
        [http://dx.doi.org/10.1016/j.radonc.2017.06.003] [PMID: 28666551]

[3]   Xia P, Godley A, Shah C, Gregory MM. Videtic MDCMF, Suh J Strategies for Radiation Therapy Treatment Planning. Springer Publishing Company 2018.
        [http://dx.doi.org/10.1891/9780826122674]

[4]   Levitt SH, Brady LW, Heilmann HP, *et al.* Technical basis of radiation therapy: Practical clinical applications. Springer Berlin Heidelberg 2008.

[5]   Bortfeld T. IMRT: a review and preview. Phys Med Biol 2006; 51(13): R363-79. [published online ahead of print 2006/06/20].
        [http://dx.doi.org/10.1088/0031-9155/51/13/R21] [PMID: 16790913]

[6]   Cho B. Intensity-modulated radiation therapy: a review with a physics perspective. Radiat Oncol J 2018; 36(1): 1-10. [published online ahead of print 2018/03/30].
        [http://dx.doi.org/10.3857/roj.2018.00122] [PMID: 29621869]

[7]   http://www.icru.org/home/reports

[8]   Bomford CK. Kunkler, I H Joseph Walter, Walter and Miller's Textbook of Radiotherapy: Radiation Physics, Therapy, and Oncology. 6th ed., Churchill Livingstone 2003.

[9]   Blomgren H, Lax I, Näslund I, Svanström R. Stereotactic high dose fraction radiation therapy of extracranial tumors using an accelerator. Clinical experience of the first thirty-one patients. Acta Oncol 1995; 34(6): 861-70.
        [http://dx.doi.org/10.3109/02841869509127197] [PMID: 7576756]

[10]   Nagata Y, Takayama K, Matsuo Y, *et al.* Clinical outcomes of a phase I/II study of 48 Gy of stereotactic body radiotherapy in 4 fractions for primary lung cancer using a stereotactic body frame. Int J Radiat Oncol Biol Phys 2005; 63(5): 1427-31.
        [http://dx.doi.org/10.1016/j.ijrobp.2005.05.034] [PMID: 16169670]

[11]   Nyman J, Johansson KA, Hultén U. Stereotactic hypofractionated radiotherapy for stage I non-small cell lung cancer--mature results for medically inoperable patients. Lung Cancer 2006; 51(1): 97-103.
        [http://dx.doi.org/10.1016/j.lungcan.2005.08.011] [PMID: 16213059]

[12]   Zimmermann FB, Geinitz H, Schill S, *et al.* Stereotactic hypofractionated radiotherapy in stage I (T1-2 N0 M0) non-small-cell lung cancer (NSCLC). Acta Oncol 2006; 45(7): 796-801.
        [http://dx.doi.org/10.1080/02841860600913210] [PMID: 16982542]

[13]   Koto M, Takai Y, Ogawa Y, *et al.* A phase II study on stereotactic body radiotherapy for stage I non-small cell lung cancer. Radiother Oncol 2007; 85(3): 429-34.
        [http://dx.doi.org/10.1016/j.radonc.2007.10.017] [PMID: 18022720]

[14]   Onishi H, Shirato H, Nagata Y, *et al.* Hypofractionated stereotactic radiotherapy (HypoFXSRT) for stage I non-small cell lung cancer: updated results of 257 patients in a Japanese multi-institutional study. J Thorac Oncol 2007; 2(7) (Suppl. 3): S94-S100.
        [http://dx.doi.org/10.1097/JTO.0b013e318074de34] [PMID: 17603311]

[15]   Lagerwaard FJ, Haasbeek CJ, Smit EF, Slotman BJ, Senan S. Outcomes of risk-adapted fractionated stereotactic radiotherapy for stage I non-small-cell lung cancer. Int J Radiat Oncol Biol Phys 2008;

70(3): 685-92.
[http://dx.doi.org/10.1016/j.ijrobp.2007.10.053] [PMID: 18164849]

[16] Baumann P, Nyman J, Hoyer M, *et al.* Outcome in a prospective phase II trial of medically inoperable stage I non-small-cell lung cancer patients treated with stereotactic body radiotherapy. J Clin Oncol 2009; 27(20): 3290-6.
[http://dx.doi.org/10.1200/JCO.2008.21.5681] [PMID: 19414667]

[17] Timmerman R, Paulus R, Galvin J, *et al.* Stereotactic body radiation therapy for inoperable early stage lung cancer. JAMA 2010; 303(11): 1070-6.
[http://dx.doi.org/10.1001/jama.2010.261] [PMID: 20233825]

[18] Ricardi U, Filippi AR, Guarneri A, *et al.* Stereotactic body radiation therapy for early stage non-small cell lung cancer: results of a prospective trial. Lung Cancer 2010; 68(1): 72-7.
[http://dx.doi.org/10.1016/j.lungcan.2009.05.007] [PMID: 19556022]

[19] Taremi M, Hope A, Dahele M, *et al.* Stereotactic body radiotherapy for medically inoperable lung cancer: prospective, single-center study of 108 consecutive patients. Int J Radiat Oncol Biol Phys 2012; 82(2): 967-73.
[http://dx.doi.org/10.1016/j.ijrobp.2010.12.039] [PMID: 21377293]

[20] Lindberg K, Nyman J, Riesenfeld Källskog V, *et al.* Long-term results of a prospective phase II trial of medically inoperable stage I NSCLC treated with SBRT - the Nordic experience. Acta Oncol 2015; 54(8): 1096-104.
[http://dx.doi.org/10.3109/0284186X.2015.1020966] [PMID: 25813471]

[21] Boily G, Filion É, Rakovich G, *et al.* Stereotactic ablative radiation therapy for the treatment of early-stage non-small-cell lung cancer: CEPO review and recommendations. J Thorac Oncol 2015; 10(6): 872-82.
[http://dx.doi.org/10.1097/JTO.0000000000000524] [PMID: 26001140]

[22] Louie AV, Palma DA, Dahele M, Rodrigues GB, Senan S. Management of early-stage non-small cell lung cancer using stereotactic ablative radiotherapy: controversies, insights, and changing horizons. Radiother Oncol 2015; 114(2): 138-47.
[http://dx.doi.org/10.1016/j.radonc.2014.11.036] [PMID: 25497873]

[23] Brada M, Pope A, Baumann M. SABR in NSCLC--the beginning of the end or the end of the beginning? Radiother Oncol 2015; 114(2): 135-7.
[http://dx.doi.org/10.1016/j.radonc.2015.01.012] [PMID: 25665955]

[24] Grills IS, Mangona VS, Welsh R, *et al.* Kestin outcomes after stereotactic lung radiotherapy or wedge resection for stage I non–small-cell lung cancer. J Clin Oncol 2010; 28: 928-35.
[http://dx.doi.org/10.1200/JCO.2009.25.0928]

[25] Chang JY, Senan S, Paul MA, *et al.* Stereotactic ablative radiotherapy versus lobectomy for operable stage I non-small-cell lung cancer: a pooled analysis of two randomised trials. Lancet Oncol 2015; 16(6): 630-7.
[http://dx.doi.org/10.1016/S1470-2045(15)70168-3] [PMID: 25981812]

[26] Chi A, Liao Z, Nguyen NP, Xu J, Stea B, Komaki R. Systemic review of the patterns of failure following stereotactic body radiation therapy in early-stage non-small-cell lung cancer: clinical implications. Radiother Oncol 2010; 94(1): 1-11.
[http://dx.doi.org/10.1016/j.radonc.2009.12.008] [PMID: 20074823]

[27] Timmerman R, McGarry R, Yiannoutsos C, *et al.* Excessive toxicity when treating central tumors in a phase II study of stereotactic body radiation therapy for medically inoperable early-stage lung cancer. J Clin Oncol 2006; 24(30): 4833-9.
[http://dx.doi.org/10.1200/JCO.2006.07.5937] [PMID: 17050868]

[28] Chang JY, Bezjak A, Mornex F. Stereotactic ablative radiotherapy for centrally located early stage non-small-cell lung cancer: what we have learned. J Thorac Oncol 2015; 10(4): 577-85.
[http://dx.doi.org/10.1097/JTO.0000000000000453] [PMID: 25514807]

[29]   Senthi S, Haasbeek CJ, Slotman BJ, Senan S. Outcomes of stereotactic ablative radiotherapy for central lung tumours: a systematic review. Radiother Oncol 2013; 106(3): 276-82.
[http://dx.doi.org/10.1016/j.radonc.2013.01.004] [PMID: 23462705]

[30]   Tekatli H, Haasbeek N, Dahele M, *et al*. Outcomes of hypofractionated high-dose radiotherapy in poor-risk patients with "ultracentral" non-small cell lung cancer. J Thorac Oncol 2016; 11(7): 1081-9.
[http://dx.doi.org/10.1016/j.jtho.2016.03.008] [PMID: 27013408]

[31]   Rowell NP, Williams CJ. Radical radiotherapy for stage I/II non-small cell lung cancer in patients not sufficiently fit for or declining surgery (medically inoperable): a systematic review. Thorax 2001; 56(8): 628-38.
[http://dx.doi.org/10.1136/thorax.56.8.628] [PMID: 11462066]

[32]   Aupérin A, Le Péchoux C, Rolland E, *et al*. Meta-analysis of concomitant versus sequential radiochemotherapy in locally advanced non-small-cell lung cancer. J Clin Oncol 2010; 28(13): 2181-90.
[http://dx.doi.org/10.1200/JCO.2009.26.2543] [PMID: 20351327]

[33]   Bradley JD, *et al*. Long-term results of NRG oncology RTOG 0617: Standard- *versus* high-dose chemoradiotherapy with or without cetuximab for unresectable stage III non–small-cell lung cancer. J Clin Oncol 2019 December 16;
[http://dx.doi.org/10.1200/JCO.19.01162] [PMID: 31841363]

[34]   Bradley JD, Paulus R, Komaki R, *et al*. Standard-dose versus high-dose conformal radiotherapy with concurrent and consolidation carboplatin plus paclitaxel with or without cetuximab for patients with stage IIIA or IIIB non-small-cell lung cancer (RTOG 0617): a randomised, two-by-two factorial phase 3 study. Lancet Oncol 2015; 16(2): 187-99.
[http://dx.doi.org/10.1016/S1470-2045(14)71207-0] [PMID: 25601342]

[35]   Ahn JS, Ahn YC, Kim JH, *et al*. Multinational randomized phase III trial with or without consolidation chemotherapy using docetaxel and cisplatin after con-current chemoradiation in inoperable stage III non–small-cell lung cancer: KCSG-LU05-04. J Clin Oncol 2015; 33(24): 2660-6.
[http://dx.doi.org/10.1200/JCO.2014.60.0130] [PMID: 26150444]

[36]   Warner A, Dahele M, Hu B, *et al*. Factors associated with early mortality in patients treated with concurrent chemoradiation therapy for locally advanced non-small cell lung cancer. Int J Radiat Oncol Biol Phys 2016; 94(3): 612-20.
[http://dx.doi.org/10.1016/j.ijrobp.2015.11.030] [PMID: 26867890]

[37]   Vokes EE, Herndon JE II, Kelley MJ, *et al*. Induction chemotherapy followed by chemoradiotherapy compared with chemoradiotherapy alone for regionally advanced unresectable stage III Non-small-cell lung cancer: Cancer and Leukemia Group B. J Clin Oncol 2007; 25(13): 1698-704.
[http://dx.doi.org/10.1200/JCO.2006.07.3569] [PMID: 17404369]

[38]   Skrzypski M, Jassem J. Consolidation systemic treatment after radiochemotherapy for unresectable stage III non-small cell lung cancer. Cancer Treat Rev 2018; 66: 114-21.
[http://dx.doi.org/10.1016/j.ctrv.2018.04.001] [PMID: 29738940]

[39]   Tsujino K, Kurata T, Yamamoto S, *et al*. Is consolidation chemotherapy after concurrent chemo-radiotherapy beneficial for patients with locally advanced non-small-cell lung cancer? A pooled analysis of the literature. J Thorac Oncol 2013; 8(9): 1181-9.
[http://dx.doi.org/10.1097/JTO.0b013e3182988348] [PMID: 23883782]

[40]   Hanna N, Neubauer M, Yiannoutsos C, *et al*. Phase III study of cisplatin, etoposide, and concurrent chest radiation with or without consolidation docetaxel in patients with inoperable stage III non-smal--cell lung cancer: the Hoosier Oncology Group and U.S. Oncology. J Clin Oncol 2008; 26(35): 5755-60.
[http://dx.doi.org/10.1200/JCO.2008.17.7840] [PMID: 19001323]

[41]   Antonia SJ, Villegas A, Daniel D, *et al*. Durvalumab after chemoradiotherapy in stage III non–small-cell lung cancer. N Engl J Med 2017; 377(20): 1919-29.

[http://dx.doi.org/10.1056/NEJMoa1709937] [PMID: 28885881]

[42] Antonia SJ, Villegas A, Daniel D, *et al.* Overall survival with durvalumab after chemoradiotherapy in stage III NSCLC. N Engl J Med 2018; 379(24): 2342-50.
[http://dx.doi.org/10.1056/NEJMoa1809697] [PMID: 30280658]

[43] Postmus PE, Kerr KM, Oudkerk M, *et al.* Early and locally advanced non-small-cell lung cancer (NSCLC): ESMO Clinical Practice Guidelines for diagnosis, treatment and follow-up. Annals of Oncology 2017; 28(Supplement 4)

[44] Mauguen A, Le Péchoux C, Saunders MI, *et al.* Hyperfractionated or accelerated radiotherapy in lung cancer: an individual patient data meta-analysis. J Clin Oncol 2012; 30(22): 2788-97.
[http://dx.doi.org/10.1200/JCO.2012.41.6677] [PMID: 22753901]

[45] PORT Meta-analysis Trialists Group. Postoperative radiotherapy for nonsmall cell lung cancer. Cochrane Database Syst Rev 2005. CD002142

[46] Albain KS, Swann RS, Rusch VW, *et al.* Radiotherapy plus chemotherapy with or without surgical resection for stage III non-small-cell lung cancer: a phase III randomised controlled trial. Lancet 2009; 374(9687): 379-86.
[http://dx.doi.org/10.1016/S0140-6736(09)60737-6] [PMID: 19632716]

[47] Pless M, Stupp R, Ris HB, *et al.* Induction chemoradiation in stage IIIA/N2 non-small-cell lung cancer: a phase 3 randomised trial. Lancet 2015; 386(9998): 1049-56.
[http://dx.doi.org/10.1016/S0140-6736(15)60294-X] [PMID: 26275735]

[48] Eberhardt WE, Pöttgen C, Gauler TC, *et al.* Phase III study of surgery versus definitive concurrent chemoradiotherapy boost in patients with resectable stage IIIA(N2) and selected IIIB non–small-cell lung cancer after induction chemotherapy and concurrent chemoradiotherapy (ESPATUE). J Clin Oncol 2015; 33(35): 4194-201.
[http://dx.doi.org/10.1200/JCO.2015.62.6812] [PMID: 26527789]

[49] Glatzer M, Rittmeyer A, Müller J, *et al.* Treatment of limited disease small cell lung cancer: the multidisciplinary team. Eur Respir J 2017; 50(2)1700422
[http://dx.doi.org/10.1183/13993003.00422-2017] [PMID: 28838979]

[50] Warde P, Payne D. Does thoracic irradiation improve survival and local control in limited-stage small-cell carcinoma of the lung? A meta-analysis. J Clin Oncol 1992; 10(6): 890-5.
[http://dx.doi.org/10.1200/JCO.1992.10.6.890] [PMID: 1316951]

[51] Pignon J-P, Arriagada R, Ihde DC, *et al.* A meta-analysis of thoracic radiotherapy for small-cell lung cancer. N Engl J Med 1992; 327(23): 1618-24.
[http://dx.doi.org/10.1056/NEJM199212033272302] [PMID: 1331787]

[52] Murray N, Coy P, Pater JL, *et al.* Importance of timing for thoracic irradiation in the combined modality treatment of limited-stage small-cell lung cancer. The National Cancer Institute of Canada Clinical Trials Group. J Clin Oncol 1993; 11: 336-44.

[53] Fried DB, Morris DE, Poole C, *et al.* Systematic review evaluating the timing of thoracic radiation therapy in combined modality therapy for limited-stage small-cell lung cancer. J Clin Oncol 2004; 22(23): 4837-45.
[http://dx.doi.org/10.1200/JCO.2004.01.178] [PMID: 15570087]

[54] Pijls-Johannesma M, De Ruysscher D, Vansteenkiste J, *et al.* Timing of chest radiotherapy in patients with limited stage small cell lung cancer: a systematic review and meta-analysis of randomised controlled trials. Cancer Treat Rev 2007; 33(5): 461-73.
[http://dx.doi.org/10.1016/j.ctrv.2007.03.002] [PMID: 17513057]

[55] Spiro SG, James LE, Rudd RM, *et al.* Early compared with late radiotherapy in combined modality treatment for limited disease small-cell lung cancer: a London Lung Cancer Group multicenter randomized clinical trial and meta-analysis. J Clin Oncol 2006; 24(24): 3823-30.
[http://dx.doi.org/10.1200/JCO.2005.05.3181] [PMID: 16921033]

[56]   Turrisi AT III, Kim K, Blum R, *et al.* Twice-daily compared with once-daily thoracic radiotherapy in limited small-cell lung cancer treated concurrently with cisplatin and etoposide. N Engl J Med 1999; 340(4): 265-71.
[http://dx.doi.org/10.1056/NEJM199901283400403] [PMID: 9920950]

[57]   Faivre-Finn C, Snee M, Ashcroft L, *et al.* Concurrent once-daily versus twice-daily chemoradiotherapy in patients with limited-stage small-cell lung cancer (CONVERT): an open-label, phase 3, randomised, superiority trial. Lancet Oncol 2017; 18(8): 1116-25.
[http://dx.doi.org/10.1016/S1470-2045(17)30318-2] [PMID: 28642008]

[58]   Slotman BJ, van Tinteren H, Praag JO, *et al.* Use of thoracic radiotherapy for extensive stage small-cell lung cancer: a phase 3 randomised controlled trial. Lancet 2015; 385(9962): 36-42.
[http://dx.doi.org/10.1016/S0140-6736(14)61085-0] [PMID: 25230595]

[59]   Palma DA, Warner A, Louie AV, *et al.* Thoracic radiotherapy for extensive stage small-cell lung cancer: a meta-analysis. Clin Lung Cancer 2016; 17(4): 239-44.
[http://dx.doi.org/10.1016/j.cllc.2015.09.007] [PMID: 26498503]

[60]   Hirsch FR, Paulson OB, Hansen HH, Vraa-Jensen J. Intracranial metastases in small cell carcinoma of the lung: correlation of clinical and autopsy findings. Cancer 1982; 50(11): 2433-7.
[http://dx.doi.org/10.1002/1097-0142(19821201)50:11<2433::AID-CNCR2820501131>3.0.CO;2-E] [PMID: 6182974]

[61]   Komaki R, Cox JD, Whitson W. Risk of brain metastasis from small cell carcinoma of the lung related to length of survival and prophylactic irradiation. Cancer Treat Rep 1981; 65(9-10): 811-4.
[PMID: 6268295]

[62]   Aupérin A, Arriagada R, Pignon JP, *et al.* Prophylactic cranial irradiation for patients with small-cell lung cancer in complete remission. N Engl J Med 1999; 341(7): 476-84.
[http://dx.doi.org/10.1056/NEJM199908123410703] [PMID: 10441603]

[63]   Wolfson AH, Bae K, Komaki R, *et al.* Primary analysis of a phase II randomized trial Radiation Therapy Oncology Group (RTOG) 0212: impact of different total doses and schedules of prophylactic cranial irradiation on chronic neurotoxicity and quality of life for patients with limited-disease small-cell lung cancer. Int J Radiat Oncol Biol Phys 2011; 81(1): 77-84.
[http://dx.doi.org/10.1016/j.ijrobp.2010.05.013] [PMID: 20800380]

[64]   Zhang W, Jiang W, Luan L, Wang L, Zheng X, Wang G. Prophylactic cranial irradiation for patients with small-cell lung cancer: a systematic review of the literature with meta-analysis. BMC Cancer 2014; 14: 793.
[http://dx.doi.org/10.1186/1471-2407-14-793] [PMID: 25361811]

[65]   Le Péchoux C, Dunant A, Senan S, *et al.* Standard-dose *versus* higher-dose prophylactic cranial irradiation (PCI) in patients with limited-stage small-cell lung cancer in complete remission after chemotherapy and thoracic radiotherapy (PCI 99-01, EORTC 22003-08004, RTOG 0212, and IFCT 99-01): a randomised clinical trial. Lancet Oncol 2009; 10(5): 467-74.
[http://dx.doi.org/10.1016/S1470-2045(09)70101-9] [PMID: 19386548]

[66]   Slotman B, Faivre-Finn C, Kramer G, *et al.* Prophylactic cranial irradiation in extensive small-cell lung cancer. N Engl J Med 2007; 357(7): 664-72.
[http://dx.doi.org/10.1056/NEJMoa071780] [PMID: 17699816]

[67]   Takahashi T, Yamanaka T, Seto T, *et al.* Prophylactic cranial irradiation *versus* observation in patients with extensive-disease small-cell lung cancer: a multicentre, randomised, open-label, phase 3 trial. Lancet Oncol 2017; 18(5): 663-71.
[http://dx.doi.org/10.1016/S1470-2045(17)30230-9] [PMID: 28343976]

[68]   Suzuki R, Komaki R. Is prophylactic cranial irradiation indicated for patients with extensive-stage small cell lung cancer with a complete response to first-line treatment? Radiother Oncol 2018; 127(3): 339-43.
[http://dx.doi.org/10.1016/j.radonc.2018.03.034] [PMID: 29747874]

[69] Rodrigues G, Videtic GM, Sur R, *et al.* Palliative thoracic radiotherapy in lung cancer: An American Society for Radiation Oncology evidence-based clinical practice guideline. Pract Radiat Oncol 2011; 1(2): 60-71.
[http://dx.doi.org/10.1016/j.prro.2011.01.005] [PMID: 25740118]

[70] Spencer K, Parrish R, Barton R, Henry A. Palliative radiotherapy. BMJ 2018; 360: k821.
[http://dx.doi.org/10.1136/bmj.k821] [PMID: 29572337]

[71] Tsao MN, Rades D, Wirth A, *et al.* Radiotherapeutic and surgical management for newly diagnosed brain metastasis(es): An American Society for Radiation Oncology evidence-based guideline. Pract Radiat Oncol 2012; 2(3): 210-25.
[http://dx.doi.org/10.1016/j.prro.2011.12.004] [PMID: 25925626]

[72] Suh JH. Stereotactic radiosurgery for the management of brain metastases. N Engl J Med 2010; 362(12): 1119-27.
[http://dx.doi.org/10.1056/NEJMct0806951] [PMID: 20335588]

[73] Gondi V, Pugh SL, Tome WA, *et al.* Preservation of memory with conformal avoidance of the hippocampal neural stem-cell compartment during whole-brain radiotherapy for brain metastases (RTOG 0933): a phase II multi-institutional trial. J Clin Oncol 2014; 32(34): 3810-6.
[http://dx.doi.org/10.1200/JCO.2014.57.2909] [PMID: 25349290]

[74] Gondi V, Deshmukh S, Brown PD, *et al.* NRG Oncology CC001: A phase III trial of hippocampal avoidance (HA) in addition to whole-brain radiotherapy (WBRT) plus memantine to preserve neurocognitive function (NCF) in patients with brain metastases (BM).
https://ascopubs.org/doi/abs/10.1200/JCO.2019.37.15_suppl.2009

[75] Casamassima F, Livi L, Masciullo S, *et al.* Stereotactic radiotherapy for adrenal gland metastases: university of Florence experience. Int J Radiat Oncol Biol Phys 2012; 82(2): 919-23.
[http://dx.doi.org/10.1016/j.ijrobp.2010.11.060] [PMID: 21300473]

[76] Ahmed KA, Barney BM, Macdonald OK, *et al.* Stereotactic body radiotherapy in the treatment of adrenal metastases. Am J Clin Oncol 2013; 36(5): 509-13.
[http://dx.doi.org/10.1097/COC.0b013e3182569189] [PMID: 22781389]

[77] Gunjur A, Duong C, Ball D, Siva S. Surgical and ablative therapies for the management of adrenal 'oligometastases' - A systematic review. Cancer Treat Rev 2014; 40(7): 838-46.
[http://dx.doi.org/10.1016/j.ctrv.2014.04.001] [PMID: 24791623]

[78] The Faculty of Clinical Oncology of The Royal College of Radiologists. Stereotactic Ablative Body Radiation Therapy (SABR): A Resource SABR UK Consortium. Version 6.1, January 2019.
https://www.sabr.org.uk/

[79] Thompson RF, Valdes G, Fuller CD, *et al.* Artificial intelligence in radiation oncology: A specialty-wide disruptive transformation? Radiother Oncol 2018; 129(3): 421-6.
[http://dx.doi.org/10.1016/j.radonc.2018.05.030] [PMID: 29907338]

[80] Chi A, Chen H, Wen S, Yan H, Liao Z. Comparison of particle beam therapy and stereotactic body radiotherapy for early stage non-small cell lung cancer: A systematic review and hypothesis-generating meta-analysis. Radiother Oncol 2017; 123(3): 346-54.
[http://dx.doi.org/10.1016/j.radonc.2017.05.007] [PMID: 28545956]

[81] Common Terminology Criteria for Adverse Events CTCAE v4.0.
http://www.acrin.org/Portals/0/Administration/Regulatory/CTCAE_4.02_2009-09-15_QuickReference_5x7.pdf

[82] Quantitative Analysis of Normal Tissue Effects in the Clinic (QUANTEC). Int J Radiat Oncol Biol Phys 2010; 76(3) (Suppl.).

[83] Murray P, Franks K, Hanna G. Systematic review of outcomes following stereotactic ablative radiotherapy in the treatment of early-stage primary lung cancer. Br J Radio 2017; 90(1071)

[84]   Stam B, van der Bijl E, Peulen H, *et al.* Dose-effect analysis of radiation induced rib fractures after thoracic SBRT. Radiother Oncol 2017; 123(2): 176-81.
[http://dx.doi.org/10.1016/j.radonc.2017.01.004] [PMID: 28110960]

CHAPTER 12

The Role of Systemic Anti-Cancer Therapy in the Management of Lung Carcinoma

Alexandra R. Lewis[*] and **Laura Cove-Smith**

The Christie Hospital The Christie NHS Foundation Trust 550 Wilmslow Road, Manchester, M20 4BX, England

Abstract: The aim of this chapter is to describe the role of systemic anti-cancer therapy in the management of lung cancer. The introduction describes the different sub-types of lung cancer as this is highly pertinent to the treatment options available. We move on to discuss the main sub-types of systemic anti-cancer therapy used for lung cancer and their mechanisms of action; specifically regarding cytotoxic chemotherapy, targeted therapy including tyrosine kinase inhibitors, monoclonal antibodies and immunotherapy, namely checkpoint inhibitors. From here we move on to discuss adjuvant systemic anti-cancer therapy following surgical resection for both small cell lung cancer and non-small cell lung cancer. Following this, we move on to describe systemic anti-cancer therapy for incurable lung cancer starting with the recent historical perspective and the remarkable changes and developments that have occurred in this field over the last ten years. We discuss systemic therapy for small cell lung cancer and non-small cell lung cancer, focussing on non-mutated adenocarcinoma, EGFR and ALK mutant adenocarcinoma and squamous cell lung cancer. In conclusion, we describe future perspectives and the importance of a joined-up approach to diagnosis, investigation and management to improve outcomes for patients with lung cancer.

Keywords: ALK Mutant Lung Cancer, Adjuvant Systemic Anti-Cancer Therapy, Cytotoxic Chemotherapy, Checkpoint Inhibitors, EGFR Mutant Lung Cancer, Immunotherapy, Monoclonal Antibodies, Non-Small Cell Lung Carcinoma, Palliative Systemic Anti-Cancer Therapy, Ros-1 Mutant Lung Cancer, Systemic Anti-Cancer Therapy, Small-Cell Lung Cancer, Tyrosine Kinase Inhibitors.

INTRODUCTION

The field of systemic anti-cancer therapy (SACT) for lung cancer has widened markedly in recent years with an explosion of new treatments and treatment combinations. The field is also changing regularly. Given these rapid changes, the

[*] **Corresponding author Alexandra R Lewis:** The Christie Hospital The Christie NHS Foundation Trust 550 Wilmslow Road, Manchester, M20 4BX, England; Tel: 0161 446 3000; E-mail: Alexandra.lewis@christie.nhs.uk

Keyvan Moghissi, Jack Kastelik, Philip Barber & Peyman Sardari Nia (Eds.)

information in this chapter will become rapidly out of date. We have limited the remit of this chapter to treatments that have the European Medicines Agency (EMA) and National Institute of Clinical Excellence (NICE) approval at the time of writing.

It is also important to note that lung cancer is not one disease. There are multiple different sub-types of lung cancer and they are all treated differently. As such, this article will only be able to provide a relatively brief overview of the issues surrounding treatment for these diseases.

SUB-TYPES OF LUNG CANCER

Broadly speaking, lung cancer can be divided into small-cell lung cancer (SCLC) which accounts for 10-15% of all lung cancers and non-small cell lung cancer (NSCLC) which makes up the remaining 85-90% [1]. Non-small cell lung cancer can be further divided into squamous cell carcinoma (SCC) or non-squamous, of which the most common sub-type is adenocarcinoma (AC) which accounts for 40% of all lung cancers [2]. For the purposes of lung cancer management, we also then sub-divide AC to tumours which harbour a genetic mutation or not. These mutations include epidermal growth factor receptor (EGFR), anaplastic lymphoma kinase (ALK), ROS-1[3] and these will be discussed in more detail below. These subtypes are summarised in Fig. (**1**).

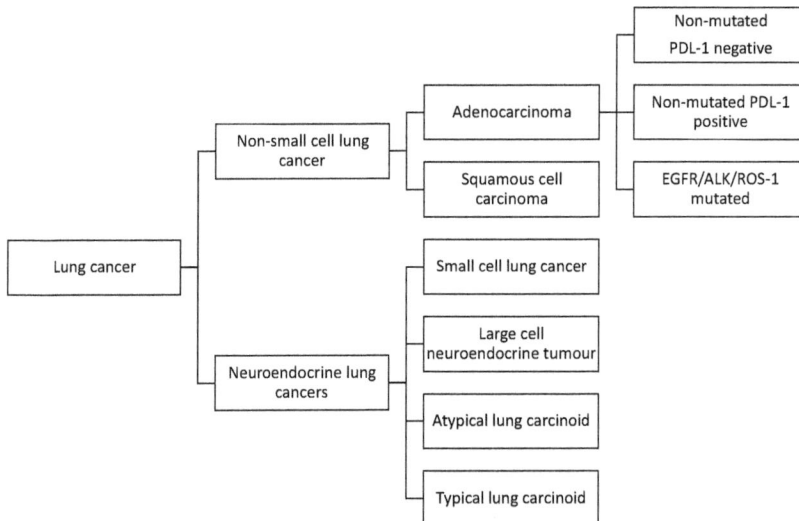

Fig. (1). Subtypes of lung cancer.

Small cell lung cancer is a form of highly aggressive, rapidly growing cancer that derives from neuroendocrine cells [4]. It exists on a spectrum of tumours that arise from the same tissue but cover a wide range of aggression and behaviours and these include typical carcinoids, atypical carcinoids and large cell neuro-endocrine tumours [5]. These tumours can arise from any site within the body, with the lung, and GI tract being most common. There are variations in practice but both nationally and internationally, as typical and atypical carcinoids are a very rare subtype, accounting for <2% of lung neoplasms and are not always treated by lung cancer physicians, they will not be covered in detail within this chapter.

EGFR, ROS-1, and ALK mutant lung cancers are more common in younger patients, women, and never smokers, they are almost invariably adenocarcinoma and are treated differently to non-mutated NSCLC [6]. They tend to be slow growing and patients can have a large volume of disease, with relatively few symptoms. They are also much more likely than patients with non-mutated NSCLC to develop metastases within the brain with around 50% of patients with EGFR or ALK mutations eventually developing brain metastases [7].

BASIC PRINCIPLES OF SYSTEMIC ANTI-CANCER THERAPY

It could have been argued that chemotherapy and systemic anti-cancer therapy (SACT) were synonyms. However, given the popular perception of chemotherapy as relating to cytotoxic chemotherapy and the rapid rise in the use of targeted or immunotherapy, the term SACT has become more often used to encompass all drug therapy for cancer treatment and we will use this term within this chapter.

There are three main groups of SACT used for the treatment of lung cancer; cytotoxic chemotherapy, targeted agents (either monoclonal antibodies (mABs) or tyrosine kinase inhibitors (TKIs) and immunotherapy.

Cytotoxic Chemotherapy

Cytotoxic chemotherapy is the oldest of these groups of drugs. Their mechanism of action is to disrupt cell growth by interrupting the process of DNA replication and cell division [8,9]. However, their action, though preferentially targeting rapidly dividing cancer cells is non-specific and thus other cells with high turnovers such as the bone marrow and gastrointestinal tract may also be affected. Cytotoxic chemotherapy can be associated with significant toxicity, such as hair loss, vomiting and bone marrow suppression, peripheral neuropathy, hearing loss and some drugs can cause pneumonitis. Clinicians, therefore, need to carefully balance the risks and benefits of chemotherapy and this is particularly important in lung cancer populations, due to the relatively low efficacy and significant effects on quality of life.

Targeted Agents

These drugs can have different mechanisms of actions; however, those most commonly used in lung cancer; TKIs are generally oral drugs that disrupt intracellular signalling to inhibit functions required for cancer growth and spread such as angiogenesis and proliferation.

Many cancers will have mutations in genes coding for receptors or proteins in the cell signalling pathway (often gain of function mutations) which will then be the main driver for the development, growth and spread of cancer (known as oncogenic mutations).

As they are targeting specific mutated proteins, the hope when developing these agents was for effective cancer treatment without the toxicity traditionally associated with cytotoxic chemotherapy. Targeted agents are associated with toxicity, it is usually different from the toxicity of cytotoxic chemotherapy, such as rashes, derangement of liver function tests and diarrhoea. Sometimes this toxicity can be significant. Similarly, these drugs are usually taken daily until the development of drug resistance and disease progression and as such relatively low level but persistent toxicity over many months can have a significant impact on the patient's quality of life.

Immunotherapy

Although some forms of immunomodulatory SACT have been available for many years, the recent revolution in lung cancer treatment has been driven by the development of a family of drugs commonly called immunotherapy or checkpoint inhibitors. They have proven efficacy in several cancers and most importantly in some patients, these responses appear to be long-lasting and involve total disappearance of visible disease, even in patients with metastatic cancer [10].

These drugs block innate immune-suppressive mechanisms (essentially immune system self-regulation processes) and allow the immune system of the patient to act against cancer. There are two main types of immunotherapy, those blocking the checkpoint CTLA-4 found on T cells and those blocking either programmed death-1 (PD-1) expressed on T cells and natural killer cells or programmed death receptor ligand-1 (PDL-1) expressed on tumours cells. When antigen-presenting cells present tumour antigen to T cells, activation of the T cell-mediated immune response can be suppressed by the PD1-PDL1 checkpoint. Therefore, inhibition of this blockade allows an uninhibited T cells response against the tumour [11]. In some cancers, the proportion of PDL-1 present on tumour cells is a biomarker for response to PD1 inhibitors.

The drugs are all given on an intravenous basis and currently are given for 2 years or until the point of disease progression (whichever comes sooner). They are generally well tolerated with relatively few side-effects. When side effects do arise, they are immune-mediated and can occur in any tissue within the body. The commonest are thyroiditis, colitis, hepatitis, dermatitis and pneumonitis [12]. These toxicities will usually resolve following treatment with corticosteroids, an exception is endocrine toxicities, most commonly thyroiditis leading to long-term hypothyroidism requiring long-term thyroid hormone replacement. A particular problem when treating patients with lung cancer with immunotherapy is the diagnosis of pneumonitis. Pneumonitis does not appear to be common in patients with lung cancer although in a recent case-series, 75% of cases identified were patients with lung cancer [13]. However, it may be difficult to diagnose in patients who often have co-morbidities such as chronic obstructive pulmonary disease causing overlapping symptoms, or previous treatment effects such as radiation pneumonitis making radiological diagnosis more challenging. Pneumonitis does appear to be frequent in previous smokers and rates [14] of treatment-associated mortality due to pneumonitis are higher in patients with lung cancer.

TREATMENT SETTINGS

SACT may be given in the neo-adjuvant, adjuvant (either pre- or post-definitive surgical management) or palliative setting. In the case of lung cancer, there has not to date been an identified role for neo-adjuvant treatment, although several studies are ongoing using different combinations of chemotherapy, immunotherapy and radiotherapy pre and post-surgery and will report over coming years.

Adjuvant treatment post-surgery is indicated as will be discussed below, and more recently maintenance immunotherapy following chemoradiotherapy has been approved (as is discussed in further detail in the chapter on radiotherapy). However the majority of SACT is given in the palliative setting for patients with either metastatic disease, or disease which is locally advanced and not amenable to radical chemo-radiotherapy either due to the size of the radiotherapy field or patient fitness.

Adjuvant Chemotherapy Following Surgery

Adjuvant Chemotherapy for Small Cell Lung Cancer

Only ~5% of patients with SCLC will present with stage I/II disease amenable to surgery [4] and as such, there is limited data supporting the use of adjuvant chemotherapy. It has been recommended in guidelines, extrapolating from the evidence of more advanced disease, on the basis that small cell lung cancer, though aggressive is also a very chemo-sensitive disease. A retrospective case study of >1400 patients with stage I resected lung cancer found that those receiving adjuvant chemotherapy had a 5-year overall survival (OS) of 52.7% *vs* 40.4% for those receiving surgery alone [15]. Thus for those patients who do have a resected stage I/II SCLC, 4 cycles of platinum-based chemotherapy should be a standard option (with consideration given to prophylactic cranial irradiation as discussed within the chapter on radiotherapy).

Adjuvant Chemotherapy for Non-small Cell Lung Cancer

Adjuvant chemotherapy is recommended for resected stage II-III NSCLC [16] as per the TNM 8th edition. For reference, the TNM staging for I-III disease is included in Table **1**. However, at the time of recruitment to most of the studies discussed below, the TNM 6th staging was in use and this contained some differences. It should be noted that the preferred treatment for patients with stage III lung cancer is concurrent or sequential chemoradiotherapy rather than surgery; however, patients with pre-operative stage II disease may be upstaged on resection pathology and this was more frequently the case in the past when there was less use of endobronchial ultrasounds (EBUS) and positron emission tomography (PET) scanning for staging.

Table 1. Tumour Node Metastasis (TNM) staging 8th Edition (simplified version).

Tumour		Node		Metastasis	
X	• Tumour not assessable but presence of malignant cells confirmed	X	• Regional lymph nodes cannot be assessed		
0/is	• No evidence primary tumour • Carcinoma in situ	0	• No regional lymph node metastasis	0	No distant metastasis
1	• Tumour <3cm in maximum diameter	1	• Metastasis in ipsilateral peribronchial • and/or ipsilateral hilar lymph nodes and intrapulmonary nodes,	1	Distant metastasis present
2	• Tumour >3cm but < 5cm in maximum diameter	2	• Metastasis in ipsilateral mediastinal • and/or subcarinal lymph node(s)		
3	• Tumour >5cm but < 7cm in maximum diameter • or invading ≥1 of chest wall (including superior sulcus tumours), phrenic nerve, parietal pericardium; • or associated separate tumour nodule(s) in the same lobe as the primary	3	• Metastasis in contralateral mediastinal, or hilar nodes • Or ipsilateral or contralateral scalene • or supraclavicular lymph node(s)		

(Table 1) cont.....

4	• Tumour > 7 cm in maximum diameter • or invading any of the following: diaphragm, mediastinum, heart, great vessels, trachea, recurrent laryngeal nerve, oesophagus, vertebral body, carina; • or separate tumour nodule(s) in a different ipsilateral lobe to that of the primary			
Staging				
1A	T1 N0 M0			
1B	T2a N0 M0			
2A	T2b N0 M0			
2B	T1/2 N1 M0 or T3 N0 M0			
3A	T1/2 N2 M0 or T3 N1 M0 or T4 N0/1 M0			
3B	T1/2 N3 M0, or T3/4 N2 M0			
3C	T3/4 N3 M0			
4	Any T, any N, M1			

There has been some debate over what stage of lung cancer should receive adjuvant chemotherapy; The International Adjuvant Lung cancer Trial (IALT) trial treated > 1800 patients with cisplatin-based chemotherapy (with choice of mitomycin, etoposide, vinorelbine or vinblastine) or observation after surgical resection. The study included patients with stage II-III lung cancer. It demonstrated a 44.5% *vs* 40.4% benefit in survival at 5 years. There was a chemotherapy-related death rate of 0.8%. The benefit of chemotherapy was most pronounced in patients with stage III disease [17]. There was a greater benefit for patients with stage III disease in this study.

The ANITA trial published two years later included 840 patients with stage Ib-IIIa resected NSCLC and compared a combination of cisplatin-vinorelbine with observation alone [18]. This study noted a larger, 8.7%, benefit in disease-free survival (DFS) at 5 years. The benefit was 2% for those with stage Ib disease, 13% for those with stage II disease and 16% for patients with stage IIIa disease. The study also reported a 2% toxic death rate.

A further study in 2005 compared cisplatin vinorelbine with observation post-surgical resection in 482 patients with stage Ib-II disease (with a 45% stage Ib - 55% stage II split) [19]. A relapse-free survival (RFS) rate at 5 years was 69% for the chemotherapy arm *vs* 54% in the observation group, although this value was significant (p 0.03), it appeared to be driven by the patients with stage II disease. The hazard ratio for survival for stage Ib patients was not significant p 0.79 compared with p 0.004 for those with stage II disease.

Based on these studies, the recommendation is to offer adjuvant chemotherapy only to fit patients with stage II-III resected NSCLC [16]. It should be noted that the impact of thoracic surgery, particularly where the patient has undergone a pneumonectomy, can be significant. The recommendation based on trial criteria is to commence adjuvant chemotherapy within 16 weeks of treatment and many patients are not sufficiently well enough to undergo relatively toxic treatment at this point.

A final point to note is that for all of the trials that have studied adjuvant chemotherapy, even for those with early, stage Ib disease, between 40-60% of patients still relapse despite surgery and chemotherapy and there is a real need for more effective adjuvant therapies for these patients.

Systemic Anti-cancer Therapy for Metastatic Disease

A (Recent) Historical Perceptive

As recently as 4 or 5 years ago, when this author first started treating patients with lung cancer, the treatment options available were relatively limited. For the majority of patients with both SCLC and NSCLC, there were only 1-2 lines of therapy available and the median OS was within 12 months.

The explosion of potential treatment options means that treatment pathways are more complex now, and survival has improved, although sadly, for many patients remains limited.

Systemic Anti-cancer Therapy for Advanced Small Cell Lung Cancer

Small cell lung cancer is a rapidly progressing, aggressive disease. Unfortunately, many patients present with advanced disease and with a history of a rapidly deteriorating performance status.

Until very recently the standard of care first-line chemotherapy for advanced SCLC has been 4 cycles of chemotherapy with cisplatin and etoposide [4]. Multiple regimens have been trialled but a meta-analysis of 36 trials found a benefit for combinations combining platinum and etoposide [20]. Response rates to this combination can be as high as 70% but unfortunately, despite this, responses are short-lived and the median progression-free survival (PFS) is just 5.5 months and OS of less than 10 months. A further meta-analysis confirmed that carboplatin has similar response rates and overall survival to cisplatin and has lower renal and neurotoxicity rates (though higher haematological toxicity) and therefore carboplatin may be used in place of cisplatin [21].

In 2018, the IMpower 133 study reported on a combination of the PDL-1 inhibitor atezolizumab with carboplatin and etoposide for first-line treatment of metastatic small cell lung cancer *vs* carboplatin, etoposide and placebo. Patients received 4 cycles of the triplet combination and then continued on maintenance treatment with either atezolizumab or placebo until the point of progression or unacceptable toxicity.

The study reported a 2 month OS benefit of 12.3 compared with 10.3 months, p0.007 [22] and an acceptable toxicity profile and the combination is likely to receive approval. This is the first trial to demonstrate a significant benefit for metastatic SCLC in over 20 years; however, it remains to be seen, at least in the UK, how many patients actually benefit from it. The funding for the drug will almost certainly demand that patients be of sufficient fitness to tolerate combination chemotherapy and the extra potential toxicity of immunotherapy and sadly, due to the aggressive nature of the disease, only a relatively small proportion of patients present still well.

For patients who progress on first-line treatment or relapse within 6 weeks, further chemotherapy is unlikely to be of benefit and patients should be offered the best supportive care. Various second-line treatment options are available, including re-challenge with carboplatin etoposide for patients who had a longer than average PFS. Other recommended options are oral or IV topotecan or CAV; cyclophosphamide, doxorubicin, vincristine [4], both of these options demonstrate response rates of around 20% and OS of approximately 6 months.

Systemic Anti-cancer Therapy for Advanced Non-small Cell Lung Cancer

Adenocarcinoma

The first line for metastatic, non-mutated adenocarcinoma until the last 2-3 years was combination chemotherapy. Several combinations are available, most commonly used include cisplatin pemetrexed [23] and carboplatin paclitaxel. Carboplatin paclitaxel and the monoclonal antibody vascular endothelial growth factor (VEGF) inhibitor bevacizumab did show a two month OS benefit of 12.3 months compared to 10.3 months (p0.03) with carboplatin paclitaxel, but given associated toxicities (including hypertension and proteinuria) and cost associated it was never funded for routine use in the UK.

A meta-analysis demonstrated a survival benefit to cisplatin pemetrexed compared to other platinum combinations with a hazard ratio for death of 0.91, p0.004. Unlike SCLC, a further meta-analysis showed that cisplatin and carboplatin are not equivalent in efficacy [24] for NSCLC and therefore cisplatin pemetrexed was the preferred standard of care in the UK (though carboplatin may be used if the patient was ineligible for cisplatin, for example, concerns over renal function or specific toxicity such as the impact on hearing or peripheral neuropathy).

A 2016 study compared the immunotherapy drug pembrolizumab to chemotherapy in the first-line setting for patients with a tumour proportion score (TPS) of PDL1 expression of >50%. This demonstrated a strong benefit in PFS of 10.4 *vs* 6.0 months 25. Approximately ~1/3 of patients in previous clinical trials had a TPS of >50% [26,28].

Keynote 189 published in 2018 compared chemotherapy with a platinum agent (either cisplatin or carboplatin) in combination with pemetrexed and either pembrolizumab or placebo, they received 4 cycles of the triplet combination and then continued pembrolizumab/placebo plus pemetrexed maintenance for up to two years or disease progression. Patients included in the trial could have any TPS (including a negative score). Patients were excluded from this trial if they had active brain metastases, autoimmune conditions requiring steroids or other immunosuppression, if they had previously received >30Gy radiotherapy to the lung or if their tumour expressed an EGFR or ALK mutation.

At 12 months, 69.2% of patients in the pembrolizumab group were still alive compared with 49.4% in the placebo arm. The median PFS was 8.8 *vs* 4.9 months [29]. This is in line with other immunotherapy trials which tend to show small PFS benefits but a much larger OS benefit. The published follow-up on this study was only 21 months and it remains to be seen whether this OS benefit develops, and whether the combination leads to some long-term responders.

This combination of chemotherapy and immunotherapy was the current first-line standard of care for non-mutated, metastatic adenocarcinoma lung cancer until just weeks before this chapter was written. The IMpower 150 study published in 2018 combined atezolizumab and bevacizumab with carboplatin and paclitaxel (ABCP), comparing to bevacizumab carboplatin, paclitaxel (BCP). Patients with any PDL-1 status were included, patients with EGFR/ALK mutations were excluded. The theory behind this combination is that VEGF inhibition would have immunomodulatory effects. The trial demonstrated a significant PFS benefit of 8.3 *vs* 6.8 months (for those PDL-1 0% PFS was 8.0 *vs* 6.8 months). Overall survival showed a similar prolonged benefit of 19.2 months for *vs* 14.7 months [30]. At the time of writing, this combination had just received NICE approval as first-line therapy.

It will, however, not be suitable for all patients. All trials only recruit patients with an Eastern Co-operative Oncology group (ECOG) performance score (PS) of 0-1. That is to say, patients who are fit enough to be working, or managing significant day to day activities such that they are capable of light work. The combination of platinum comes with significant toxicity and many patients presenting with metastatic lung cancer are not fit for this, let alone the addition of immunotherapy and VEGF inhibition toxicity. The funding for the drug from NICE requires that patients be fit enough for the combination. Furthermore, patients who have relapsed after radical chemoradiotherapy will not be eligible if they have previously received immunotherapy, and for those with autoimmune conditions (other than hypothyroidism and diabetes mellitus which do not seem to be affected by immunotherapy) due to the risk of worsening these other conditions, they are unfortunately ineligible for these drugs.

For patients not eligible for either combination chemotherapy and immunotherapy regimen then standard chemotherapy (potentially with a single agent regimen), or single-agent immunotherapy if they have a TPS >50% remain other options. For patients with specific contraindications to, or a desire to avoid chemotherapy, and a TPS >50%, single-agent pembrolizumab is an attractive option for this trial demonstrated a PFS of 10.6 months *vs* 6.0 months for chemotherapy and mOS of 30.0 *vs* 14.2 months [25].

For patients who have received a combination of a PD1 inhibitor and chemotherapy in the first-line setting then the only option at the time of disease progression is a combination of the taxane cytotoxic docetaxel with the oral angiogenesis tyrosine kinase inhibitor nindetanib nindetanib. This combination demonstrated a small but significant benefit of docetaxel alone (the previous second-line standard of care) of 12.6 *vs* 10.3 months. There is no evidence to support the use of 2nd line PD1/PDL1 inhibitors after progression on 1st line checkpoint inhibition.

For patients who have not received immunotherapy in the first-line setting then they may receive immunotherapy as a single-agent regimen. The drugs nivolumab, pembrolizumab, and atezolizumab have all been licensed and funded. Nivolumab was the first of these to show efficacy, reporting in 2015, demonstrating an mOS of 12.2 months compared with 9.4 for the docetaxel group (which was standard second-line therapy at the time) [26]. Although the trial enrolled patients regardless of PDL-1 expression it only demonstrated a significant benefit for those with some expression ≥1%. Pembrolizumab, reporting later the same year as Nivolumab, was trialled only on patients with PDL-1 expression ≥1%, again mOS was 12.4 months compared to 8.4 months with docetaxel [27]. Both of these drugs are licensed and funded for patients who have previously received platinum chemotherapy (with no previous checkpoint inhibitor therapy) if they have a TPS of ≥1%. Atezolizumab, which is a PDL-1 inhibitor (as opposed to PD-1 inhibitor), has demonstrated efficacy in the second line for patients with any degree of PDL-1 expression, including those with a TPS of 0%, mOS was 13.8 months *vs* 9.6 for docetaxel in the whole trial population, and 12.6 months *vs* 8.9 months in the PDL-1 undetectable group [28]. Atezolizumab is licensed and funded in the UK for patients with any TPS including 0%.

Given that the efficacy and toxicity of these drugs are similar, the choice of the agent may depend on patient or physician preference, practicalities and cost. Pembrolizumab and atezolizumab are both given 3 weekly, whereas nivolumab was initially trialled two weekly. This naturally has a significant impact both on the patient but also on treatment centre capacity. More recently, pharmacokinetic studies have demonstrated that nivolumab and atezolizumab can be given 4 weekly and pembrolizumab 6 weekly with similar efficacy [31]. There is also a cost consideration in that atezolizumab is available at a much lower cost.

These patients may then receive docetaxel nindetanib in the third-line setting.

Such was the paucity of effective treatments for metastatic lung cancer, that docetaxel gained its' approval for second-line therapy 20 years ago from a trial which compared it to best supportive care (with a median survival of 7 months compared to 4) [32]. It is hopefully evident that treatment options are now much more plentiful. These options are summarised in Fig. (**2**).

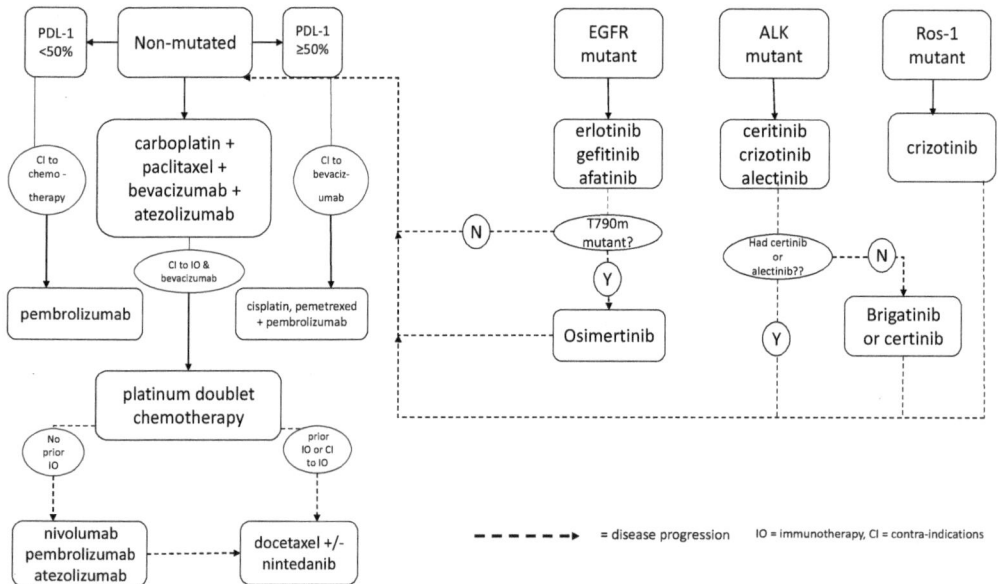

Fig. (2). Treatment options for incurable adenocarcinoma.

EGFR and ALK Mutant Disease

All patients with a new diagnosis of advanced NSCLC should be tested for EGFR, ALK and Ros-1 mutations. Tyrosine kinase inhibitors targeting sensitising EGFR mutations are recommended first-line treatment for patients with EGFR mutant disease. For patients with EGFR and ALK mutations, these drugs have better RR, PFS, OS and lower toxicity than chemotherapy [33 - 35]. EGFR mutations were the first to be identified after it was noted that a subset of patients responded much better to these drugs than the rest of the population. Gefitinib was the first drug to prove efficacy in this setting and when tested in a cohort of patients with either a proven EGFR mutation or who were non-smokers or light former smokers, it demonstrated an impressive 12-month PFS rate of 24.9% compared with 6.7% for patients treated with carboplatin paclitaxel [36]. This trial led to further work that identified ALK and Ros-1 mutations and changed treatment for this subset of patients with lung cancer.

EGFR TKIs have not demonstrated activity against EGFR wild-type lung cancer and should not be used in this setting [37].

At the point of progression, patients receiving treatment with a first-line EGFR TKI can be tested for the development of a known resistance mutation; T790M. Should this be present, the patient can receive second-line TKI therapy with osimertinib [38]. Should it not be present, the patient may receive other standards of care options as available to patients with EGFR wildtype lung cancer.

There is debate about the optimal sequencing of EGFR TKIs and the recent FLAURA study compared the use of osimertinib first-line compared to a first-generation EGFR TKI and demonstrated an improved PFS of 18 months compared with 10 months. Overall survival data is immature but may lead to a change in first-line treatment.

For patients with ALK or ROS-1 mutated lung cancer, the standard of care has been the TKI crizotinib which demonstrated a PFS of 7.7 months compared to 3.3 months with chemotherapy in the initial trial [39]. An alternative option is ceritinib which showed a PFS of 16.6 months *vs* 8.1 months for platinum combination chemotherapy, it has not been compared directly against crizotinib [40]. A direct comparison against crizotinib was made for alectinib. At the time of the initial report, median PFS had not been reached but a 12-month event-free survival rate was 68.4% for alectinib compared with 48.7% for crizotinib. Patients with ALK and EGFR mutations are at increased risk of brain metastases and both ceritinib and alectinib have increased CNS penetrance compared to crizotinib. The rate of CNS progression was 12% for alectinib compared with 48% for crizotinib.

Following progression from first-line therapy, ceritinib has demonstrated efficacy after crizotinib though it has not been tested after alectinib. Brigantinib, another 2nd generation ALK inhibitor has demonstrated efficacy after crizotinib in a phase II study with a median PFS of 12.3 months [41]. Following the progression of all available TKIs patients with ALK, positive patients also have the available treatment options for non-mutated NSCLC including chemotherapy and immunotherapy. The benefit of immunotherapy seems to be less significant in EGFR and ALK mutant cancers, most likely reflecting the different biology of these diseases. These options are also summarised in Fig. (**2**).

BRAF Mutant Carcinoma

BRAF is a serine/threonine protein kinase included in the mitogen-activated protein kinase pathway. This pathway is involved in cell signalling and mutations in the genes coding this pathway are common in cancer patients.

The most common mutation is BRAF V600E and this was first recognised as a common driver mutation in patients with metastatic melanoma. The mutation is found in 2-4% of patients with NSCLC [42] and most commonly older patients and smokers. Approval was granted for the use of a combination of drugs that BRAF mutations and another protein kinase within the same pathway MEK following results of a phase 2 trial of BRAF mutant NSCLC patients. The primary end-point of the study was the response rate and it showed an overall response rate of 33% and a disease control rate of 58%. The PFS within the study was 5.5 months and mOS 12.7 months. The drug is not currently available in the UK [43].

Squamous Cell Carcinoma

The options for patients with squamous cell carcinoma are slightly more limited than for those with adenocarcinoma.

In the first line, pembrolizumab demonstrated efficacy patients with squamous histology and a TPS >50% similar to that of those with adenocarcinoma [25]. For those that have a lower TPS, the only first-line option is combination chemotherapy as the trial combining pembrolizumab and chemotherapy only recruited patients with non-squamous histology. Pemetrexed has only shown significant efficacy in those with non-squamous histology [44] and is therefore not recommended. Common first-line chemotherapy regimens include cisplatin/carboplatin in combination with either vinorelbine or gemcitabine.

In the second line patients who have received pembrolizumab first line could receive platinum combination chemotherapy second line. Those who received platinum combination can receive immunotherapy (pembrolizumab or nivolumab if PDL-1 positive, or atezolizumab if PDL-1 negative) as all of these drugs have been trialled in patients with squamous histology [27, 45, 46].

The third line option for patients with squamous histology is docetaxel. Docetaxel nintedanib showed significant efficacy only in those with adenocarcinoma histology [47]. These options are summarised in Fig. (**3**).

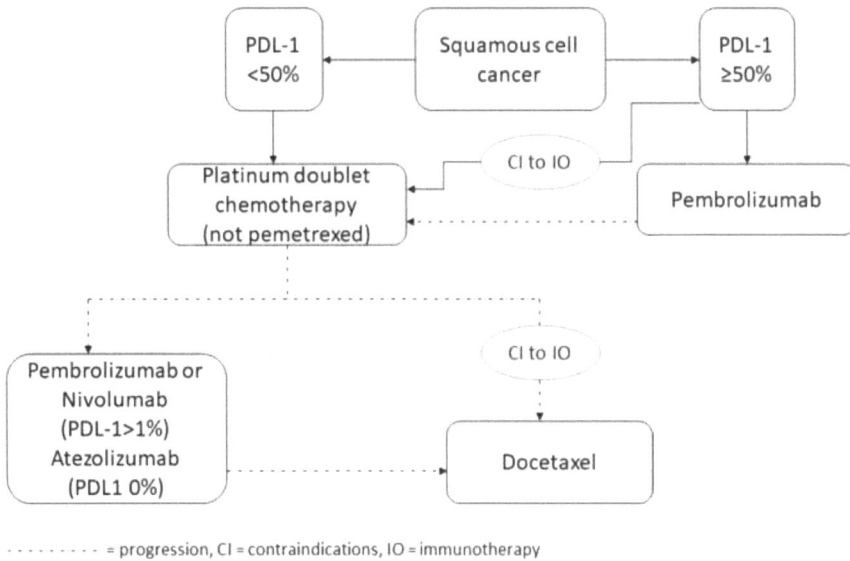

- - - - - - - - = progression, CI = contraindications, IO = immunotherapy

Fig. (3). Treatment options for metastatic squamous cell cancer.

CONCLUSION

It is an exciting time to be a thoracic oncologist, with multiple new emerging therapeutic options over recent years. There is still a long way to go though, most promising data is for survival in the region of 24-30 months but there is still a significant group of patients who live < 12 months following a diagnosis of metastatic lung cancer. Many patients still present not fit for any SACT, whether due to co-morbidities, or the advanced state of their disease.

The development of effective SACT for lung cancer is certainly changing the outlook for patients with lung cancer. However, to truly improve outcomes for lung cancer patients, we need a joined-up approach that includes improvements to prevention, screening, diagnosis and support of patients so that we can identify the right treatment, for the right patients, at the right time.

LIST OF ABBREVIATIONS

EGFR	epidermal growth factor receptor
AC	adenocarcinoma
ALK	anaplastic lymphocyte kinase
CNS	central nervous system
CLTA-4	cytotoxic T-lymphocyte-associated protein 4
DFS	disease-free survival
DNA	deoxyribonucleic acid
EBUS	endobronchial ultrasound
ECOG	Eastern Co-operative Oncology Group
EMA	European Medicines Agency
GI	gastrointestinal
mABs	monoclonal antibodies
NICE	National Institute for Clinical Excellence
NSCLC	non-small cell lung cancer
OS	overall survival
PD-1/PDL-1	programmed cell death protein-1 / programmed cell death ligand-1
PET-	positron emission tomography
PFS	progression-free survival
PS	performance status
RFS	relapse-free survival
ROS-1	tyrosine kinase receptor ROS-1
RR	response rate
SACT	systemic anti-cancer therapy
SCC	squamous cell carcinoma
SCLC	squamous cell carcinoma
TKI	tyrosine kinase inhibitor
TNM	tumour node metastasis
TPS	tumour proportion score
UK	United Kingdom
VEGF	vascular endothelial growth factor

CONSENT FOR PUBLICATION

Not applicable.

CONFLICT OF INTEREST

The author declares that there is no conflict of interest in this chapter.

ACKNOWLEDGEMENTS

Declared none.

REFERENCES

[1]   Jemal A, Bray F, Center MM, *et al.* Global cancer statistics. CA Cancer J Clin 2011; 61(2): 69-90.
        [http://dx.doi.org/10.3322/caac.20107] [PMID: 21296855]

[2]   Reck M, Popat S, Reinmuth N, De Ruysscher D, Kerr KM, Peters S. Metastatic non-small-cell lung
        cancer (NSCLC): ESMO Clinical Practice Guidelines for diagnosis, treatment and follow-up. Ann
        Oncol 2014; 25 (Suppl. 3): iii27-39.
        [http://dx.doi.org/10.1093/annonc/mdu199] [PMID: 25115305]

[3]   Travis WD, Brambilla E, Noguchi M, *et al.* International association for the study of lung
        cancer/american thoracic society/european respiratory society: International multidisciplinary
        classification of lung adenocarcinoma: executive summary. Proc Am Thorac Soc 2011; 8(5): 381-5.
        [http://dx.doi.org/10.1513/pats.201107-042ST] [PMID: 21926387]

[4]   Früh M, De Ruysscher D, Popat S, *et al.* Small-cell lung cancer (SCLC): ESMO Clinical Practice
        Guidelines for diagnosis, treatment and follow-up. Ann Oncol 2013; 24 (Suppl. 6): vi99-vi105.
        [http://dx.doi.org/10.1093/annonc/mdt178] [PMID: 23813929]

[5]   Gustafsson BI, Kidd M, Chan A, Malfertheiner MV, Modlin IM. Bronchopulmonary neuroendocrine
        tumors. Cancer 2008; 113(1): 5-21.
        [http://dx.doi.org/10.1002/cncr.23542] [PMID: 18473355]

[6]   Kerr KM, Bubendorf L, Edelman MJ, *et al.* Second ESMO consensus conference on lung cancer:
        pathology and molecular biomarkers for non-small-cell lung cancer. Ann Oncol 2014; 25(9): 1681-90.
        [http://dx.doi.org/10.1093/annonc/mdu145] [PMID: 24718890]

[7]   Rangachari D, Yamaguchi N, VanderLaan PA, *et al.* Brain metastases in patients with EGFR-mutated
        or ALK-rearranged non-small-cell lung cancers. Lung Cancer 2015; 88(1): 108-11.
        [http://dx.doi.org/10.1016/j.lungcan.2015.01.020] [PMID: 25682925]

[8]   Sessa CGL, Garassino M, van Halteren H. ESMO Handbookof clinical pharmacology of anti-cancer
        agents Vigaello-Lugano. European Society for Medical Oncology Press 2012.

[9]   Sessa C, Gianni L, Garassino M, van Halteren H. Clinical Pharmacology of Anti-Cancer Agents
        Viganello-Lugano. ESMO Press 2012.

[10]   Ribas A, Wolchok JD. Cancer immunotherapy using checkpoint blockade. Science 2018; 359(6382):
        1350-5.
        [http://dx.doi.org/10.1126/science.aar4060] [PMID: 29567705]

[11]   Suresh K, Naidoo J, Lin CT, Danoff S. Immune checkpoint immunotherapy for non-small cell lung
        cancer: benefits and pulmonary toxicities. Chest 2018; 154(6): 1416-23.
        [http://dx.doi.org/10.1016/j.chest.2018.08.1048] [PMID: 30189190]

[12]   Haanen JBAG, Carbonnel F, Robert C, Kerr KM, Peters S, Larkin J, *et al.* Management of toxicities
        from immunotherapy: ESMO Clinical Practice Guidelines for diagnosis, treatment and follow-up. Ann
        Oncol 2017; 2828(suppl_4): iv119 - iv42..

[13]   Delaunay M, Cadranel J, Lusque A, *et al.* Immune-checkpoint inhibitors associated with interstitial
        lung disease in cancer patients. Eur Respir J 2017; 50(2)1700050
        [http://dx.doi.org/10.1183/13993003.00050-2017] [PMID: 28798088]

[14] Khunger M, Rakshit S, Pasupuleti V, *et al.* Incidence of pneumonitis with use of programmed death 1 and programmed death-ligand 1 inhibitors in non-small cell lung cancer: a systematic review and meta-analysis of trials. Chest 2017; 152(2): 271-81.
[http://dx.doi.org/10.1016/j.chest.2017.04.177] [PMID: 28499515]

[15] Yang CF, Chan DY, Speicher PJ, *et al.* Role of adjuvant therapy in a population-based cohort of patients with early-stage small-cell lung cancer. J Clin Oncol 2016; 34(10): 1057-64.
[http://dx.doi.org/10.1200/JCO.2015.63.8171] [PMID: 26786925]

[16] Vansteenkiste J, Crinò L, Dooms C, *et al.* 2nd ESMO consensus conference on lung cancer: Early-stage non-small-cell lung cancer consensus on diagnosis, treatment and follow-up. Ann Oncol 2014; 25(8): 1462-74.
[http://dx.doi.org/10.1093/annonc/mdu089] [PMID: 24562446]

[17] Arriagada R, Bergman B, Dunant A, *et al.* Cisplatin-based adjuvant chemotherapy in patients with completely resected non-small-cell lung cancer. N Engl J Med 2004; 350(4): 351-60.
[http://dx.doi.org/10.1056/NEJMoa031644] [PMID: 14736927]

[18] Douillard JY, Rosell R, De Lena M, *et al.* Adjuvant vinorelbine plus cisplatin versus observation in patients with completely resected stage IB-IIIA non-small-cell lung cancer (Adjuvant Navelbine International Trialist Association [ANITA]): a randomised controlled trial. Lancet Oncol 2006; 7(9): 719-27.
[http://dx.doi.org/10.1016/S1470-2045(06)70804-X] [PMID: 16945766]

[19] Winton T, Livingston R, Johnson D, *et al.* Vinorelbine plus cisplatin *vs.* observation in resected non-small-cell lung cancer. N Engl J Med 2005; 352(25): 2589-97.
[http://dx.doi.org/10.1056/NEJMoa043623] [PMID: 15972865]

[20] Mascaux C, Paesmans M, Berghmans T, *et al.* A systematic review of the role of etoposide and cisplatin in the chemotherapy of small cell lung cancer with methodology assessment and meta-analysis. Lung Cancer 2000; 30(1): 23-36.
[http://dx.doi.org/10.1016/S0169-5002(00)00127-6] [PMID: 11008007]

[21] Rossi A, Di Maio M, Chiodini P, *et al.* Carboplatin- or cisplatin-based chemotherapy in first-line treatment of small-cell lung cancer: the COCIS meta-analysis of individual patient data. J Clin Oncol 2012; 30(14): 1692-8.
[http://dx.doi.org/10.1200/JCO.2011.40.4905] [PMID: 22473169]

[22] Horn L, Mansfield AS, Szczęsna A, *et al.* First-line atezolizumab plus chemotherapy in extensive-stage small-cell lung cancer. N Engl J Med 2018; 379(23): 2220-9.
[http://dx.doi.org/10.1056/NEJMoa1809064] [PMID: 30280641]

[23] Scagliotti GV, Parikh P, von Pawel J, *et al.* Phase III study comparing cisplatin plus gemcitabine with cisplatin plus pemetrexed in chemotherapy-naive patients with advanced-stage non-small-cell lung cancer. J Clin Oncol 2008; 26(21): 3543-51.
[http://dx.doi.org/10.1200/JCO.2007.15.0375] [PMID: 18506025]

[24] Ardizzoni A, Boni L, Tiseo M, *et al.* Cisplatin- versus carboplatin-based chemotherapy in first-line treatment of advanced non-small-cell lung cancer: an individual patient data meta-analysis. J Natl Cancer Inst 2007; 99(11): 847-57.
[http://dx.doi.org/10.1093/jnci/djk196] [PMID: 17551145]

[25] Reck M, Rodríguez-Abreu D, Robinson AG, *et al.* Updated analysis of KEYNOTE-024: Pembrolizumab *versus* platinum-based chemotherapy for advanced non-small-cell lung cancer with PD-L1 tumor proportion score of 50% or greater. J Clin Oncol 2019; 37(7): 537-46.
[http://dx.doi.org/10.1200/JCO.18.00149] [PMID: 30620668]

[26] Borghaei H, Paz-Ares L, Horn L, *et al.* Nivolumab *versus* docetaxel in advanced nonsquamous non-small-cell lung cancer. N Engl J Med 2015; 373(17): 1627-39.
[http://dx.doi.org/10.1056/NEJMoa1507643] [PMID: 26412456]

[27]   Herbst RS, Baas P, Kim DW, *et al.* Pembrolizumab versus docetaxel for previously treated, PD-L-
       -positive, advanced non-small-cell lung cancer (KEYNOTE-010): a randomised controlled trial.
       Lancet 2016; 387(10027): 1540-50.
       [http://dx.doi.org/10.1016/S0140-6736(15)01281-7] [PMID: 26712084]

[28]   Rittmeyer A, Barlesi F, Waterkamp D, *et al.* Atezolizumab versus docetaxel in patients with
       previously treated non-small-cell lung cancer (OAK): a phase 3, open-label, multicentre randomised
       controlled trial. Lancet 2017; 389(10066): 255-65.
       [http://dx.doi.org/10.1016/S0140-6736(16)32517-X] [PMID: 27979383]

[29]   Gandhi L, Rodríguez-Abreu D, Gadgeel S, *et al.* Pembrolizumab plus chemotherapy in metastatic
       non-small-cell lung cancer. N Engl J Med 2018; 378(22): 2078-92.
       [http://dx.doi.org/10.1056/NEJMoa1801005] [PMID: 29658856]

[30]   Socinski MA, Jotte RM, Cappuzzo F, *et al.* Atezolizumab for first-line treatment of metastatic
       nonsquamous NSCLC. N Engl J Med 2018; 378(24): 2288-301.
       [http://dx.doi.org/10.1056/NEJMoa1716948] [PMID: 29863955]

[31]   Long GV, Tykodi SS, Schneider JG, *et al.* Assessment of nivolumab exposure and clinical safety of
       480 mg every 4 weeks flat-dosing schedule in patients with cancer. Ann Oncol 2018; 29(11): 2208-13.
       [http://dx.doi.org/10.1093/annonc/mdy408] [PMID: 30215677]

[32]   Shepherd FA, Dancey J, Ramlau R, *et al.* Prospective randomized trial of docetaxel versus best
       supportive care in patients with non-small-cell lung cancer previously treated with platinum-based
       chemotherapy. J Clin Oncol 2000; 18(10): 2095-103.
       [http://dx.doi.org/10.1200/JCO.2000.18.10.2095] [PMID: 10811675]

[33]   Maemondo M, Inoue A, Kobayashi K, *et al.* Gefitinib or chemotherapy for non-small-cell lung cancer
       with mutated EGFR. N Engl J Med 2010; 362(25): 2380-8.
       [http://dx.doi.org/10.1056/NEJMoa0909530] [PMID: 20573926]

[34]   Sequist LV, Yang JC, Yamamoto N, *et al.* Phase III study of afatinib or cisplatin plus pemetrexed in
       patients with metastatic lung adenocarcinoma with EGFR mutations. J Clin Oncol 2013; 31(27): 3327-
       34.
       [http://dx.doi.org/10.1200/JCO.2012.44.2806] [PMID: 23816960]

[35]   Rosell R, Carcereny E, Gervais R, *et al.* Erlotinib versus standard chemotherapy as first-line treatment
       for European patients with advanced EGFR mutation-positive non-small-cell lung cancer (EURTAC):
       a multicentre, open-label, randomised phase 3 trial. Lancet Oncol 2012; 13(3): 239-46.
       [http://dx.doi.org/10.1016/S1470-2045(11)70393-X] [PMID: 22285168]

[36]   Mok TS, Wu YL, Thongprasert S, *et al.* Gefitinib or carboplatin-paclitaxel in pulmonary
       adenocarcinoma. N Engl J Med 2009; 361(10): 947-57.
       [http://dx.doi.org/10.1056/NEJMoa0810699] [PMID: 19692680]

[37]   Lee SM, Khan I, Upadhyay S, *et al.* First-line erlotinib in patients with advanced non-small-cell lung
       cancer unsuitable for chemotherapy (TOPICAL): a double-blind, placebo-controlled, phase 3 trial.
       Lancet Oncol 2012; 13(11): 1161-70.
       [http://dx.doi.org/10.1016/S1470-2045(12)70412-6] [PMID: 23078958]

[38]   Goss G, Tsai CM, Shepherd FA, *et al.* Osimertinib for pretreated EGFR Thr790Met-positive advanced
       non-small-cell lung cancer (AURA2): a multicentre, open-label, single-arm, phase 2 study. Lancet
       Oncol 2016; 17(12): 1643-52.
       [http://dx.doi.org/10.1016/S1470-2045(16)30508-3] [PMID: 27751847]

[39]   Shaw AT, Kim DW, Nakagawa K, *et al.* Crizotinib versus chemotherapy in advanced ALK-positive
       lung cancer. N Engl J Med 2013; 368(25): 2385-94.
       [http://dx.doi.org/10.1056/NEJMoa1214886] [PMID: 23724913]

[40]   Soria JC, Tan DSW, Chiari R, *et al.* First-line ceritinib versus platinum-based chemotherapy in
       advanced ALK-rearranged non-small-cell lung cancer (ASCEND-4): a randomised, open-label, phase

3 study. Lancet 2017; 389(10072): 917-29.
[http://dx.doi.org/10.1016/S0140-6736(17)30123-X] [PMID: 28126333]

[41]   Kim DW, Tiseo M, Ahn MJ, *et al.* Brigatinib in patients with crizotinib-refractory anaplastic lymphoma kinase-positive non-small-cell lung cancer: a randomized, multicenter phase II trial. J Clin Oncol 2017; 35(22): 2490-8.
[http://dx.doi.org/10.1200/JCO.2016.71.5904] [PMID: 28475456]

[42]   Comprehensive molecular profiling of lung adenocarcinoma. Nature 2014; 511(7511): 543-50.
[http://dx.doi.org/10.1038/nature13385] [PMID: 25079552]

[43]   Planchard D, Besse B, Groen HJM, *et al.* Dabrafenib plus trametinib in patients with previously treated BRAF(V600E)-mutant metastatic non-small cell lung cancer: an open-label, multicentre phase 2 trial. Lancet Oncol 2016; 17(7): 984-93.
[http://dx.doi.org/10.1016/S1470-2045(16)30146-2] [PMID: 27283860]

[44]   Scagliotti G, Hanna N, Fossella F, *et al.* The differential efficacy of pemetrexed according to NSCLC histology: a review of two Phase III studies. Oncologist 2009; 14(3): 253-63.
[http://dx.doi.org/10.1634/theoncologist.2008-0232] [PMID: 19221167]

[45]   Fehrenbacher L, Spira A, Ballinger M, *et al.* Atezolizumab versus docetaxel for patients with previously treated non-small-cell lung cancer (POPLAR): a multicentre, open-label, phase 2 randomised controlled trial. Lancet 2016; 387(10030): 1837-46.
[http://dx.doi.org/10.1016/S0140-6736(16)00587-0] [PMID: 26970723]

[46]   Brahmer J, Reckamp KL, Baas P, *et al.* Nivolumab *versus* docetaxel in advanced squamous-cell non-small-cell lung cancer. N Engl J Med 2015; 373(2): 123-35.
[http://dx.doi.org/10.1056/NEJMoa1504627] [PMID: 26028407]

[47]   Reck M, Kaiser R, Mellemgaard A, *et al.* Docetaxel plus nintedanib versus docetaxel plus placebo in patients with previously treated non-small-cell lung cancer (LUME-Lung 1): a phase 3, double-blind, randomised controlled trial. Lancet Oncol 2014; 15(2): 143-55.
[http://dx.doi.org/10.1016/S1470-2045(13)70586-2] [PMID: 24411639]

CHAPTER 13

The Role of Palliative Care in Lung Cancer

Elaine G. Boland[1,*] and **Jason W. Boland**[2]

[1] *Consultant & Honorary Senior Lecturer in Palliative Medicine, Hull University Teaching Hospitals NHS Trust, Queen's centre for Oncology and Haematology, Castle Hill Hospital, Castle Road, Cottingham, UK*

[2] *Senior Clinical Lecturer and Honorary Consultant in Palliative Medicine, Hull York Medical School, University of Hull, Hull, UK*

Abstract: Patients with lung cancer are often diagnosed late and the disease in such cases is often advanced. Common symptoms include breathlessness, haemoptysis and pain and these can have an impact on their quality of life. Patients might have challenging palliative and supportive care needs and in order to address these, palliative care should be offered earlier in the disease trajectory. An interdisciplinary approach, working jointly with the oncologists, respiratory teams and palliative care teams provide a holistic, comprehensive assessment in response to their changing needs. Advance care planning is best to be started early on especially in patients with a prognosis of about a year, in a sensitive manner, in order to involve the patient in discussion about their future wishes and priorities for care. It is important to recognise dying to be able to communicate with the patient and their family, recognise any symptoms and manage them proactively and achieve preferred place of care and death; a patient-centred approach is needed.

Keywords: End of life, Interdisciplinary approach, Palliative care, Quality of life, Supportive care, Symptom management.

INTRODUCTION

Lung cancer is the 2nd most common cancer in both males and females, and the most common cause of cancer death in the UK [1]. It is more common in patients living in areas of socioeconomic deprivation [1].

Worldwide, there were 2 million new cases and 1.7 million deaths in 2018 [2, 3]. The National Lung Cancer Audit in England reported that 19% of patients who are diagnosed with non-small cell lung cancer (NSCLC) present as an emergency

---

[*] **Corresponding author Elaine G. Boland:** Consultant & Honorary Senior Lecturer in Palliative Medicine, Hull University Teaching Hospitals NHS Trust, Queen's centre for Oncology and Haematology, Castle Hill Hospital, Castle Road, Cottingham; Tel: 01482461147; E-mail: elaine.boland@hey.nhs.uk

Keyvan Moghissi, Jack Kastelik, Philip Barber & Peyman Sardari Nia (Eds.)

to hospital [4]. There was a strong association between emergency presentation and more advanced disease, older age and poor performance status in these patients; they were also more likely to be dead within 1 year of diagnosis [4].

Lung cancer is often diagnosed at an advanced stage, but this is often not what patients understand. Patients are most commonly (49-53%) diagnosed with lung cancer at stage IV, with 72-76% being diagnosed at stage III or IV [5]. In a study of patients with newly diagnosed metastatic NSCLC, almost 70% thought that the aim of treatment was to get rid of all the cancer [6].

A large Irish retrospective observational study (n=14,228) found that one in five patients newly diagnosed with lung cancer died within 30 days of diagnosis; 75% died in hospital [7]. Patients who were ≥80 years old, admitted as an emergency to hospital and then diagnosed with lung cancer, and patients with co-morbidities were more likely to die within 30 days of diagnosis [7].

Palliative Care

Palliative care is a holistic, multidisciplinary approach, aiming to relieve the suffering of patients and support families/loved-ones, by identifying problems such as symptoms, including physical, spiritual and psychosocial in patients with advanced life-limiting illness [8, 9]. Supportive care is delivered throughout the disease cancer trajectory, from diagnosis onwards and is fully integrated in management and treatment [10].

A systematic review (8 randomized controlled trials and 32 observational or quasi-experimental studies) looked at specialist palliative care in the hospital, home, or inpatient settings for patients with cancer and found that pain and symptom control, and anxiety had significantly improved whilst these patients also had reduced hospital admissions [11]. Early palliative care in patients with advanced NSCLC is associated with better patient-reported outcomes and a longer survival [12] (see section: EVIDENCE FOR EARLY PALLIATIVE CARE). Palliative care should be offered to patients with advanced life-limiting illnesses with the aim to diagnose and treat symptoms early thus improving their quality of life. There still remain misconceptions about the role of palliative care and although oncologists refer patients to palliative care services, these referrals are often late in the disease trajectory and patients tend to have uncontrolled symptoms [13, 14]. As patients have historically been referred to palliative care services late, the World Health Organization declared that patients with a poor prognosis at diagnosis should be considered for referral to palliative care and palliative care should be part of the integrated care they receive [15]. Referrals to specialist palliative care should be based on needs rather than prognosis.

SYMPTOMS AND QUALITY OF LIFE

Patients might develop symptoms, which can be caused by the primary cancer itself, metastasis, from cancer treatment or co-morbidities. Lung cancer can metastasise to different sites, including bone and brain, can cause spinal cord compression (from spinal metastasis), superior vena cava obstruction, trachea-oesophageal fistulas and airway stenosis; these can lead to an array of symptoms [16]. Common symptoms include pain in chest, back or shoulder, persistent cough, breathlessness, haemoptysis, weight loss, fatigue and headaches [17]. Pain, breathlessness and haemoptysis are covered in more detail below. Other symptoms like anorexia, cachexia, fatigue, depression and insomnia might be harder to identify unless the patient reports them or if these symptoms are diagnosed by the treating team if systematically assessed [16, 18]. Questionnaires (from the Short-Form 8 health survey) from 2205 patients with newly diagnosed lung cancer showed a significant association between emotional problems and worse quality of life (QoL) and a high symptom burden (pain severity and frequency, cough, shortness of breath, and fatigue) [19].

Supportive Care Needs

Patients with lung cancer face substantial burden and challenges. A systematic review of 59 articles looked at the experiences and supportive care needs of patients with lung cancer and reported on 9 domains [20]. This has been summarised in Table **1**.

Table 1. Experiences and supportive care needs of patients with lung cancer [20].

Supportive Care Needs Domain	Reported Issues/Concerns and Explanation
Distressing *Physical needs*	Loss of energy, breathlessness, pain and sleeplessness. Pain and digestive problems were more common as patients approached the end of their life.
Daily living needs	Dictated by treatment and results of tests. Patients were trying to live as normally as possible and were concerned about not being able to work, do the housework and do things they used to do and struggled with loss of independence.
Emotional problems	Anxiety, panic attacks, sadness. Patients were worried about being unable to control effects of treatment, the cancer spreading and feeling a burden.

(Table 1) cont.....

Supportive Care Needs Domain	Reported Issues/Concerns and Explanation
Spiritual and existential needs	Highest at diagnosis, at discharge (after completion of treatment), at disease progression, and during end of life care. 13 to over 70% of patients reported uncertainty about the future including failure to find meaning and purpose in life, worries about prioritizing their time left alive and reported the importance of powers such as God or fate.
Information giving	Consistent need where patients wanted to know about their diagnosis, results, and lifestyle factors in a timely manner, and how to manage their disease and side-effects of treatment and also prolonged survival. Patients reported that they would like information to be given in the presence of a relative.
Communication needs	Patients wanted clinicians to be available and care for them in a sensitive manner.
Practical needs	Financial issues, getting affairs in order, household and/or work-related problems, access to the healthcare system out-of-hours, funeral arrangements or making a living will/advance directive.
Social and family-related needs	Associated with increased clinical distress and patients reported worries about the impact of illness and their death on family members and they felt responsible for taking care of their families.
Distressing *Cognitive needs*	Forgetfulness, poor thinking, and confusion

A cross-sectional study of 89 patients with lung cancer reported that 78% of patients had at least 1 unmet need and the mean number of unmet needs was 8 [21]. The highest proportion of needs was psychological (anxiety, depression, and concerns about cancer recurrence and death) and physical. Younger patients, patients with more advanced disease, and those who had worse QoL were more likely to have a greater number of unmet needs [21]. It is also important to assess the needs of family/carers and the impact of the patients' disease and symptoms on them [22, 23].

Assessment of Symptoms

Symptom assessment includes a detailed history and physical examination followed by specific investigations depending on the findings of the history and examination (Table **2**). Investigations need to be appropriate, based on the likely clinical outcomes, patient's wishes, goals of care, stage of disease and prognosis. Sometimes assessment tools are used to measure dyspnoea such as modified Borg scale, Cancer Dyspnea Scale, Visual Analogue Scale, and Numerical Rating Scale and Dyspnea-12 Questionnaire.

Table 2. An approach to symptom management.

Assessment (history, examination and appropriate investigations)	Impact, goals of care and cause of symptoms
Explanation to patient/family/carers	Communication honestly and openly
Reverse the reversible (treat the underlying cause of symptoms)	If consistent with the goals of care/patients' wishes
Stop unnecessary medications (and medications causing potential harms)	Medications might become unnecessary as someone becomes less well
Disease directed approaches	A Multidisciplinary Team (MDT) approach: as systemic anticancer therapy and/or radiotherapy, might help symptoms
Symptom directed approaches	To reduce severity and/or impact of symptoms. This includes: non-pharmacological and pharmacological management of symptoms
May need symptom directed approaches while addressing the underlying cause	Symptom and disease directed approaches can be used together
Review effect and side effects of medications	Need a net overall benefit to continue
Re-Assessment	Of the symptom, effect of management strategies, and their impact on the patient

MANAGEMENT

Patients want their physical symptoms to be managed in discussion with healthcare professionals, they would like to discuss possible treatment options, as well as access to self-help and support groups [10]. They would like professionals to listen to and understand their concerns and offer emotional support accordingly [10]. Despite unmet needs in patients with lung cancer, not everyone wants help. One study reported that 45% to 58% of patients with lung cancer indicated they did not want help from their cancer centre for some of their needs despite significant distress arising (from lack of energy, fears about spread of the cancer and not being able to do the things you used to do) [24]. Another study reported that the availability of hospital staff to speak about all aspects of care was frequently recognised as an asset by patients with lung cancer to help resolve their unmet needs [21]. This emphasises the need for an individualised approach.

Breathlessness

As breathlessness is a multi-factorial sensation, non-pharmacological and pharmacological interventions are usually used in combination for patients with shortness of breath. The British Thoracic Society suggests that in the palliative care setting, oxygen should only be used for symptom management in patients with oxygen saturation consistently <90% or in patients who report that oxygen therapy significantly relieves their breathlessness [25]. Breathlessness often impacts on activities of daily living, work, and sleep and might lead to psychological distress including anxiety, fear and social isolation and will likely have a negative impact on the carer [22].

Low dose regular opioids are usually prescribed for breathlessness [26]. A Cochrane review on opioids for refractory breathlessness in adults with advanced disease and terminal illness reported a small benefit of opioids [27]. However this meta-analyses was re-analysed to account for crossover data and the authors report that opioids decreased breathlessness, which represented a clinically meaningful significance and concluded that the evidence supporting regular low-dose systemic opioids is moderate [28].

Patients with breathlessness can have concomitant anxiety and in such cases benzodiazepines can be trialled. Commonly used benzodiazepines are sublingual lorazepam, or subcutaneous midazolam (injection/infusion) for patients at end of life [26]. However a Cochrane review (8 studies, 214 participants) in patients with Chronic Obstructive Pulmonary Disease (COPD) or advanced cancer on benzodiazepines compared to placebo, morphine, or promethazine showed that there was no significant improvement in breathlessness regardless of the type of benzodiazepine, dose, route and frequency of delivery, duration of treatment and caused more adverse effects [29]. Therefore, benzodiazepines should not be used routinely for breathlessness but can be considered when it is refractory to other treatments.

Non-pharmacological Treatment for Breathlessness

A hand-held fan is often recommended to alleviate the sensation of breathlessness. There are mixed results in the literature, a phase 2 trial did not show benefit of the use of hand-held fan in patients with breathlessness due to advanced cancer or COPD whilst another randomised single-centre study in terminally ill patients with cancer who had dyspnoea showed that there was a significant difference in the mean scores of dyspnoea intensity in the fan-to-face group versus the fan-to-legs group (P<0.001) [30]. A mixed method feasibility study to test the effect of the handheld fan on physical activity and carer anxiety in patients with refractory breathlessness reported that patients found the fan helpful for self-management and assists in recovery; this study found no harms [31]. There is an on-going Cochrane review: 'Respiratory interventions for breathlessness in adults with advanced diseases' which aims to evaluate the effects and safety of interventions [32].

In a single-blind randomised trial, 105 adults with advanced disease (21 with cancer) and refractory breathlessness were consecutively enrolled to either breathlessness support service or usual care [33]. The breathlessness service included physiotherapy, occupational therapy, and respiratory and palliative care clinicians involvement to assess physical, psychological, emotional and spiritual concerns and hand information of guidance for breathlessness, self-management and exercise and plan for crisis, together with a home visit to help with adaptations. The results showed that at 6 weeks patients in the breathlessness service group had an average of 16% improvement in breathlessness mastery (the patients' feeling of control over their breathlessness and its effects on quality of life and function) compared to controls [33].

Palliative interventions for breathlessness should also include spiritual and psychological support together with breathing control and coping strategies such as meditation and relaxation; these are usually delivered by an interdisciplinary team consisting of different experts from palliative care teams including palliative medicine physicians, specialist nurses, physiotherapists, occupational therapists, pharmacists, social workers and psychologists [34].

Interventional Management of Breathlessness

In patients with breathlessness due to mechanical issues such as airway obstruction in central lung cancer or endobronchial metastatic disease, interventional bronchoscopy might be appropriate. Although this is an invasive procedure it can still be appropriate for some patients, even those with advanced disease and it can achieve good symptom control. It is important to discuss with an oncologist to see if a short course of palliative radiation therapy might also be appropriate at this time.

Haemoptysis

Haemoptysis is common in lung cancer but a life-threatening bleed is rare and has been reported as occurring in 3% of patients with lung cancer in a retrospective case-series of 877 patients [35]. Life-threatening haemoptysis has been described as a bleed >100 mL/24 hour; causes airway obstruction and abnormal gas exchange, or haemodynamic instability [36]. The prognosis is very poor in patients with life-threatening haemoptysis. A more recent retrospective study in France showed that stopping of bleeding was achieved in 108/125 (87%) patients with NSCLC who had haemoptysis >100ml on admission; and fatal haemoptysis occurred in 22/125 (18%) patients [37]. If a life-threatening bleed is predictable, discussions about possible treatment options need to take place early on in order to manage the patient and forewarn the family. If the aim of care is to keep the patient comfortable (preferably in their current place of care) and not resuscitated, then anxiolytic medication such as midazolam could be prescribed in anticipation and administered if needed (however the priority is for staff to stay with, and support, the patient/family). It is important the family/carers are aware of the goals of care and are given appropriate information and supportive strategies (eg: to use dark towels in the event of a bleed).

Advanced cancer, mechanical ventilation and poor performance status were independent predictors of in-hospital mortality; overall in-hospital survival rates of 69% has been reported [37]. Haemoptysis due to a tumour usually can be controlled by radiotherapy, endobronchial treatment, interventional radiology, chemotherapy and occasionally by bronchial artery embolization. Antifibrinolytic agents (such as tranexamic acid) act by inhibiting the process that dissolves clots, thus reduces bleeding. A Cochrane review reported that the bleeding time was reduced significantly with the use of tranexamic acid but when reviewed at 7 days after starting it, there was no difference to the number of patients who were still suffering from haemoptysis [38].

Pain

Pain can be caused by the lung cancer itself invading pleura, ribs, brachial plexus or vertebral bodies, or metastasis especially to bone, and also due to anti-cancer treatment including surgery, chemotherapy, and radiotherapy (often as a single fraction). Cryoablation is another technique that could be considered for controlling cancer pain [39]. Cancer-related pain is thought to be a combination of nociceptive, inflammatory and neuropathic mechanisms [40]. Both patients and their carers are often anxious about pain and the impact pain has on their quality of life. A review reported that the overall weighted mean pain prevalence of pain in patients with lung cancer was 47% with pain being caused by cancer in 73% of cases and cancer treatment in 11% [41].

International guidelines are available based on systematic review data for the use of opioids for cancer pain [42]. Opioids are often used in the treatment of cancer-related pain and it is important to communicate with the patient the benefit and side effects of opioids, as well as exploring any fears they might have [43]. Recommendations suggest starting low doses of slow release oral morphine with immediate release oral morphine available for breakthrough pain in patients with normal renal function and who are able to swallow medications. The doses then titrated according to response and side effects. Specialist advice should be available if needed. However a systematic review showed that cancer pain is still being under-treated in about 30% of patients [44]. In such cases, especially if neuropathic pain is present, a combination of adjuvant analgesics such as anticonvulsants (gabapentin/pregabalin) or tricyclic antidepressants (amitriptyline) might be required for optimising pain control and, in some instances, pain that is refractory may require input from specialists and interventional procedures [45, 46].

Non-pharmacological management of pain

Non-pharmacological management to help control pain can be used alongside medications, these include complementary therapies, transcutaneous electrical nerve stimulation (TENS), acupuncture and psychosocial support. A recent systematic review (26 RCTs, 4735 patients) looked at the effectiveness of patient-based educational interventions to improve cancer-related pain and reported that in 31% of the studies significant difference in pain intensity in the intervention group compared to the control group was found, however the interventions varied widely in content, duration and intensity [47].

As pain is usually multifactorial an interdisciplinary approach is necessary to ensure that the pain is managed.

INTERDISCIPLINARY APPROACH

A prospective, quasi-experimental study included 491 ambulatory patients with lung cancer who were enrolled in an interdisciplinary palliative care intervention or control group; the intervention group included a nurse assessment, presentation of assessment at a interdisciplinary team meeting and recommendations made for palliative care consultations and/or referrals to supportive care services [48]. The interdisciplinary team consisted of nurses, palliative medicine physicians, thoracic surgeons, medical oncologists, geriatric oncologist, pulmonologist, social worker, chaplain, dietitian, and physical therapist. This study found that the intervention group scored better for symptom control and QoL ($P<0.001$), spiritual well-being ($P=0.001$), they had less psychological distress ($P<0.001$), and had more advance care directives completed ($P<0.001$) compared to the control group [48]. The same research group studied 366 family caregivers of patients with lung cancer who received interdisciplinary palliative care intervention and found significant positive results for social well-being ($p=0.010$), and less psychological distress ($p<0.001$) and less caregiver burden ($p=0.008$) compared the group receiving usual care [49].

ADVANCE CARE PLANNING

Advance care planning is a process of discussion about future care including a range of voluntary discussions between health care providers and the patient (and if they wish, their family and friends). This explores their preferences and wishes for types of care or treatment that may be beneficial in the future and the availability of these; advantages/disadvantages of future treatments, resuscitation (including Do Not Attempt Cardiopulmonary Resuscitation), where their preference is to be cared for and die, ceilings of care, antibiotics (oral and/or intravenous) [50, 51]. These discussions need to be handled with skill and sensitivity and should ideally be done when the patient is well enough to participate. Advance care plans are of utmost importance when the patient loses capacity which usually happens as patient approaches the last days of life, but can also happen suddenly due to infection, metabolic disturbances etc [52]. The outcomes of such discussions should be documented, regularly reviewed and communicated to other relevant people, with the patients' agreement. However some patients might not want to discuss future plans as this reminds them on their deteriorating condition; they might however give permission to discuss with a relative.

END OF LIFE CARE IN PATIENTS WITH LUNG CANCER

Recognising dying is vital in order to reduce unnecessary investigations, treatments, to prepare the patient and the family, and also to recognise changes in the patient's condition that may lead to new symptoms or changes in their existing ones. It also enables expressed preferences for care to be achieved and allows the dying person to prioritise their time and spend it with family/friends. Towards the end of life, the patient might be unable to swallow their oral symptom management medications and thus alternative routes of administration must be used. This is usually subcutaneous injection or if medications are regularly needed a syringe pump delivering medications continuously via a subcutaneous needle/catheter is used. Common symptoms that may develop in the last hours to days of life include pain, delirium, agitation, noisy upper respiratory tract secretions, breathlessness, nausea and vomiting. Patients who are approaching the end of their life should be prescribed subcutaneous anticipatory medicines with individualised indications for use and dosage [9]. Patients, relatives and clinicians are sometimes worried about the effect of opioids on survival however; a systematic review which included 13 studies (all low quality) of patients with days or weeks to live, did not find a consistent association between opioid analgesic use and survival [53]. Regular assessment of pressure areas, urine and bowel continence, mouth care are needed as well as assessing and supporting the psychological, cultural and spiritual care needs of the patient and family. Ensure that Do Not Attempt Cardiopulmonary Resuscitation/ Recommended Summary Plan for Emergency Care and Treatment (ReSPECT) forms decision has been made to allow the person to die with dignity.

A prospective study in terminally ill patients showed that once certain symptoms develop, death was imminent; the mean time from the onset of upper respiratory secretions to death was 57 hours, respiration with mandibular movement to death was 7.6 hours, cyanosed extremities to death was 5.1 hours however the authors reported that patients who had lung primary or metastatic lung neoplasms had significantly longer time from the onset of respiration with mandibular movement and cyanosis to death compared to other patients with cancer not involving the lung [54].

It is important to assess the level of hydration on a daily basis and support the patient to drink if able to do so and provide mouth care; if clinically assisted hydration is indicated or being asked for, the risks and benefits of hydration options needs to be discussed [9, 55].

A patient-centred approach is needed, reviewing the individualised care plan and taking into account the patient's wishes. Ensure that the patient (if they want to be informed) and the family are aware of the short prognosis and communicate with them about any anxieties or fears they might have. The patient and the family should be given opportunities to discuss their concerns.

EVIDENCE FOR EARLY PALLIATIVE CARE

A recent systematic review (5 studies) assessed (or evaluated) whether early palliative care for advanced NSCLC patients on anticancer treatment was beneficial when compared to standard oncological care and found that overall survival and patient-reported outcomes were better in patients receiving early palliative care [56].

A project ENABLE (Educate, Nurture, Advise, Before Life Ends) looked at delivering a specific telephone palliative care intervention by a trained nurse (4 weekly educational sessions and monthly follow-up) to patients with newly diagnosed advanced cancer [57]. On-going assessment, advice about problem-solving, communication strategies, advance care planning, symptom management and crisis prevention, and timely referral to palliative care services were provided [57]. 322 participants were randomly assigned to receive usual oncology care (N=161) or the telephone intervention (N=161), 36% had a lung cancer diagnosis. The results showed that the intervention group had higher QOL (P=0.02) and less depressed mood (P=0.02), a trend toward lower symptom intensity (P=0.06), but no statistical difference in hospital days (P=0.14), ICU stays (P=1.00) or emergency department visits (P=0.53) [57].

A randomised controlled study of newly diagnosed patients with metastatic NSCLC showed that integrating early palliative care (patients were reviewed as an outpatient by palliative care physicians and advanced-practice nurses, within 3 weeks after enrolment and at least monthly thereafter until death) had a beneficial effect on their QoL compared to the standard oncological care (P=0.03). Patients receiving early palliative care had less depressive symptoms when compared to only receiving standard oncological care (16% vs. 38%, P=0.01). Less patients in the early palliative care group received aggressive end of life (33% vs. 54%, P=0.05), and patients in the early palliative care group survived longer (11.6 months vs. 8.9 months, P=0.02) [12]. A more recent randomized clinical trial had a group of patients with a diagnosis of incurable lung cancer (small-cell, NSCLC, or mesothelioma) who were randomised to receive either early integrated palliative care and oncology care or usual oncological care, showed that the early integrated palliative care group continued to have improvements in QoL until death and less depression, whereas usual care patients with lung cancer reported deterioration in QoL [58]. The patients in the group receiving early integrated palliative care reported a better understanding of their prognosis which helped them make decisions about their treatment, assisted them cope with the disease, and had discussed their end of life wishes with their oncologist [58].

A qualitative analysis of clinical documentation from 20 patients with advanced lung cancer who received early palliative care, showed that the clinics helped with symptoms and coping, built rapport, assisted with understanding of the disease and EoL advance care planning, and ensured family members were involved; the content of discussions varied over time [59].

CONCLUSION

Patients with lung cancer have a high symptom burden and unmet physical, psychological, spiritual and social needs. Patients with lung cancer should receive supportive and palliative care by general and specialist palliative care providers and referrals to specialist palliative care services should be done early if the patient has needs that could be met by the interdisciplinary team. There is evidence that early referrals to palliative care and an integrated approach benefit the patient and family.

CONSENT FOR PUBLICATION

Not applicable.

CONFLICT OF INTEREST

The author declares that there is no conflict of interest in this chapter.

ACKNOWLEDGEMENTS

Declared none.

REFERENCES

[1]   Cancer Research UK. Lung cancer statistics. 2018. Available from: https://www.cancerrese archuk.org/health-professional/cancer-statistics/statistics-by-cancer-type/lung-cancer-heading-Zero.

[2]   World Cancer Research Fund International. Lung cancer statistics 2018. https://www.wcrf.org/ dietandcancer/cancer-trends/lung-cancer-statistics

[3]   International Agency for Research on Cancer. GLOBOCAN 2018 2018. Available from: https://gco.iarc.fr/today/online-analysis-table?v=2018&mode=cancer&mode_population=continents &population=900&populations=900&key=asr&sex=0&cancer=39&type=1&statistic=5&prevalence= 0&population_group=0&ages_group%5B%5D=0&ages_group%5B%5D=17&nb_items=5&group_ca ncer=1&include_nmsc=1&include_nmsc_other=1.

[4]   Beckett P, Tata LJ, Hubbard RB. Risk factors and survival outcome for non-elective referral in non-small cell lung cancer patients--analysis based on the National Lung Cancer Audit. Lung Cancer 2014; 83(3): 396-400.
[http://dx.doi.org/10.1016/j.lungcan.2013.10.010] [PMID: 24457105]

[5]   Cancer Research UK. Lung cancer incidence statistics 2017. https://www.cancerresearchuk.org/ health-professional/cancer-statistics/statistics-by-cancer-type/lung-cancer/incidence

[6]   Temel JS, Greer JA, Admane S, *et al.* Longitudinal perceptions of prognosis and goals of therapy in patients with metastatic non-small-cell lung cancer: results of a randomized study of early palliative care. J Clin Oncol 2011; 29(17): 2319-26.
[http://dx.doi.org/10.1200/JCO.2010.32.4459] [PMID: 21555700]

[7]   Kelly M, O'Brien KM, Lucey M, Clough-Gorr K, Hannigan A. Indicators for early assessment of palliative care in lung cancer patients: a population study using linked health data. BMC Palliat Care 2018; 17(1): 37.
[http://dx.doi.org/10.1186/s12904-018-0285-5] [PMID: 29482533]

[8]   World Health Organization. WHO Definition of Palliative Care 2018. https://www.who.int/cancer/ palliative/definition/en/

[9]   National Institute for Health and Care Excellence. Care of dying adults in the last days of life 2017.https://www.nice.org.uk/guidance/qs144/chapter/Quality-statement-3-Anticipatory-prescribing

[10]   National Institute for Health and Care Excellence. Improving Supportive and Palliative Care for Adults with Cancer 2004.https://www.nice.org.uk/guidance/csg4/resources/improving-supportive-a-d-palliative-care-for-adults-with-cancer-pdf-773375005

[11]   Higginson IJ, Evans CJ. What is the evidence that palliative care teams improve outcomes for cancer patients and their families? Cancer J 2010; 16(5): 423-35.
[http://dx.doi.org/10.1097/PPO.0b013e3181f684e5] [PMID: 20890138]

[12]   Temel JS, Greer JA, Muzikansky A, *et al.* Early palliative care for patients with metastatic non-smal-

-cell lung cancer. N Engl J Med 2010; 363(8): 733-42.
[http://dx.doi.org/10.1056/NEJMoa1000678] [PMID: 20818875]

[13]   Wentlandt K, Krzyzanowska MK, Swami N, Rodin GM, Le LW, Zimmermann C. Referral practices
        of oncologists to specialized palliative care. J Clin Oncol 2012; 30(35): 4380-6.
        [http://dx.doi.org/10.1200/JCO.2012.44.0248] [PMID: 23109708]

[14]   Greer JA, Jackson VA, Meier DE, Temel JS. Early integration of palliative care services with standard
        oncology care for patients with advanced cancer. CA Cancer J Clin 2013; 63(5): 349-63.
        [http://dx.doi.org/10.3322/caac.21192] [PMID: 23856954]

[15]   World Health Assembly. Strengthening of palliative care as a component of integrated treatment
        within the continuum of care. in 134th session of the World Health Assembly.

[16]   Simoff MJ, Lally B, Slade MG, Goldberg WG, Lee P, Michaud GC, *et al.* Symptom management in
        patients with lung cancer: Diagnosis and management of lung cancer, 3rd ed: American College of
        Chest Physicians evidence-based clinical practice guidelines. Chest. 2013; 143: pp. (5 Suppl)e455S-
        97S.

[17]   British Lung Foundation. Tackling emergency presentation of lung cancer: An expert working group
        report and recommendations 2015. https://www.blf.org.uk/sites/default/files/BLF_lung_cancer_
        report_2015.pdf

[18]   Boland EG, Boland JW, Ezaydi Y, *et al.* Holistic needs assessment in advanced, intensively treated
        multiple myeloma patients. Support Care Cancer 2014; 22(10): 2615-20.
        [http://dx.doi.org/10.1007/s00520-014-2231-2] [PMID: 24733635]

[19]   Morrison EJ, Novotny PJ, Sloan JA, *et al.* Emotional problems, quality of life, and symptom burden in
        patients with lung cancer. Clin Lung Cancer 2017; 18(5): 497-503.
        [http://dx.doi.org/10.1016/j.cllc.2017.02.008] [PMID: 28412094]

[20]   Maguire R, Papadopoulou C, Kotronoulas G, *et al.* A systematic review of supportive care needs of
        people living with lung cancer. Eur J Oncol Nurs 2013; 17(4): 449-64.
        [http://dx.doi.org/10.1016/j.ejon.2012.10.013] [PMID: 23246484]

[21]   Giuliani ME, Milne RA, Puts M, *et al.* The prevalence and nature of supportive care needs in lung
        cancer patients. Curr Oncol 2016; 23(4): 258-65.
        [http://dx.doi.org/10.3747/co.23.3012] [PMID: 27536176]

[22]   Williams AC, Grant M, Tiep B, Kim JY, Hayter J. Dyspnea management in early stage lung cancer: a
        palliative perspective. J Hosp Palliat Nurs 2012; 14(5): 341-2.
        [http://dx.doi.org/10.1097/NJH.0b013e318258043a] [PMID: 24058283]

[23]   Boland JW, Reigada C, Yorke J, *et al.* The adaptation, face, and content validation of a needs
        assessment tool: progressive disease for people with interstitial lung disease. J Palliat Med 2016;
        19(5): 549-55.
        [http://dx.doi.org/10.1089/jpm.2015.0355] [PMID: 26840603]

[24]   Fitch MI, Steele R. Supportive care needs of individuals with lung cancer. Can Oncol Nurs J 2010;
        20(1): 15-22.
        [http://dx.doi.org/10.5737/1181912x2011522] [PMID: 20369641]

[25]   O'Driscoll BR, Howard LS, Earis J, Mak V. BTS guideline for oxygen use in adults in healthcare and
        emergency settings. Thorax 2017; 72 (Suppl. 1): ii1-ii90.
        [http://dx.doi.org/10.1136/thoraxjnl-2016-209729] [PMID: 28507176]

[26]   Star A, Boland JW. Updates in palliative care - recent advancements in the pharmacological
        management of symptoms. Clin Med (Lond) 2018; 18(1): 11-6.
        [http://dx.doi.org/10.7861/clinmedicine.18-1-11] [PMID: 29436433]

[27]   Barnes H, McDonald J, Smallwood N, Manser R. Opioids for the palliation of refractory
        breathlessness in adults with advanced disease and terminal illness. Cochrane Database Syst Rev 2016;
        3CD011008

[http://dx.doi.org/10.1002/14651858.CD011008.pub2] [PMID: 27030166]

[28] Ekström M, Bajwah S, Bland JM, *et al.* One evidence base; three stories: do opioids relieve chronic breathlessness? Thorax 2018; 73(1): 88-90.
[http://dx.doi.org/10.1136/thoraxjnl-2016-209868] [PMID: 28377491]

[29] Simon ST, Higginson IJ, Booth S, *et al.* Benzodiazepines for the relief of breathlessness in advanced malignant and non-malignant diseases in adults. Cochrane Database Syst Rev 2016; 10: CD007354.
[http://dx.doi.org/10.1002/14651858.CD007354.pub3] [PMID: 27764523]

[30] Kako J, Morita T, Yamaguchi T, *et al.* Fan therapy is effective in relieving dyspnea in patients with terminally Ill cancer: a parallel-arm, randomized controlled trial. J Pain Symptom Manage 2018; 56(4): 493-500.
[http://dx.doi.org/10.1016/j.jpainsymman.2018.07.001] [PMID: 30009968]

[31] Johnson MJ, Booth S, Currow DC, Lam LT, Phillips JL. A mixed-methods, randomized, controlled feasibility trial to inform the design of a phase III trial to test the effect of the handheld fan on physical activity and carer anxiety in patients with refractory breathlessness. J Pain Symptom Manage 2016; 51(5): 807-15.
[http://dx.doi.org/10.1016/j.jpainsymman.2015.11.026] [PMID: 26880253]

[32] Bolzani A. Bolzani A, R.S., Kalies H, Maddocks M, Rehfuess E, Swan F, Gysels M, Higginson IJ, Booth S, Bausewein C, Respiratory interventions for breathlessness in adults with advanced diseases (Protocol). 2017, Cochrane Database of Systematic Reviews.

[33] Higginson IJ, Bausewein C, Reilly CC, *et al.* An integrated palliative and respiratory care service for patients with advanced disease and refractory breathlessness: a randomised controlled trial. Lancet Respir Med 2014; 2(12): 979-87.
[http://dx.doi.org/10.1016/S2213-2600(14)70226-7] [PMID: 25465642]

[34] National Institute for Health and Care Excellence. Lung cancer in adults 2019. Available from: https://www.nice.org.uk/guidance/qs17

[35] Miller RR, McGregor DH. Hemorrhage from carcinoma of the lung. Cancer 1980; 46(1): 200-5.
[http://dx.doi.org/10.1002/1097-0142(19800701)46:1<200::AID-CNCR2820460133>3.0.CO;2-V] [PMID: 6248189]

[36] Ibrahim WH. Massive haemoptysis: the definition should be revised. Eur Respir J 2008; 32(4): 1131-2.
[http://dx.doi.org/10.1183/09031936.00080108] [PMID: 18827169]

[37] Razazi K, Parrot A, Khalil A, *et al.* Severe haemoptysis in patients with nonsmall cell lung carcinoma. Eur Respir J 2015; 45(3): 756-64.
[http://dx.doi.org/10.1183/09031936.00010114] [PMID: 25359349]

[38] Prutsky G, Domecq JP, Salazar CA, Accinelli R. Antifibrinolytic therapy to reduce haemoptysis from any cause. Cochrane Database Syst Rev 2016; 11CD008711
[http://dx.doi.org/10.1002/14651858.CD008711.pub3] [PMID: 27806184]

[39] Ferrer-Mileo L, Luque Blanco AI, González-Barboteo J. Efficacy of cryoablation to control cancer pain: a systematic review. Pain Pract 2018; 18(8): 1083-98.
[http://dx.doi.org/10.1111/papr.12707] [PMID: 29734509]

[40] Kane CM, Mulvey MR, Wright S, *et al.* Opioids combined with antidepressants or antiepileptic drugs for cancer pain: Systematic review and meta-analysis. Palliat Med 2018; 32(1): 276-86.
[http://dx.doi.org/10.1177/0269216317711826] [PMID: 28604172]

[41] Potter J, Higginson IJ. Pain experienced by lung cancer patients: a review of prevalence, causes and pathophysiology. Lung Cancer 2004; 43(3): 247-57.
[http://dx.doi.org/10.1016/j.lungcan.2003.08.030] [PMID: 15165082]

[42] Caraceni A, Hanks G, Kaasa S, *et al.* Use of opioid analgesics in the treatment of cancer pain: evidence-based recommendations from the EAPC. Lancet Oncol 2012; 13(2): e58-68.

[http://dx.doi.org/10.1016/S1470-2045(12)70040-2] [PMID: 22300860]

[43]   National Institute for Health and Care Excellence. Palliative care for adults: strong opioids for pain relief 2016.https://www.nice.org.uk/guidance/cg140

[44]   Greco MT, Roberto A, Corli O, *et al.* Quality of cancer pain management: an update of a systematic review of undertreatment of patients with cancer. J Clin Oncol 2014; 32(36): 4149-54.
[http://dx.doi.org/10.1200/JCO.2014.56.0383] [PMID: 25403222]

[45]   Simmons CP, Macleod N, Laird BJ. Clinical management of pain in advanced lung cancer. Clin Med Insights Oncol 2012; 6: 331-46.
[http://dx.doi.org/10.4137/CMO.S8360] [PMID: 23115483]

[46]   Wood H, Dickman A, Star A, Boland JW. Updates in palliative care - overview and recent advancements in the pharmacological management of cancer pain. Clin Med (Lond) 2018; 18(1): 17-22.
[http://dx.doi.org/10.7861/clinmedicine.18-1-17] [PMID: 29436434]

[47]   Oldenmenger WH, Geerling JI, Mostovaya I, *et al.* A systematic review of the effectiveness of patient-based educational interventions to improve cancer-related pain. Cancer Treat Rev 2018; 63: 96-103.
[http://dx.doi.org/10.1016/j.ctrv.2017.12.005] [PMID: 29272781]

[48]   Ferrell B, Sun V, Hurria A, *et al.* Interdisciplinary palliative care for patients with lung cancer. J Pain Symptom Manage 2015; 50(6): 758-67.
[http://dx.doi.org/10.1016/j.jpainsymman.2015.07.005] [PMID: 26296261]

[49]   Sun V, Grant M, Koczywas M, *et al.* Effectiveness of an interdisciplinary palliative care intervention for family caregivers in lung cancer. Cancer 2015; 121(20): 3737-45.
[http://dx.doi.org/10.1002/cncr.29567] [PMID: 26150131]

[50]   National End of Life Care Programme Capacity, Care Planning And Advance Care Planning In Life Limiting Illness 2011.

[51]   Boland J, Owen J, Ainscough R, Mahdi H. Developing a service for patients with very severe chronic obstructive pulmonary disease (COPD) within resources. BMJ Support Palliat Care 2014; 4(2): 196-201.
[http://dx.doi.org/10.1136/bmjspcare-2012-000393] [PMID: 24644174]

[52]   Mullick A, Martin J, Sallnow L. An introduction to advance care planning in practice. BMJ 2013; 347: f6064.
[http://dx.doi.org/10.1136/bmj.f6064] [PMID: 24144870]

[53]   Boland JW, Ziegler L, Boland EG, McDermid K, Bennett MI. Is regular systemic opioid analgesia associated with shorter survival in adult patients with cancer? A systematic literature review. Pain 2015; 156(11): 2152-63.
[http://dx.doi.org/10.1097/j.pain.0000000000000306] [PMID: 26207652]

[54]   Morita T, Ichiki T, Tsunoda J, Inoue S, Chihara S. A prospective study on the dying process in terminally ill cancer patients. Am J Hosp Palliat Care 1998; 15(4): 217-22.
[http://dx.doi.org/10.1177/104990919801500407] [PMID: 9729972]

[55]   Boland E, Johnson M, Boland J. Artificial hydration in the terminally ill patient. Br J Hosp Med (Lond) 2013; 74(7): 397-401.
[http://dx.doi.org/10.12968/hmed.2013.74.7.397] [PMID: 24159642]

[56]   Ambroggi M, Biasini C, Toscani I, *et al.* Can early palliative care with anticancer treatment improve overall survival and patient-related outcomes in advanced lung cancer patients? A review of the literature. Support Care Cancer 2018; 26(9): 2945-53.
[http://dx.doi.org/10.1007/s00520-018-4184-3] [PMID: 29704108]

[57]   Bakitas M, Lyons KD, Hegel MT, *et al.* The project ENABLE II randomized controlled trial to improve palliative care for rural patients with advanced cancer: baseline findings, methodological challenges, and solutions. Palliat Support Care 2009; 7(1): 75-86.

[http://dx.doi.org/10.1017/S1478951509000108] [PMID: 19619377]

[58]   Temel JS, Greer JA, El-Jawahri A, *et al.* Effects of early integrated palliative care in patients with lung and GI cancer: a randomized clinical trial. J Clin Oncol 2017; 35(8): 834-41.
[http://dx.doi.org/10.1200/JCO.2016.70.5046] [PMID: 28029308]

[59]   Yoong J, Park ER, Greer JA, *et al.* Early palliative care in advanced lung cancer: a qualitative study. JAMA Intern Med 2013; 173(4): 283-90.
[http://dx.doi.org/10.1001/jamainternmed.2013.1874] [PMID: 23358690]

CHAPTER 14

Lasers and Photodynamic Therapy (PDT) in Lung Cancer

Keyvan Moghissi[*]

The Yorkshire Laser Centre, Goole & District Hospital, Goole, UK

Abstract: Laser application for lung cancer was introduced early in the 1980s to remove malignant obstructive lesion of the lower trachea and main bronchi. The main indication was in patients with inoperable central lung cancer. Intraoperative use of Thermal laser began later. In the early and mid-1980s, Photodynamic Therapy (PDT) became available.

In this chapter, the laser and laser light physics are briefly described prior to their applications and indications in lung cancer. The Nd;YAG laser, which is the most commonly employed thermal laser and its effects on lung tissue, is described, followed by its brief indication in the clinical practice of lung cancer.

The principle and mechanisms of PDT in destroying cancer tissues have also been discussed in this chapter. PDT indications in a variety of lung cancer are also discussed to some extent.

Keywords: Effects of Nd:YAG laser on the lung, Indications of lasers in lung Cancer, PDT and its role in Lung Cancer, What is laser.

INTRODUCTION

The term laser has two different connotations, namely:

Laser Device, which produces and emits the laser light and the laser light energy.

LASER DEVICE

Laser is a device that produces and emits a specific light, the laser light, through the process of stimulated emission followed by optical amplification.

---

[*] **Corresponding author Keyvan Moghissi:** The Yorkshire Laser Centre, Goole & District Hospital, Goole, UK; Tel: 01724 290456; E-mail: kmoghissi@yorkshirelasercentre.org

Keyvan Moghissi, Jack Kastelik, Philip Barber & Peyman Sardari Nia (Eds.)

Essential components of a Laser Device are:

1. Optical Resonant Cavity, which consists of an arrangement of mirrors within a metal box (or a cavity).
2. Gain medium, which is the lasing medium.
3. Laser pumping energy. This refers to the energy, which is to initiate stimulated emission.
4. High reflector: This consists of mirrors within the cavity.

Basically, stimulated emission results in the production of Photons (unit of light energy) which after amplification in the resonator, are emitted from one end of the cavity as the laser light (Fig. **1**).

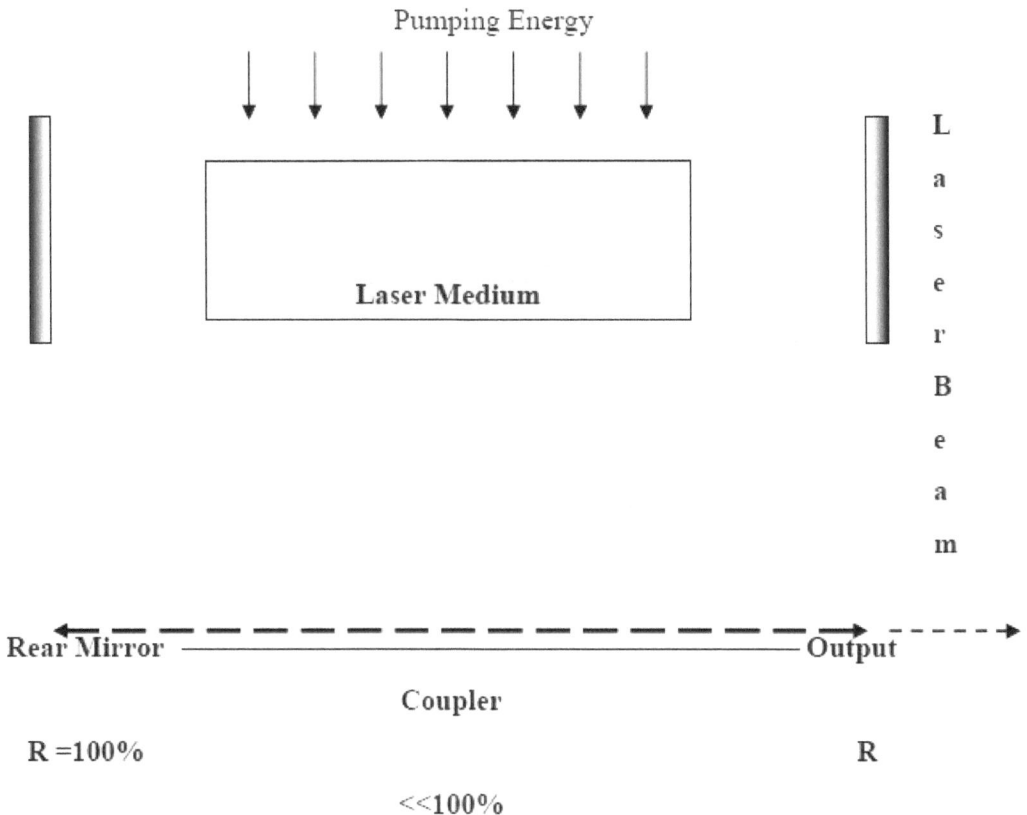

Fig. (1). Schematic of an optical resonant cavity.

Laser Light

The word 'laser' is an acronym of Light Amplification by Stimulated Emission of Radiation. In a nutshell, it describes the phenomenon in which a light, that is, the laser light is produced by "Stimulated Emission". It denotes that following absorption of light (photon) energy by an atom or molecule, an excited state is created, which is usually related to a change in electron orbit, from lower to a higher energy level of that atom. This unstable excited state can return spontaneously to the lower (equilibrium) energy level, (return of the electron to their original orbit) with the emission of a photon (the unit of light).

The rate of such stimulated emission is dependent upon the number of excited states created; in order for an amplification process to proceed, it is, therefore, necessary that the number of excited states be increased at the expense of the equilibrium state. This is referred to as a population inversion and can only be achieved by a method of pumping, which involves the delivery of sufficient energy to the medium. The method of pumping (as well as the wavelength of laser output) depends upon the laser medium.

Classification of Lasers

Lasers are named according to the specific laser medium which can take many forms:

Solid-state Lasers

This consists of ions contained within a host medium of solid crystal or glass.

Examples of this type are Ruby laser (694.3 nm), Nd-YAG (1064 nm), Ho-YAG (2.1 μm) lasers.

Nd-YAG consists of a medium of Yttrium Aluminium Garnet doped with Neodymium (Nd$^{3)}$ and is in common usage in pulmonology and thoracic surgery.

Gas Lasers

This consist of an atomic or molecular species in the gaseous, vapour or plasma state. Lasing action can be stimulated by passing an electric current through the laser medium. Examples of these are Argon ion laser (principal emission lines at 488 and 514 nm).

Carbon dioxide (CO_2) laser (10.6 μm).

Dye Lasers

This comprises organic dyes in solution or suspension, which are optically pumped by flash tube or by another laser. Each dye may be tuned over a limited wavelength range (~30 nm), and a wide range of dyes is available, allowing, with the appropriate choice of pumping source, laser emission from ultra-violet through to infrared wavelengths.

Diode Lasers

This employs suitably doped semiconducting materials, which are pumped by the passage of an electric current.

CHARACTERISTICS OF LASER LIGHT

Three fundamental properties characterise laser emission:

- Coherence is the term used to describe the relationship between the two waveforms, and it may be discussed in terms of both time (temporal coherence) and space (spatial coherence).
- Monochromaticity: This is a consequence of temporal coherence and implies a single output wavelength.
- Colimitation: This is a consequence of spatial coherence and represents the directionality of the beam as defined by the angular beam divergence.

The combination of very low divergence and narrow bandwidth results in an output that has a very high spectral intensity. Even low-power devices (such as the HeNe laser) exhibit a spectral intensity of much greater magnitude than can be obtained from a non-laser light source. One of the principle benefits of laser light in medical applications is the ability to focus the beam to a spot of small diameter. This is useful in allowing efficient light delivery via a narrow optical fibre.

LASER-TISSUE INTERACTION

The effect of an incident laser light upon tissue depends on a number of factors, principally the output characteristics of the laser (wavelength, average power, pulse energy and duration and spot-size) and the optical properties of the tissue. Briefly, incident laser light can be reflected, scattered or absorbed. Reflection is a type of scattering that occurs at the tissue surface; irradiation of a reflective tissue surface results in a loss that demands the input of a higher laser power to achieve the desired effect. Scattering below the surface has the effect of diffusing the incident beam so that biological effects may be induced at sites other than the target resulting in collateral damage.

THE BIOLOGICAL EFFECTS OF LASERS

Many lasers affect tissue through a thermal effect. The laser energy is absorbed by the tissue and is converted into heat. Other lasers affect tissue by photochemical effects in combination with a photosensitising chemical, which interferes with cell and tissue metabolism. These are dye lasers or diode lasers of specific wavelengths used in Photodynamic Therapy. It is therefore convenient, if somewhat simplistic, to classify medical lasers into:

Thermal Lasers

The most suitable Thermal Laser for use in endobronchial tumour photo-radiation and in pulmonary surgery is Laser. The visible and tangible evidence of the effects of Nd:YAG thermal lasers [1] are:

- Coagulation: This results from denaturisation of tissue protein, causing destruction and necrosis.
- Haemostasis: Arrest of haemorrhage caused by the laser is partially due to fibrin formation (clotting) and also from vasoconstriction sealing of small vessels.
- Vaporisation: High power laser energy produces total burn and evaporation of water, thus creating a crater in the target tissue, the border of which is formed by charred and totally and partially necrosed tissue. When vaporisation occurs over a narrow area, the effect is similar to surgical incision

Metabolic/Dye Lasers & Diodes

The effects of these lasers are:

- Interference with tissue/cell metabolism by a number of mechanisms which affect cell respiration and produce cytotoxic agents.
- Ischemia and necrosis due to the release of vasoactive substances affecting small vessels.

The wavelength produced by a dye laser is dependent on the type of dye used. In Photodynamic Therapy, a photochemical/photosensitizer needs to be incorporated into the target tissue, which is referred to as *"Pre-sensitization."* The pre-sensitized tissue is then exposed to the laser light of a specific wavelength

(Illumination). The interaction between the light whose wavelength matches the absorption band of the chemical, usually in the presence of oxygen produces, what is known as photodynamic reaction (PDR). This is responsible for the photochemical effects with the release of "singlet oxygen" and other cytotoxic species, which in turn bring about necrosis (cell death) and destruction of the target tissues [2].

LASER EQUIPMENT FOR CLINICAL APPLICATION

This comprises 3 essential components:

1. Laser generator: This generates laser light of a specific wavelength.

2. Delivery system: To transmit the emitted laser light to the patient.

3. Applicators: These are the devices which carry the delivered laser light to a specific site in the body. Applicators are part of the delivery system manipulated by the clinician.

Types of Lasers Used Specifically for Lung Cancer

Amongst a variety of currently available lasers, the most commonly used in thoracic surgery and for lung cancer are:

CO_2 lasers

Nd YAG and Ho YAG lasers

Diode lasers employed in Photodynamic Therapy

Carbon Dioxide (CO_2) Laser

This laser emits light at a wavelength of 10.6 micrometers (10600 nm) in the infrared range of the electromagnetic spectrum. Its properties are:

• Strong absorption by water.

• Great cutting power.

• Weak haemostatic activity.

The great disadvantage of this laser is that it cannot be delivered through optical fibres, which thus restricts its endoscopic application. At the present time, the application of the CO_2 laser in lung cancer is limited to its application to the cancers which have expanded or has metastasised to the upper trachea.

Nd:YAG Laser

This is the most extensively used laser in thoracic surgery and in lung cancer. Its prominent properties are:

- Emits light at a wavelength of 1064 nm.
- Will transmit through water.
- Good haemostatic effect.
- Can be delivered through optical fibres.
- Can be used in either contact or non-contact mode

Nd:YAG, being a colourless light, is usually coupled with a Helium-Neon red light laser, the beam of which acts as an aiming red light as a guide to target. In lung cancer Nd;YAG laser is used endoscopically and/or intraoperatively.

Diode Laser

The introduction of the high-power gallium-arsenide (GaAs) diode array allows the possibility of a much more compact and easily applied laser system. There is a range of Diode lasers which can emit light within the visible spectrum (380 – 740 nm) and also near Infrared (800 – 1000 nm). The latter induces a comparable clinical effect to the Nd YAG source and can be used as a Contact Mode at the point of delivery.

ND YAG LASER INDICATIONS IN LUNG CANCER

ND-YAG in Central Lung Cancer/Bronchoscopic YAG Laser Radiation

Tracheo-bronchoscopic laser therapy using Nd YAG laser begun in the 1970's [3, 4], and its methodology was consolidated in the 1980's [5 - 7]. Since then, the method has received universal acceptance for the treatment of endoluminal projecting lesions in the tracheobronchial tree.

Its main indications are:

- Inoperable lung cancer with tumour component obstructing trachea, main or lobar bronchi. The obstructed airway leads to collapse (atelectasis) of the portion of the lung, which is ventilated by the obstructed bronchial branch. This causes dyspnoea (breathing difficulties). Thermal lasers applied through the bronchoscope relieves the obstruction and in a matter of minutes, can also relieve the dyspnoea.

• Haemoptysis (bleeding from airway). This can be from endobronchial cancer, which is ulcerated. The arrest of Haemorrhage by thermal laser application is very prompt and effective.

Bronchoscopic NdYAG laser can be carried out with the use of the flexible fibreoptic instrument under local anaesthesia as was originally practiced. However, the safest and most reliable method, which is also the least distressing for the patient, is to carry out tracheo-bronchoscopic YAG laser therapy under general anaesthesia with the use of the rigid bronchoscope [4 - 8].

The task is greatly facilitated if a specially designed instrument is used. Alternatively, the rigid instrument may be used through which ventilation is maintained. The Flexible Fibreoptic Bronchoscope (FFB) instrument is then passed through the rigid bronchoscope to localise the target. FFB also provides a route through its biopsy channel for the laser delivery fibre to reach targeted cancer.

The laser radiation is of non-contact mode and is carried out by directing the fibre towards the target. The Helium-Neon (He-Ne) aiming beam is then focused on cancer, but not touching it. The Helium beam will be seen as a red circle (Fig. **2**). The smaller the diameter of the circle, the more focused is the beam at the target. Therefore, less power (in watts) will be needed to achieve evaporation. A power of 20-40 watts for 2-4 seconds is sufficient to ablate (evaporate) the tumour, small portion at the time. This is repeated several times until the lesion is totally evaporated.

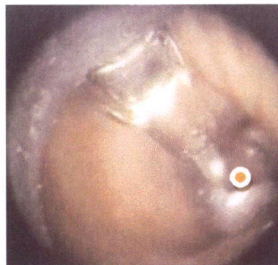

Fig. (2). Laser invisible light coupled with visible light (Helium-Neon Laser) to add precision to target the lesion.

If charring rather than evaporation is required, the same power may be used, but the tip of the laser fibre kept further away from the target.

Following the completion of therapy, pieces of tumour and debris should be removed with biopsy forceps through the rigid bronchoscope and thorough cleansing and lavage of the bronchial tree carried out. This is important because distal to the point of obstruction, there is often a collection of pus and infected material. It is also logical in such cases to obtain a sample of secretions for microbiological studies.

Results

The mortality of bronchoscopic Yag laser therapy is reported to be between 1-3% [7]. In the author's series of just over 700 patients, no procedure-related mortality was observed [8].

Complications

There are a variety of reported complications associated with tracheobronchial laser therapy in the literature:

Major fatal haemorrhage approx. 1%

Minor haemorrhage 4 – 6%

Pneumothorax/fistula <1%

Fire <1%

Others (infection) 1-2%

- Symptomatic and functional results expressed as a reduction of dyspnoea and improved ventilation are reported worldwide.

- Survival: depends almost entirely on the histology, topography and stage of the tumour, as well as the performance status of the patients.

Nd YAG in Early Central Lung Cancer: Early Superficial Endo-bronchial superficial cancers may be treated by Nd YAG laser. However, since the development of PDT, this has been abandoned. This is because of the specific anti-neoplastic effect of PDT and its precision targeting compared with Nd YAG laser.

Intraoperative Use of YAG Laser

A pilot study carried out by Moghissi *et al*. which started in 1985 and completed in 1988 [8 - 10], showed the potentials of Nd YAG laser in pulmonary surgery. It was shown that low power, 10-15 Watts, for a couple of seconds of laser energy radiation promoted clotting and seals air leaks from alveoli and the high power, 40-50 Watts, for 3-5 seconds evaporated tissue and incise the lung tissues with little bleeding or air leak (Fig. **3**). Later both experimental and clinical work showed that YAG laser may be used to locally excise coin (nodular pulmonary) lesions.

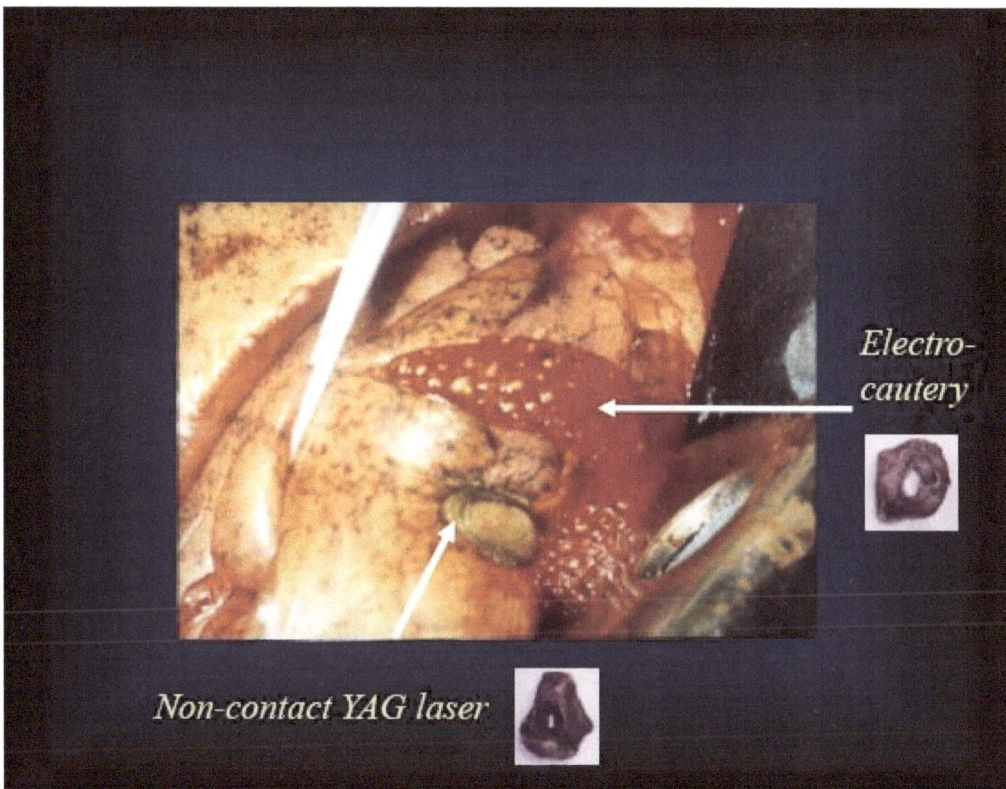

Fig. (3). Comparison between the effect of the YAG laser and electro diathermy on lung tissue. An incision on the lung by laser produces no air leak or bleeding, whereas an incision made by electrocautery is attended by bleeding as well as air leak (bubble) as shown by arrows.

In practice, Nd YAG laser can be used intra-operatively for a variety of purposes:

- Local excision of nodular lesions [10, 11]
- Pulmonary metastasectomy [9, 12 - 14].

• In conjunction with conventional pulmonary surgery [9, 12]

When its use is envisaged for local excision of pulmonary nodular lesions, the patient should be fully investigated as per usual standard for lung cancer.

The lesion can be primary cancer and or a metastatic secondary tumour. We performed the first pulmonary metastasectomy with the use of NdYAG laser in 1985. The lesion was a single pulmonary nodule (secondary breast tumour) in a female with the previous mastectomy for breast cancer and rather poor cardio-respiratory function.

Metatstatectomy was carried out through a mini-thoracotomy. The patient could be discharged 3 days after the operation and the case was presented at the first meeting of the European Association in Vienna (September 1986).

In suitable candidates and with the use of mini-thoracotomy, a single secondary lesion is attended by a simple postoperative course. A drainage tube may not even be required because of the lack of air leak. The hospital stay is between 2-4 days. More importantly, there is no loss of function resulting from the operation symptomatically and objectively post-operative ventilation figures are not significantly altered in comparison with the pre-operative ones [11] (Figs. **4** and **5**).

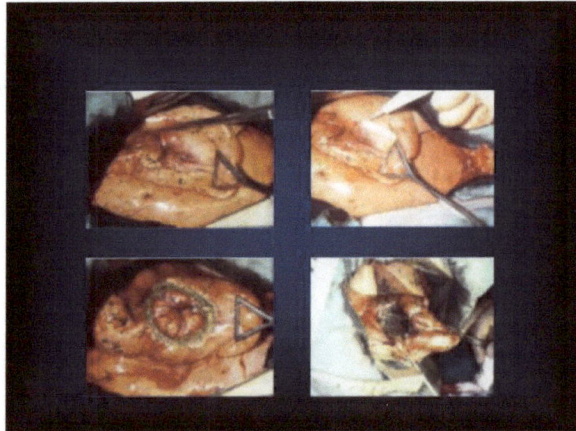

Fig. (4). Sequence in local excision of a pulmonary nodular lesion using YAG laser.
Top left: The tumour showing on the surface of the lung.
Top right: Tumour demarcation by laser light.
Bottom left: Circulator incision made by laser around the tumour area.
Bottom right: The tumour has been excised and a crater left in the lung, which although is inflated neither bleeds or has an air leak.

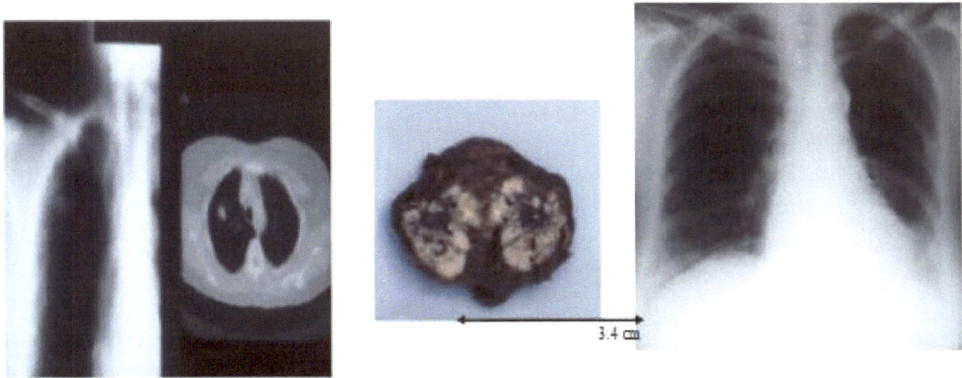

Fig (5). A Case of a 72 years lady with a single pulmonary metastasis from a breast cancer.
Left: Pre-operative chest X ray and CT scan, the latter showing a small nodule in the right lung.
Middle: Specimen excised with a minimum of healthy lung using Nd YAG laser.
Right: Chest radiograph 8 weeks post laser excision of the tumour.
Hospital stay: 3 days

Limited, muscle-sparing thoracotomy with an appropriately placed incision usually suffices to expose the tumour. Local excision is carried out by using high power 70-90 watts of energy. A circular incision is made some 2 cm away from the visible border of the tumour. The incision is deepened, and the tumour removed. Only small sub-segmental arteries and sub-segmental bronchi require stitching or clipping (Fig. **4**).

Some authors [14] feel it is totally justifiable to remove multiple metastatic tumours bilaterally. In exceptional circumstances (colon cancer metastases) we have excised up to 5 secondary lung metastases.

Working within a multidisciplinary team is important. Many patients' secondary tumours become unaffected by chemotherapy, even when the primary lesion still shows signs of positive response.

- Nd YAG in conjunction with standard pulmonary surgery can be used for dissection of segments to prevent excessive air leak, for haemostasis and for reducing lymphatic leaks following excision of lymph nodes.

Photodynamic Therapy (PDT)

The basis of PDT is photosensitisation of tissue by a chemical photosenitizer (PS) with a defined absorption band for a specific wavelength of laser light. When such sensitised tissue is exposed to the appropriate light (of a specific wavelength) in the presence of oxygen, injury and necrosis of the treated tissues will occur. Formation of singlet oxygen and the release of other cytotoxic species are mechanisms of necrosis and tissue destruction. Several photosensitizers have been used experimentally and clinically such as Photofrin and mTHPC (mesotetra hydroxy phenol phthalocyanine) 5-ALA (Amino Levulinic Acid), each requiring a specific laser light wavelength for their activation. ALA is a naturally occurring precursor in the process of Heme (hemoglobin) biosynthesis pathway. It is converted to the endogenous photosensitizer protoporphyrin IX. This can be activated by red, green and blue light.

The commonest photosensitiser in use for clinical PDT for is Photofrin requiring a matching 630 nm laser light (red). A variety of laser light sources have also emerged, the latest being Diode lasers combining efficiency with manageability and mobility of the equipment.

In 1975 Dougherty and colleagues [15] showed that by administering haematoporphyrin derivatives (HPD) systemically as a photosensitiser in mice with transplanted mammary tumours, eradication of the tumour was achieved with little damage to the surrounding tissue. This was also shown to be the case in a variety of other tumours [16]. The first PDT treatment in human lung cancer was carried out by Hayata and colleagues in 1982 [16].

At the same time Balchum *et al* [17] and Cortese *et al* (1982 and 1986) demonstrated the feasibility and potential benefits of endobronchial PDT in cases of bronchial carcinoma. Since then a number of authors have shown total response and long survival of patients with early stage carcinoma treated by endoscopic PDT. Others have also demonstrated benefit in terms of palliation of symptoms as well as survival benefit in those patients with inoperable tumours when treated by endoscopic interstitial PDT [17 - 19].

Bronchoscopic PDT for Lung Cancer

Clinical practice PDT is carried out as a two-step procedure:

In the first called "Pre-sensitisation", the photosensitiser (PS) is administered intravenously

The steps of the procedure are (Fig. **6**):

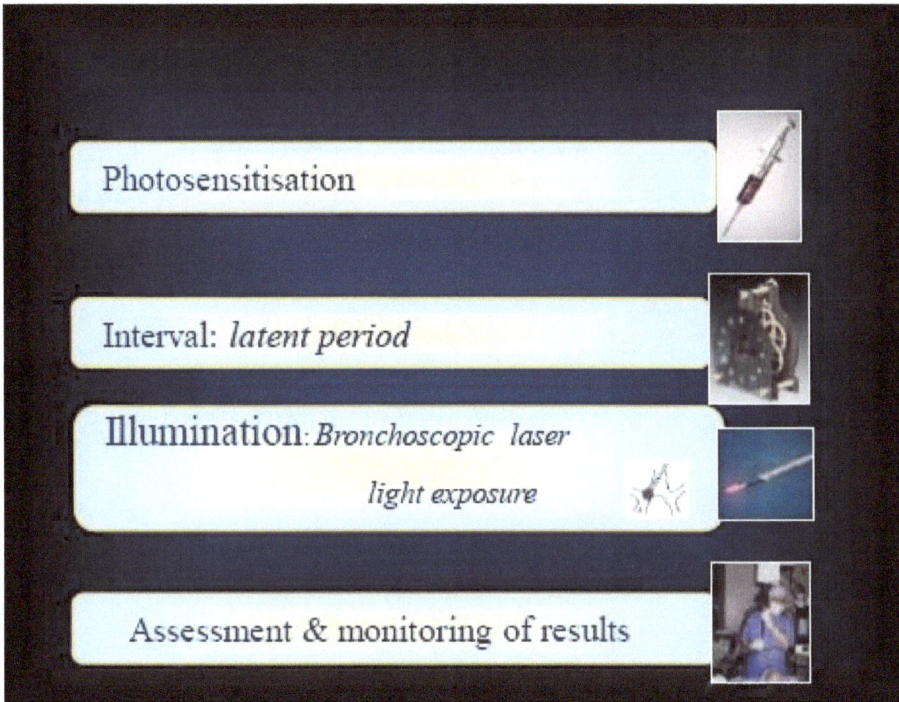

Fig. (6). Scheme of bronchoscopic PDT (See text).

- Currently the most commonly used photosensitiser is Photofrin administered 2 mg/kg bw.
- The second step is referred to as "Illumination". This is exposure of the tumour to the laser light and is carried out 24 – 72 hours after pre-sensitisation. Two methods of illumination are:
    a. Interstitial for bulky tumours when the diffuser end after laser fibre is inserted into the mass of the tumour.
    b. Superficial, where a fibre used with a diffuser with a "Micro lens" which projects the light forward and superficially (Fig. 7).

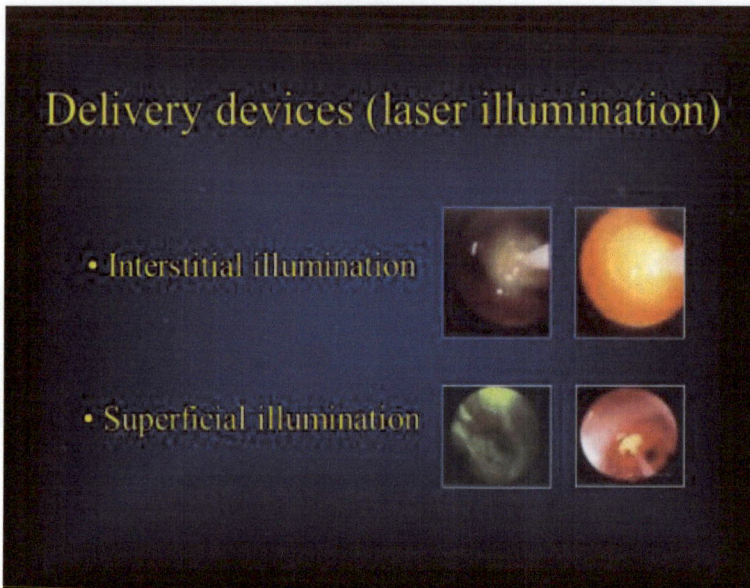

Fig. (7). Methods of Illuminations in PDT for Central Lung Cancer: Top: Interstitial Illumination Bottom: Surface/ Superficial Illumination.

The Light and Light Dose

The wavelength of light used with Photofrin is a red light at 630 nm.

Many investigators, including the authors, use a dose of 200 joules per cm of tumour tissue (400-mw output/cm of the diffuser for 500 seconds). Experience is needed to optimise time and energy to achieve necrosis of the tumour in its entirety.

Post-operative Management

Patients with bulky tumour occupying main bronchi require a repeat bronchoscopy 4 – 6 days later in order to rid the bronchus of necrotic debris and to carry out further illumination of residual tumour, if required. Clearly, this debridement in larger obstructive tumours cannot be carried out satisfactorily via FFB with its narrow aspiratory channel and the minute cup biopsy forceps. Rigid open-ended bronchoscope with its larger biopsy device is the instrument of choice.

Patients are monitored at 2 – 3 monthly intervals and additional PDT, Nd YAG laser or other treatment is given as appropriate.

Indications

PDT for Central Lung Cancer

This is essentially an endobronchial disease and PDT for central lung cancer is carried out bronchoscopically (see chapter on Bronchoscopy).

Over 95% of patients with lung cancer treated by PDT the treatment is currently carried out bronchoscopically. The indications are:

- In locally advanced disease, symptom improvement can be expected for over 70% of patients provided that the malignant obstruction is within the lumen of the main bronchus and there are no metastatic extra thoracic secondary tumours.
- In early endobronchial cancer PDT is given with curative intent [19, 21] indicated to achieve complete response at long term amounting to cure of the disease locally.

A review of the literature shows that in early endobronchial cancer PDT can achieve 60 -70% 5 years survival depending on the age and performance status of the patient at the time of therapy [22 - 24] (Fig. **8**).

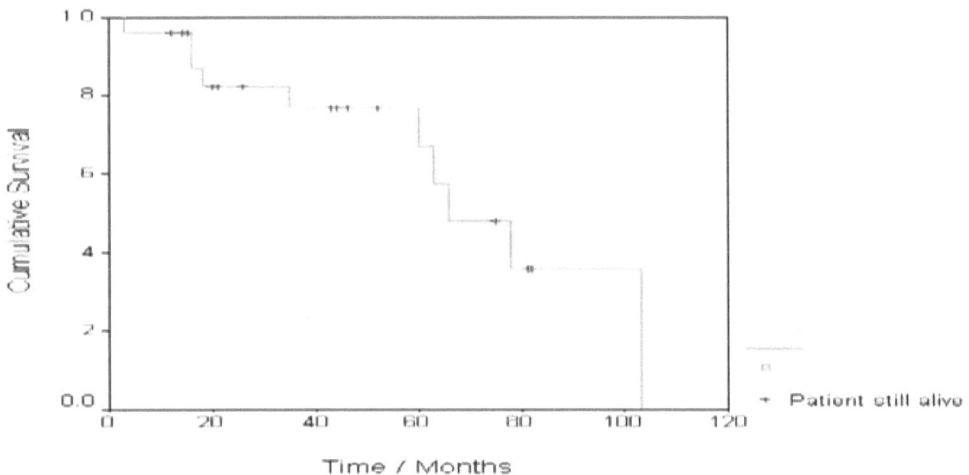

Fig. (8). Results of bronchoscopic PDT in early stage lung cancer.
Mean survival: 68.91 +8.35 months – Median survival: 66.00 + 9.96 months Taken from Moghissi *et al* Thorax 2007;62(5): 391-395.

- PDT can also be carried out bronchoscopically as a new adjuvant therapy for down staging (T factor) in resectable lung cancer.

PDT for Peripheral Lung Cancer

Rarely and occasionally, PDT can be applied for a peripheral malignant nodular lesion. In such cases, pre-sensitization is carried out intravenously. The illumination is then performed either by image-guided CT scan [25] or under vision thoracoscopically [26] (Fig. **9**).

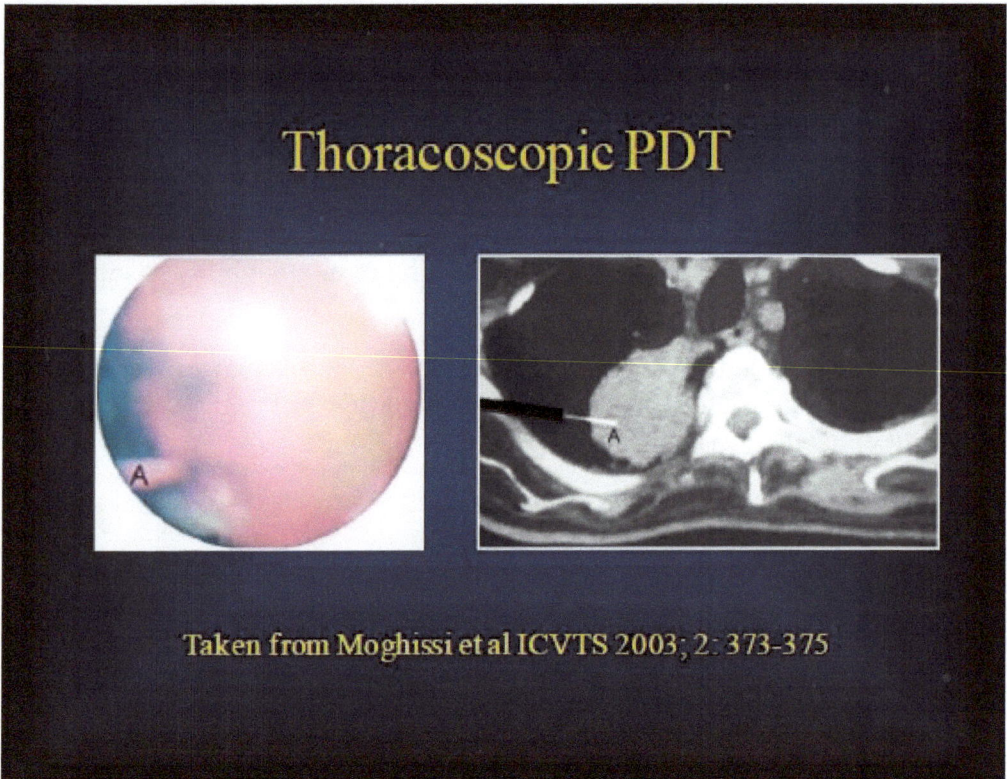

Fig. (9). Left interstitial illumination of a tumour I the right lung A = the laser optical light delivery fibre in the tumour.
Right CT scan with optical fibre insert in the tumour just prior to Illumination/activation of laser light.

PDT for Unusual Lung Cancer

There are a number of situations in which PDT can be considered as the prime indication, in some of them it is almost the only solution to a clinical problem. These include:

• Typical carcinoid tumour [28] (Fig. **10a** and Fig. **10b**).

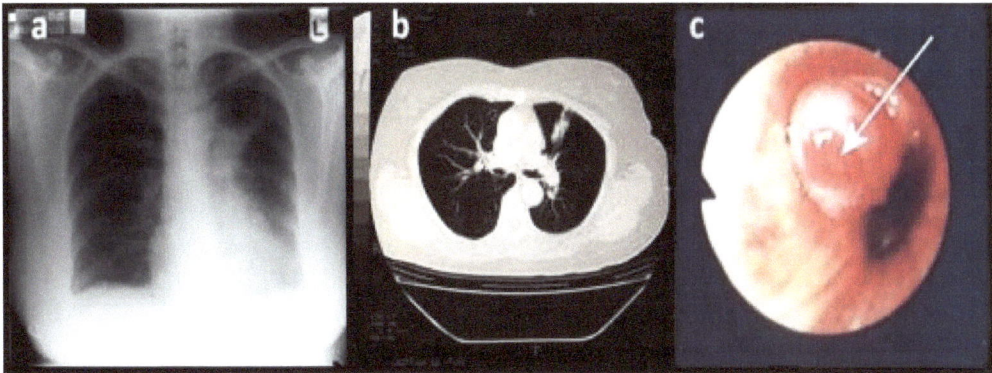

Fig. (10a). Pre PDT Chest x-ray, CT and Bronchoscopic picture of a patient (Mrs AS) with a typical carcinoid involving left upper lobe and extending to the left main stem bronchus.

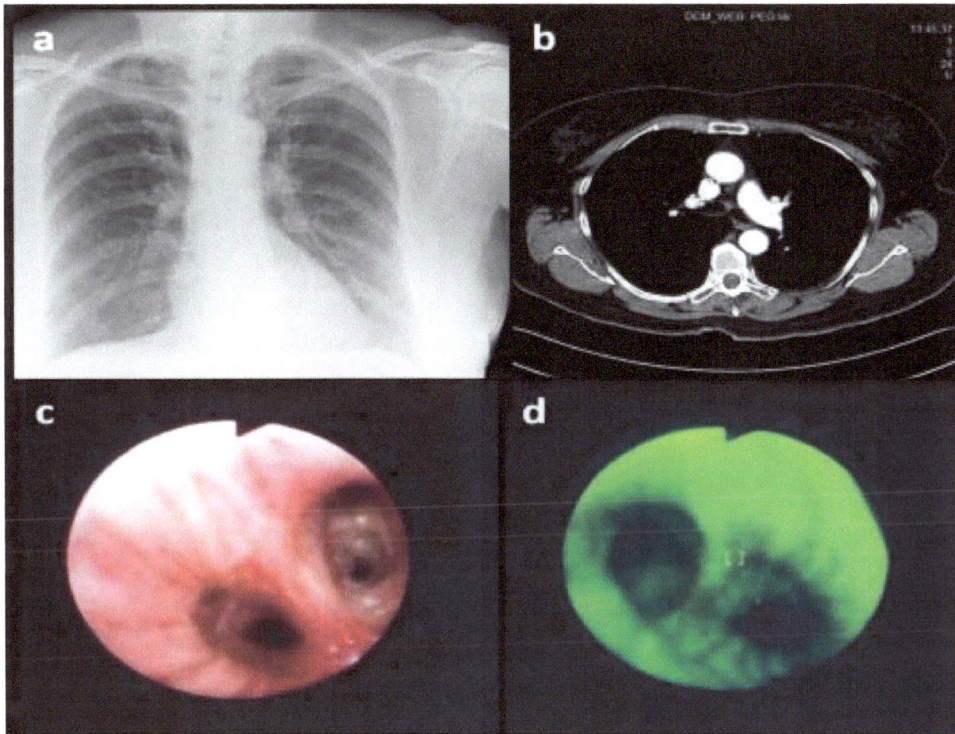

Fig. (10b). Post endo bronchial PDT of the same patient 15 years later showing (**a**) clear chest x-ray, (**b**) clear CT scan, (**c**) white light bonchoscopy and (**d**) autofluorescence bonchoscopy. Both these endoscopic examinations show total normality.
The case was published in 2013;43:54-1256.

- Endobronchial recurrence of cancer after lobectomy.
- Metachronous tumour after pneumonectomy in the residual lung

• Synchronous endobronchial tumour (in the left and the right).

Complications

The following complications have been reported:

• Photosensitivity skin reaction: The incidence is dependent on patient's compliance in avoiding sunlight and upon rigour of counselling. Although this has the potential to be an important drawback, its incidence can be reduced (<4%) by thorough counselling and education of the patient [19, 20].

• Haemorrhage has been reported when treatment was undertaken in patients with bulky inoperable tumours [17]. However, more recent reports of a large series have not shown such complication [18-20, 27].

• Post-treatment dyspnoea and breathlessness. This is a rare event but can occur in patients with severe obstructive lesion due to a bulky endoluminal tumour. After treatment debris and secretions may be retained in the bronchus, thus obliterating the lumen. In such patients, repeat bronchoscopy for debridement 3 – 5 days later should be routine. Further rebronchoscopy/ aspiration should be carried out as appropriate.

• Infective complication due to retention of secretion. This can be prevented by carrying out thorough aspiration and cleansing of the bronchial tree at the conclusion of bronchoscopic PDT. Active physiotherapy and prophylactic antibiotic should be given in those with severe bronchial obstruction and distal infection.

CONCLUSION

In this chapter, the principles of laser and laser light production have been described. Attention is paid to the classification of lasers, which is useful to clinicians. The principles of targeting and the specific role of PDT in targeting cancer have been stressed. Attention is drawn to the fact that Photodynamic Therapy (PDT), which uses lasers in the case of lung cancer, is the only specific procedure in which laser does not only target the lesion through the intervention of the operator (clinician) but that the laser light targets specifically its matching photosensitizer.

Nd:YAG laser is a rapid reaction tool in laser technology, which can bring great relief to patients with locally advanced tumours in the airway. PDT is a slow reaction but sustained and specific to cancer tool, which, although is used for locally advanced tumours, its main interest is within the early local tumour in which a cure can be achieved.

Bronchoscopic use of Nd:YAG laser is an established treatment for endobronchial malignant obstructive lesions throughout the world but its practice is confined to a few centres in the developed countries. It requires appropriate resources and manpower not affordable by some other countries.

In recent years Local Excision of Primary and Metastatic lung cancer has received renewed interest in a number of countries in Europe. The cost is a prohibitive factor, not efficacy or clinical benefit, which has been shown in many trials and thousands of patients.

PDT for lung cancer has not had as widespread expansion as was expected; nevertheless, in every developed country centres for lung cancer using the method in selected cases. Japan has always led these advances.

In Britain, the National Institute for Care Excellence (NICE) and the British Thoracic Society (BTS) have published guidelines for its use for Central Lung Cancer.

In Russia and China, the financial assistance of the state has been a driving force in PDT use in lung cancer. The problem in many countries is finance and education, particularly amongst Oncologists and Respiratory Physicians.

FURTHER READING

Principles of Lasers. Fifth Edition 2010. Orazio Svelton. Springer ISBN 978144191312.

Basics of Laser Physics. Kan F Renk 2018. Springer, Heidelber,: Dordrecht, London:, New York. ISSN 1868 -4513

CONFLICT OF INTEREST

The author declares that there is no conflict of interest in this chapter.

CONSENT FOR PUBLICATION

Not applicable.

ACKNOWLEDGEMENTS

Kate Dixon & Janet Melvin

REFERENCES

[1]   Moghissi K, Dench M, Neville E. Effects of non-contact mode of YAG laser on pulmonary tissue and its comparison with electrodiathermy; an anatomopathological study. Lasers Med Sci 1989; 4: 17-23.

[http://dx.doi.org/10.1007/BF02032505]

[2]   Allison RR, Moghissi K. Photodynamic therapy (PDT): PDT mechanisms. Clin Endosc 2013; 46(1): 24-9.
        [http://dx.doi.org/10.5946/ce.2013.46.1.24] [PMID: 23422955]

[3]   Toty L, Personne CL, Hertzog P, *et al.* Utilisation d'un faisceau laser (YAG) à conducteur souple, pour le traitement endoscopique de certaines lésions trachéo-bronchiques. Rev Fr Mal Respir 1979; 7(5): 475-82.
        [PMID: 575806]

[4]   Toty L, Personne C, Colchin A. Vourch. Bronchoscopic management of tracheal lesions using the NdYag laser. Thorax 1981; 36: 175-8.
        [http://dx.doi.org/10.1136/thx.36.3.175] [PMID: 7197061]

[5]   Moghissi K, Jessop T, Dench M. A new bronchoscopy set for laser therapy. Thorax 1986; 41(6): 485-6.
        [http://dx.doi.org/10.1136/thx.41.6.485] [PMID: 3787525]

[6]   Moghissi K, Budd A. Laser treatment for tracheobronchial tumours: local or general anesthesia? Thorax 1988; 43(3): 218.
        [http://dx.doi.org/10.1136/thx.43.3.218] [PMID: 3406910]

[7]   Personne C, Colchen A, Leroy M, Vourc'h G, Toty L. Indications and technique for endoscopic laser resections in bronchology. A critical analysis based upon 2,284 resections. J Thorac Cardiovasc Surg 1986; 91(5): 710-5.
        [http://dx.doi.org/10.1016/S0022-5223(19)35991-4] [PMID: 3009998]

[8]   Moghissi K, Dench M, Goebells P. Experience in non-contact Nd YAG laser in pulmonary surgery. A pilot study. Eur J Cardiothorac Surg 1988; 2(2): 87-94.
        [http://dx.doi.org/10.1016/S1010-7940(88)80004-6] [PMID: 3272211]

[9]   Moghissi K, Dixon K. Bronchoscopic Nd YAG laser treatment in lung cancer, 30 years on: an institutional review Lasers Med Sci 2006; 21(4): 186-91.

[10]   Moghissi K. Local excision of pulmonary nodular (coin) lesion with noncontact yttrium-aluminu--garnet laser. J Thorac Cardiovasc Surg 1989; 97(1): 147-51.
        [http://dx.doi.org/10.1016/S0022-5223(19)35140-2] [PMID: 2911192]

[11]   Moghissi K, Dixon K. Neodymium-yttrium-aluminium-garnet laser for excision of pulmonary nodules: an institutional review. Lasers Med Sci 2009; 24(2): 252-8.
        [http://dx.doi.org/10.1007/s10103-007-0538-7]

[12]   Moghissi K. Experience in limited lung resection with the use of laser. 1990; pp. 1103-9.
        [http://dx.doi.org/10.1007/BF02718250]

[13]   Branscheid D, Krysa S, Wollkopf G, *et al.* Does ND-YAG laser extend the indications for resection of pulmonary metastases? Eur J Cardiothorac Surg 1992; 6(11): 590-6.
        [http://dx.doi.org/10.1016/1010-7940(92)90132-H] [PMID: 1280452]

[14]   Rolle A, Pereszlenyi A, Koch R, Richard M, Baier B. Is surgery for multiple lung metastases reasonable? A total of 328 consecutive patients with multiple-laser metastasectomies with a new 1318-nm Nd:YAG laser. J Thorac Cardiovasc Surg 2006; 131(6): 1236-42.
        [http://dx.doi.org/10.1016/j.jtcvs.2005.11.053] [PMID: 16733151]

[15]   Dougherty TJ, Grindey GB, Fiel R, Weishaupt KR, Boyle DG. Photoradiation therapy. II. Cure of animal tumors with hematoporphyrin and light. J Natl Cancer Inst 1975; 55(1): 115-21.
        [http://dx.doi.org/10.1093/jnci/55.1.115] [PMID: 1159805]

[16]   Hayata Y, Kato H, Konaka C, *et al.* Bronchoscopic photoradiation for tumour localisation in lung cancer. Chest 1982; 82: 10-3.
        [http://dx.doi.org/10.1378/chest.82.1.10] [PMID: 6282545]

[17] Balchum OJ, Doiron DR. Photoradiation therapy of obstructing endobronchial lung cancer. Lasers Med Surg 1982; 357: 53-5.
[http://dx.doi.org/10.1117/12.976073]

[18] McCaughan JS Jr, Hawley PC, Bethel BH, Walker J. Photodynamic therapy of endobronchial malignancies. Cancer 1988; 62(4): 691-701.
[http://dx.doi.org/10.1002/1097-0142(19880815)62:4<691::AID-CNCR2820620408>3.0.CO;2-I]
[PMID: 2969279]

[19] Moghissi K, Dixon K, Stringer M, *et al.* The place of bronchoscopic photodynamic therapy in advanced unresectable lung cancer: experience of 100 cases. Eur J Cardiothorac Surg 1999; 15(1): 1-6.
[http://dx.doi.org/10.1016/S1010-7940(98)00295-4] [PMID: 10077365]

[20] McCaughan JS Jr, Williams TE. Photodynamic therapy for endobronchial malignant disease: a prospective fourteen-year study. J Thorac Cardiovasc Surg 1997; 114(6): 940-6.
[http://dx.doi.org/10.1016/S0022-5223(97)70008-4] [PMID: 9434689]

[21] Hayata Y, Kato H, Konaka C, *et al.* Photoradiation therapy with hematoporphyrin derivative in early and stage 1 lung cancer. Chest 1984; 86(2): 169-77.
[http://dx.doi.org/10.1378/chest.86.2.169] [PMID: 6235103]

[22] Cortese DA. Bronchoscopic photodynamic therapy of early lung cancer. Chest 1986; 90(5): 629-31.
[http://dx.doi.org/10.1378/chest.90.5.629b] [PMID: 3769558]

[23] Kato H, Okunaka T, Shimatani H. Photodynamic therapy for early stage bronchogenic carcinoma. J Clin Laser Med Surg 1996; 14(5): 235-8.
[http://dx.doi.org/10.1089/clm.1996.14.235] [PMID: 9612188]

[24] Moghissi K, Dixon K, Thorpe JA, Stringer M, Oxtoby C. Photodynamic therapy (PDT) in early central lung cancer: a treatment option for patients ineligible for surgical resection. Thorax 2007; 62(5): 391-5.
[http://dx.doi.org/10.1136/thx.2006.061143] [PMID: 17090572]

[25] Okunaka T, Kato H, Tsutsui H, Ishizumi T, Ichinose S, Kuroiwa Y. Photodynamic therapy for peripheral lung cancer. Lung Cancer 2004; 43(1): 77-82.
[http://dx.doi.org/10.1016/j.lungcan.2003.08.016] [PMID: 14698541]

[26] Moghissi K, Dixon K, Thorpe JA. A method for video-assisted thoracoscopic photodynamic therapy (VAT-PDT). Interact Cardiovasc Thorac Surg 2003; 2(3): 373-5.
[http://dx.doi.org/10.1016/S1569-9293(03)00073-2] [PMID: 17670074]

[27] Moghissi K, Dixon K, Gibbins S. A surgical view of photodynamic therapy in oncology: A review. Surg J (N Y) 2015; 1(1): e1-e15.
[http://dx.doi.org/10.1055/s-0035-1565246] [PMID: 28824964]

[28] Moghissi K, Dixon K, Gibbins SV. Case report: PDT for bronchial carcinoid tumours: report of a case with 10 year follow up. EJCTS 2013; 43: 1254-6.
[PMID: 23284100]

CHAPTER 15

Image-guided Surgery and Therapy for Broncho-pulmonary (Lung) Cancer

Keyvan Moghissi[*]

The Yorkshire Laser Centre, Goole & District Hospital, Goole, UK

Abstract: An important issue in the treatment of malignant tumours is concerned with the completeness of the resection/or destruction destruction of cancer and pre-cancerous lesions, without which no curative intent can be contemplated. In lung cancer, be it central or peripheral, the pre-cancerous lesions, usually at the margin of cancer itself, will have to be treated.

Image-guided lung cancer surgery and/or therapy is a method in which intraoperative real-time and updated images are provided to the operator, to allow him to access not only the tumour but also provide him with the outline of pre-cancerous lesions. As such, image-guided surgery and therapy provide navigational tools and real insight to perform complete treatment of cancer.

In this chapter, the various methods to identify small lesions within the wide field of the lung tissue are referred to and some of the methods which are currently under translational studies are explored.

Keywords: Fluorescence guided operations for lung cancer, Intraoperative localization of a pulmonary nodule, Image-guided intra-operative navigation for lung cancer.

INTRODUCTION

Image-Guided Surgery and Therapy (IGS/IGT) refer to operations undertaken for surgical and non-surgical treatment of lung cancer under the guidance of repeatedly updated intra-operative real-time images, facilitating navigation and access to the lesion.

From a therapeutic perspective, the variety of lung cancers are best considered as two closely related topographical entities: central and peripheral lesions (Fig. **1**).

[*] **Corresponding author Keyvan Moghissi:** The Yorkshire Laser Centre, Goole & District Hospital, Goole, UK; Tel: 01724 290456; E-mail: kmoghissi@yorkshirelasercentre.org

Keyvan Moghissi, Jack Kastelik, Philip Barber & Peyman Sardari Nia (Eds.)

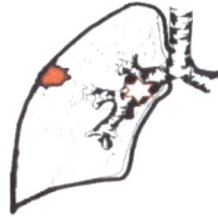

Fig. (1). Topographical classification of lung lesions: Solid red-peripheral, clear red-Central.

Peripheral lung cancers (PLC) develop in the substance of the pulmonary parenchyma. At their early stage, they can be imaged radiologically but not usually visualized bronchoscopically with the use of the standard technology.

Central lung cancers (CLC) develop from bronchial mucosa. These can usually be visualized bronchoscopically provided that the lesion is projecting from the mucosa into the lumen (*i.e.*, an exophytic tumour). However, an early CLC, such as a superficial *carcinoma in situ,* may not be imaged radiologically due to its mass size in relation to the resolution of the x-ray or CT scan.

Surgery, radiotherapy and chemotherapy (the trio) are currently considered the standard methods of therapy for lung cancer. They are employed individually or in concert to treat a given case of cancer.

In recent years, a number of *non-standard* cancer therapies - such as thermal lasers, photodynamic therapy (PDT) and radiofrequency have been developed; these are available for use in specific indications. They contribute considerably to the management of some patients with lung cancer.

The ultimate aim of lung cancer treatment is a long period of cancer free survival (CFS), amounting to the cure of the disease. At the present time, surgical resection has the best potential for achieving this objective. In suitable subjects with an early-stage cancer (stage IA), surgical resection can provide 70.9–81.5% 5-year CFS depending on the size of the lesion [1, 2].

However, overall, the majority of patients with lung cancer are oncologically and/or surgically inoperable at presentation, non-surgical and non-standard treatments play an important role in their management [3].

IGS/IGT SCHEME (FIG. 2)

IGS/IGT incorporates 3 steps:

Step 1

Preoperative: this is concerned with the use of a variety of imaging modalities to determine baseline parameters related to topography, the local extent of the lesion and its metastases. It must be emphasized that imaging, at best, offers the possibility of cancer diagnosis but cannot convey the actual diagnosis in its pathological meaning. This is an important issue not to be ignored.

Step 2

Marking or tagging cancer at an appropriate time prior to surgery (or non-surgical therapy), which would facilitate targeting and intraoperative identification of the lesion. In practice, an early PLC which has been radiologically imaged pre-operatively by CT may not be easily located at operation particularly if VATS (with no possibility of intra-operative palpation) is being used. An early CLC may also defy imaging by radiology (CT scan) and escape visual identification using standard bronchoscopic technology - *i.e.*, using white light. The reasons are that such a tumour can fall short of the discriminative power of the CT and can, equally, be outside the visual acuity of the observer.

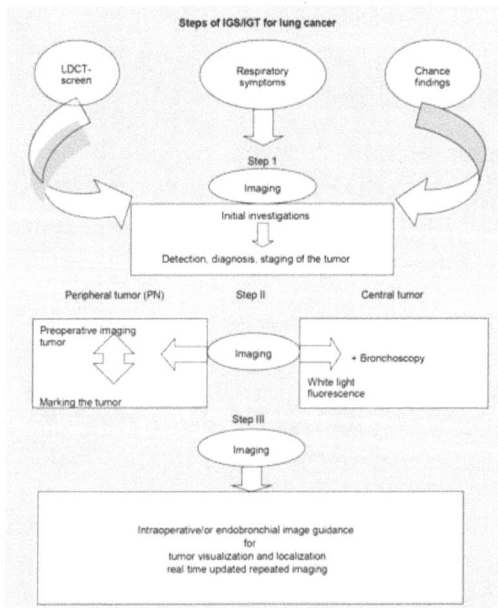

Fig. (2). Steps of image-guided surgery/image-guided therapy for lung cancer. IGS/IGT: Image-guided surgery/therapy; LDCT: Low dose computerized tomography. Taken from Moghissi K, Dixon K. Image guided surgery and therapy for lung cancer: a critical review.

Marking/Tagging of a PLC

Identification of small PLC (pulmonary nodule) at operation, within the vast parenchyma, can be extremely difficult - akin to seeking a needle in a haystack. Another issue in cancer surgery, especially that of lung cancer, is that healthy pulmonary parenchyma is a precious commodity. It is not reasonable to sacrifice a lobe of the lung for a small lesion merely because the true extent of cancer (with its precancerous zone) cannot be evaluated at operation. It follows that the aim should be to target cancer and to excise it totally, together with sufficient - but not excessive - healthy lung tissue.

In the absence of accurate methods to conventionally image pre-cancerous changes in the perimeter of the main tumour, a 50 mm visible or palpable clear margin is deemed sufficient.

Currently, there are a number of methods of marking a small lesion within the lung fields so that they can be easily identified at operation with the help of imaging methods. These markers are inserted in or around the lesion, prior to the surgical or endoscopic approach to the treatment of cancer. These markers may be grouped into:

1. Metallic coils and wires: These are usually placed pre-operatively under a CT scan shortly before the patient is anesthetized for surgery. They are then imaged fluoroscopically in the operating theatre (OT). Sometimes they can also be identified by palpation at thoracotomy [4 - 9].
2. X Ray-Contrast agents: Lipiodol or similar contrast agents are injected a couple of days pre-operatively under CT guidance into or around the lesion. These are then imaged fluoroscopically at operation [10, 11].
3. Dye material; Methylene Blue staining: This is injected in and around the lesion pre-operatively under CT guidance; the area may then be picked up at operation with the naked eye. A variant of this is Methylene Blue with antilogous blood. This gives extra precision at operation [12 - 14].
4. Isotope (TC - 99m) Scintigraphic method: This radioactive substance is injected pre-operatively under CT guidance; at operation, scintigraphy is carried out to navigate to the area of the lesion [15, 16].
5. Chemical Photosensitizing (PS) agents: The method is a fluorescence-guided (FG) identification of neoplastic lesions. In the first place, these photosensitizing chemicals are injected in the area of the lesion under CT guidance. At operation, the area is exposed to appropriate laser light to generate specific fluorescence, allowing navigation towards the tumour and its complete excision/treatment. Indocyanine green is one such chemical PS which is activated by a near infra-red- light laser. This is an accurate method of locating

the lesion as well as imaging pre-cancerous changes at its margin. At the present time, the method is under clinical translational study [17, 18].

6. Ultrasonography: This is entirely intra-operative. The ultrasound-guided intraoperative navigation does not require pre-operative marking. The ultrasound device is used at operation - either at thoracotomy or through VATS. Its success is, however, tied up with the specialist's interpretation, which, in ordinary circumstances, may be a cumbersome practice [19, 20].

It is important to note that none of the methods have been universally adopted to be ranked as 'standard'.

Marking/Tagging of a CLC

In CLCs, bronchoscopy is a fundamental requirement for diagnosis. Nevertheless, standard white-light bronchoscopy (WLB) may be unable to visualize and locate early neoplastic changes. Autofluorescence bronchoscopy (AFB), with its considerably higher sensitivity than WLB, may visualize precancerous lesions [21 - 23].

AFB is the only imaging method which can display an early CLC. It can localize the lesion for targeted biopsy and demonstrate the extent of the endobronchial disease for non-surgical interventional therapies such as PDT, cryotherapy and thermal lasers. Additionally, by registering and dynamic recording of the topography of the lesion, AFB can provide useful information for the conservation of the pulmonary parenchyma through economic lung resection or bronchoplastic operation such as sleeve resection of the right upper lobe.

In practice, pre-treatment images of AFB record the topography and extent of the lesion to be used for planning bronchoscopic treatment.

Step 3

This step is the final station of the IGS/IGT path, where a range of medical imaging technologies (MITs) are used to provide updated real-time information to navigate toward the lesion, allowing surgical excision or appropriate non-surgical treatment.

Intra-operative Image Guidance for PLC

A number of MITs may be used for this step, depending on the type of markers which have been used at step 2 above. Each centre uses a method according to the availability of imaging equipment and the experience of the operator - physician or surgeon. At the present time, the use of intra-operative radiology (Fluoroscopy and CT scan) is the most commonly used method, employed intra-operatively to image some of the markers which have been placed preoperatively [24, 25]. However, the method has a number of deficiencies. These include:

•Inability to image precancerous margins of the lesion.
•Problems with real-time imaging - unless fluoroscopy continues throughout the treatment procedure.
•Displacement of the markers, thus conveying misleading information.

The fluorescence-guided method is unique in imaging the totality of cancer with its precancerous components [26 - 29].

Image-Guided Therapy for CLC

An early CLC confined to the bronchial mucosa can be imaged by AFB, for localization and mapping, just before the start of therapeutic interventional bronchoscopy (TIB). However, AFB cannot be used to provide continuing real-time or frequently updated information. This is because intra treatment trauma will provide false-positive fluorescence images which defeat the objective of guided therapy. It is, though, possible to generate fluorescent images (FI) for the purpose, based on the use of a fluorescent chemical agent (FCA), which is activated by appropriate laser light. This is being tried for endobronchial lesions using PDT as the treatment method.

The use of an exogenous chromophore (FCA) and its appropriate light of a higher wavelength permits fluorescence emission, thus changing the paradigm and allowing better light penetration as well as the possibility of FI in the presence of hemoglobin. FCA can also be used as a photosensitizer (PS) for PDT.

The principle is to use a PS, which can be activated to fluoresce with a different wavelength to that which initiates photodynamic reaction (PDR), which is the basis of PDT.

Akopov and his colleagues [29] demonstrated the feasibility of guided endobronchial PDT. Their group has used a chlorine-based PS, which, when exposed to the light of 662 nm, achieves a photodynamic reaction - PDT. Alternatively, when the tumor containing PS is exposed to the light of 408 nm, the lesion generates fluorescence emission. Following pre-sensitization with the PS, they use two different lasers alternately; one laser emits light of 408 nm for tumor detection for FI, the other emits light of 662 nm for PDT.

We used an alternative method of fluorescence-guided bronchoscopic PDT [30].

In the first place, we carried out WLB and AFB to map out the extent of the tumor and precancerous lesions. Then at a separate session, after intravenous pre-sensitization with Photofrin" porfimer sodium" - we used a 630 nm laser light for endoscopic PDT, intermittently switching the wavelength to filtered 440 nm blue light for FI (Fig. **3**).

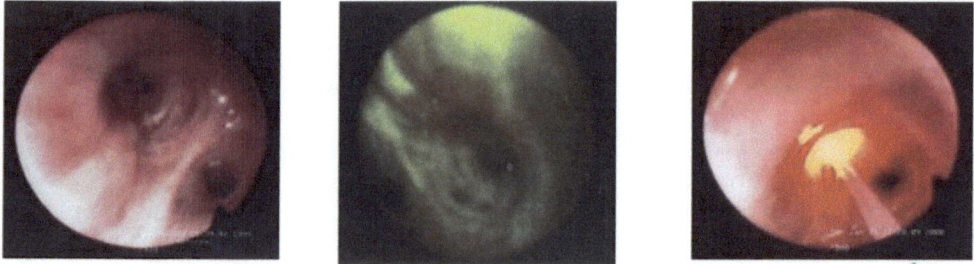

Fig. (3). Fluorescence Guided PDT for an Early Endobronchial Cancer. Left: WLB image. Middle: AFB image. Right. Cancer exposure to Laser light (L.F.= Laser fibre).

Perspective

IGS/IGT in lung cancer is in its infancy and there is plenty of scope for further development. Progress in MITs needs to address a number of challenges:

- Firstly, the invisible precancerous lesions at the margin of the visible tumour need to be identified and excised or be destroyed by a non-surgical method, in order to achieve treatment with curative intent.
- Secondly, the method of IGS/IGT should provide continuing updated dynamic live images throughout the operation, allowing the operator to navigate to the lesion for treatment.
- Thirdly IGS/IGT method should be operator friendly and not cumbersome in interfering with the smooth running of the OT and the operative procedure.

The use of FI in IGS is relatively recent and is still in its experimental and translational study stages [18, 31]. However, FI is by far the most intelligent of the imaging technologies and could, potentially, be the ideal method for IGS [18, 32].

Ultimately IGS/IGT can be best utilized within a Hybrid Operating Theatre (HOT) furnished with a range of imaging devices as well as surgical - or other treatment facilities.

CONCEPT OF HOT FOR IGS/IGT OF LUNG CANCER

A hybrid operating theatre (HOT) is a surgical operating room which is equipped with a variety of medical imaging devices in addition to surgical and anesthetic facilities allowing IGS/IGT.

HOTs, in thoracic and pulmonary oncology, should aim to facilitate: detection, localization and delineation of the extent of a CLC (endobronchial) and PLC (pulmonary nodules), especially at their pre- and early stages of development. It should accommodate equipment for biopsy procedures under CT and/or ultrasound imaging, as well as IGS within the standard, minimal access (VATS) and endoscopic procedures, such as PDT under image guidance.

In addition, HOTs should have the potential of incorporating research and deploying new technologies for targeted therapies within translational studies. A review of the literature concerned with minimal access/ minimal invasive therapies suggests that lung cancer surgery and/or interventional endoscopic therapy can best be carried out within HOTs. However, thoracic oncology in general and lung cancer surgery/therapy, in particular, can only be a stakeholder of HOTs in a hospital or institution. HOTs require to be multipurpose and multidisciplinary in structure and function [33, 34].

CONCLUSION

The main message of this chapter is that the evolutionary processes in cancer surgery of the lung, since its beginning in the first half of the 20th century, have been aiming to achieve an optimal resection.

In practice, this means excision of the totality of cancer (and its precancerous component) with a minimum of the health pulmonary parenchyma. For as long as the extent of cancer cannot be determined with certainty at operation and its perimeter determined with accuracy, the aim of an 'optimal resection' cannot be achieved.

The preoperative marking of the lesion in the lung, for identification at operation, is only a step towards surgical targeting. However, intra-operative real-time imaging - a dynamic process - is required to enable continuous imaging of the lesion, guiding the surgeon's navigation throughout the operative procedure. Radiological and most other methods of imaging, other than fluorescence imaging, cannot provide real-time images to assess cancer and precancerous lesions at the margin of the main neoplasm.

This chapter discusses image-guided surgery as it is practiced currently in some centres and also refers to the principle and possible ways of use of FI in lung cancer.

Fluorescence image-guided bronchoscopic photodynamic therapy (PDT), to treat some early endobronchial lesions, as it is practiced in one or two centres in the world, is explained.

CONSENT FOR PUBLICATION

Not applicable.

CONFLICT OF INTEREST

The author declares that there is no conflict of interest in this chapter.

ACKNOWLEDGEMENTS

Kate Dixon and Janet Melvin.

REFERENCES

[1]   Kato H, Nakamura H, Tsuboi M, *et al.* Treatment of peripheral early stage lung cancer. Ann Thorac Cardiovasc Surg 2004; 10(1): 1-3.
[PMID: 15008690]

[2]   Gajra A, Newman N, Gamble GP, *et al.* Impact of tumor size on survival in stage IA non-small cell lung cancer: a case for subdividing stage IA disease. Lung Cancer 2003; 42(1): 51-7.
[http://dx.doi.org/10.1016/S0169-5002(03)00285-X] [PMID: 14512187]

[3]   Vergnon JM, Huber RM, Moghissi K. Place of cryotherapy, brachytherapy and photodynamic therapy in therapeutic bronchoscopy of lung cancers. Eur Respir J 2006; 28(1): 200-18.
[http://dx.doi.org/10.1183/09031936.06.00014006] [PMID: 16816349]

[4]   Gossot D, Miaux Y, Guermazi A, Celerier M, Friga J. The hook-wire technique for localization of pulmonary nodules during thoracoscopic resection. Chest 1994; 105(5): 1467-9.
[http://dx.doi.org/10.1378/chest.105.5.1467] [PMID: 8181339]

[5]   Ciriaco P, Negri G, Puglisi A, *et al.* Video-assisted thoracoscopic surgery for pulmonary nodules: rationale for preoperative computed tomography-guided hookwire localization. Eur J Cardiothorac Surg 2004; 25(3): 429-33.
[http://dx.doi.org/10.1016/j.ejcts.2003.11.036] [PMID: 15019673]

[6]   Chen S, Zhou J, Zhang J, *et al.* Video-assisted thoracoscopic solitary pulmonary nodule resection after CT-guided hookwire localization: 43 cases report and literature review. Surg Endosc 2011; 25(6): 1723-9.
[http://dx.doi.org/10.1007/s00464-010-1502-3] [PMID: 21181200]

[7]   Li W, Wang Y, He X, *et al.* Combination of CT-guided hookwire localization and video-assisted thoracoscopic surgery for pulmonary nodular lesions: Analysis of 103 patients. Oncol Lett 2012; 4(4): 824-8.
[http://dx.doi.org/10.3892/ol.2012.800] [PMID: 23205107]

[8]   Torre M, Ferraroli GM, Vanzulli A, Fieschi S. A new safe and stable spiral wire needle for thoracoscopic resection of lung nodules. Chest 2004; 125(6): 2289-93.
[http://dx.doi.org/10.1378/chest.125.6.2289] [PMID: 15189953]

[9]   Hirschburger M, Sauer S, Schwandner T, *et al.* Extratumoral spiral fixed wire marking of small pulmonary nodules for thoracoscopic resection. Thorac Cardiovasc Surg 2008; 56(2): 106-9.
[http://dx.doi.org/10.1055/s-2007-989398] [PMID: 18278687]

[10]   Watanabe K, Nomori H, Ohtsuka T, *et al.* Usefulness and complications of computed tomography-guided lipiodol marking for fluoroscopy-assisted thoracoscopic resection of small pulmonary nodules: experience with 174 nodules. J Thorac Cardiovasc Surg 2006; 132(2): 320-4.
[http://dx.doi.org/10.1016/j.jtcvs.2006.04.012] [PMID: 16872957]

[11]   Kim YD, Jeong YJ, i H, *et al.* Localization of pulmonary nodules with lipiodol prior to thoracoscopic surgery. Acta Radiol 2011; 52(1): 64-9.
[http://dx.doi.org/10.1258/ar.2010.100307] [PMID: 21498328]

[12]   Lenglinger FX, Schwarz CD, Artmann W. Localization of pulmonary nodules before thoracoscopic surgery: value of percutaneous staining with methylene blue. AJR Am J Roentgenol 1994; 163(2): 297-300.
[http://dx.doi.org/10.2214/ajr.163.2.7518642] [PMID: 7518642]

[13]   Wang YZ, Boudreaux JP, Dowling A, Woltering EA. Percutaneous localisation of pulmonary nodules prior to video-assisted thoracoscopic surgery using methylene blue and TC-99. Eur J Cardiothorac Surg 2010; 37(1): 237-8.
[http://dx.doi.org/10.1016/j.ejcts.2009.07.022] [PMID: 19700335]

[14]   McConnell PI, Feola GP, Meyers RL. Methylene blue-stained autologous blood for needle localization and thoracoscopic resection of deep pulmonary nodules. J Pediatr Surg 2002; 37(12): 1729-31.
[http://dx.doi.org/10.1053/jpsu.2002.36707] [PMID: 12483642]

[15]   Galetta D, Bellomi M, Grana C, Spaggiari L. Radio-guided localization of small or ill-defined pulmonary lesions. Ann Thorac Surg 2015; 100(4): 1175-80.
[http://dx.doi.org/10.1016/j.athoracsur.2015.04.092] [PMID: 26209481]

[16]   Ambrogi MC, Melfi F, Zirafa C, *et al.* Radio-guided thoracoscopic surgery (RGTS) of small pulmonary nodules. Surg Endosc 2012; 26(4): 914-9.
[http://dx.doi.org/10.1007/s00464-011-1967-8] [PMID: 22011947]

[17]   Schaafsma BE, Mieog JS, Hutteman M, *et al.* The clinical use of indocyanine green as a near-infrared fluorescent contrast agent for image-guided oncologic surgery. J Surg Oncol 2011; 104(3): 323-32.
[http://dx.doi.org/10.1002/jso.21943] [PMID: 21495033]

[18]   Mondal SB, Gao S, Zhu N, *et al.* Real-time fluorescence image-guided oncologic surgery. Adv Cancer Res 2014; 124: 171-211.
[http://dx.doi.org/10.1016/B978-0-12-411638-2.00005-7] [PMID: 25287689]

[19]   Kondo R, Yoshida K, Hamanaka K, *et al.* Intraoperative ultrasonographic localization of pulmonary ground-glass opacities. J Thorac Cardiovasc Surg 2009; 138(4): 837-42.
[http://dx.doi.org/10.1016/j.jtcvs.2009.02.002] [PMID: 19660350]

[20]   Rocco G, Cicalese M, La Manna C, La Rocca A, Martucci N, Salvi R. Ultrasonographic identification of peripheral pulmonary nodules through uniportal video-assisted thoracic surgery. Ann Thorac Surg 2011; 92(3): 1099-101.
[http://dx.doi.org/10.1016/j.athoracsur.2011.03.030] [PMID: 21871306]

[21]   Zeng H, McWilliams A, Lam S. Optical spectroscopy and imaging for early lung cancer detection: a review. Photodiagn Photodyn Ther 2004; 1(2): 111-22.
[http://dx.doi.org/10.1016/S1572-1000(04)00042-0] [PMID: 25048182]

[22]   Stringer M, Moghissi K. Photodiagnosis and fluorescence imaging in clinical practice. Photodiagn Photodyn Ther 2004; 1(1): 9-12.
[http://dx.doi.org/10.1016/S1572-1000(04)00004-3] [PMID: 25048059]

[23]   Moghissi K, Dixon K, Stringer MR. Current indications and future perspective of fluorescence bronchoscopy: a review study. Photodiagn Photodyn Ther 2008; 5(4): 238-46.

[http://dx.doi.org/10.1016/j.pdpdt.2009.01.008] [PMID: 19356663]

[24]   Miyoshi T, Kondo K, Takizawa H, *et al.* Fluoroscopy-assisted thoracoscopic resection of pulmonary nodules after computed tomography--guided bronchoscopic metallic coil marking. J Thorac Cardiovasc Surg 2006; 131(3): 704-10.
[http://dx.doi.org/10.1016/j.jtcvs.2005.09.019] [PMID: 16515927]

[25]   Kawakita N, Takizawa H, Kondo K, Sakiyama S, Tangoku A. Indocyanine green fluorescence navigation thoracoscopic metastasectomy for pulmonary metastasis of hepatocellular carcinoma. Ann Thorac Cardiovasc Surg 2016; 22(6): 367-9.
[http://dx.doi.org/10.5761/atcs.cr.15-00367] [PMID: 27193496]

[26]   Ujiie H, Kato T, Hu HP, *et al.* A novel minimally invasive near-infrared thoracoscopic localization technique of small pulmonary nodules: A phase I feasibility trial. J Thorac Cardiovasc Surg 2017; 154(2): 702-11.
[http://dx.doi.org/10.1016/j.jtcvs.2017.03.140] [PMID: 28495056]

[27]   Okusanya OT, Madajewski B, Segal E, *et al.* Small portable interchangeable imager of fluorescence for fluorescence guided surgery and research. Technol Cancer Res Treat 2015; 14(2): 213-20.
[http://dx.doi.org/10.7785/tcrt.2012.500400] [PMID: 24354756]

[28]   Kunshan He , Yamin Mao , Jinzuo Ye , *et al.* A novel wireless wearable fluorescence image-guided surgery system. Conf Proc IEEE Eng Med Biol Soc 2016; 2016: 5208-11.
[PMID: 28269438]

[29]   Akopov AL, Rusanov AA, Papayan GV, *et al.* Endobronchial photodynamic therapy under fluorescence control: Photodynamic theranostics. Photodiagn Photodyn Ther 2017; 19: 73-7.
[http://dx.doi.org/10.1016/j.pdpdt.2017.05.001] [PMID: 28478107]

[30]   Moghissi K, Dixon K. Image-guided surgery and therapy for lung cancer: a critical review. Future Oncol 2017; 13(26): 2383-94.
[http://dx.doi.org/10.2217/fon-2017-0265] [PMID: 29129114]

[31]   Gioux S, Choi HS, Frangioni JV. Image-guided surgery using invisible near-infrared light: fundamentals of clinical translation. Mol Imaging 2010; 9(5): 237-55.
[http://dx.doi.org/10.2310/7290.2010.00034] [PMID: 20868625]

[32]   Keereweer S, Kerrebijn JD, van Driel PB, *et al.* Optical image-guided surgery--where do we stand? Mol Imaging Biol 2011; 13(2): 199-207.
[http://dx.doi.org/10.1007/s11307-010-0373-2] [PMID: 20617389]

[33]   Zhao ZR, Lau RW, Ng CS. Hybrid theatre and alternative localization techniques in conventional and single-port video-assisted thoracoscopic surgery. J Thorac Dis 2016; 8 (Suppl. 3): S319-27.
[PMID: 27014480]

[34]   Terra RM, Andrade JR, Mariani AW, *et al.* Applications for a hybrid operating room in thoracic surgery: from multidisciplinary procedures to --image-guided video-assisted thoracoscopic surgery. J Bras Pneumol 2016; 42(5): 387-90.
[http://dx.doi.org/10.1590/S1806-37562015000000177] [PMID: 27812640]

CHAPTER 16

Lung Cancer Centre Concept: A Vision for the Future

Jack Kastelik[1] and **Keyvan Moghissi**[2,*]

[1] *Castle Hill Hospital, & Hull Royal Infirmary, Hull, UK*

[2] *The Yorkshire Laser Centre, Goole, UK*

Abstract: In this chapter, we highlight the evolution of pathways for patients with suspected undiagnosed lung cancer from presentation to treatment in the 20th Century. We focus on the pathway which is currently in progress in the UK as well as some of the developed countries. We discuss the pros and cons of the system and we then propose a concept of a Lung Cancer Unit within Primary Care, City/Region and a Supra Regional Centre for lung cancer diagnosis and treatment.

Keywords: Concept of organisation of lung cancer pathway from presentation to treatment, Primary Care Unit Regional Centre and Supra Regional Centres for lung cancer as a vision for the future.

INTRODUCTION

The management of lung cancer sufferers has been an evolving process ever since the development of Surgery, Radiotherapy and Chemotherapy in the early part of the 20th century [1 - 3]. The almost explosive advances in molecular science and medicine in the second half of the century opened the door to new discoveries and the understanding of lung cancer genesis. In the UK, during the early years of the National Health Service (NHS) during the 1950s, patients with suspected lung cancer were referred by their General Practitioner (GP) to a General/Respiratory Physician of the City Hospital and sometimes directly to the Regional Thoracic Surgery Unit for investigations leading to diagnosis and treatment; at the time, this was predominantly surgery. Investigations consisted of Chest Radiography, often added to by tomography and bronchoscopy and biopsy sampling. All patients with histology confirmed or radiologically suspected lung cancer, who were fit for thoracotomy, were offered surgery. At this time, up to one-third of all

* **Corresponding author Keyvan Moghissi:** The Yorkshire Laser Centre, Goole, UK; Tel: 01724 290456; E-mail: kmoghissi@yorkshirelasercentre.org

Keyvan Moghissi, Jack Kastelik, Philip Barber & Peyman Sardari Nia (Eds.)

thoracotomies were exploratory, with no cancer being excised [4]. They were classified as 'inoperable'. Operability in the 1950s and the 1960s meant surgical resectability. The idea of oncological inoperability was yet to be conceived.

During this period, the pathway for patients with suspected lung cancer was a simple 3 step process (Fig. **1**):

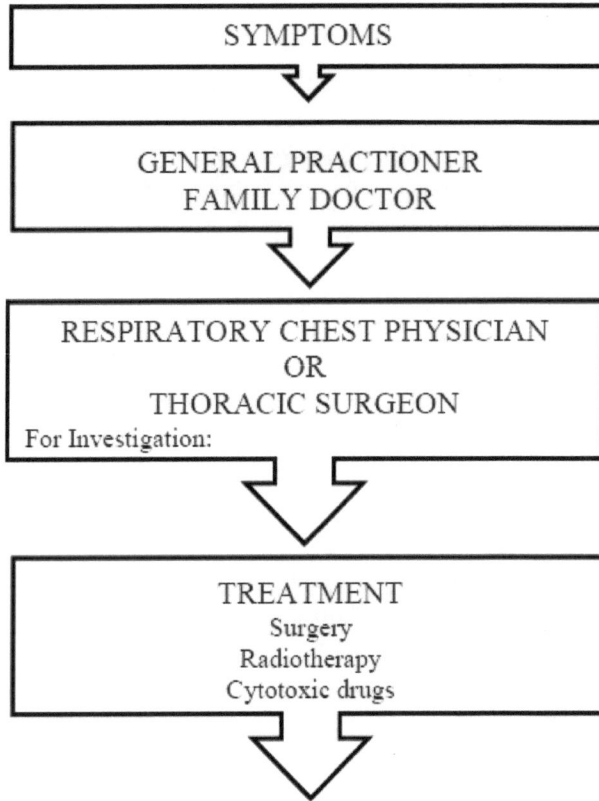

```
┌─────────────────────────────────────────┐
│              SYMPTOMS                     │
└─────────────────────────────────────────┘
                    ↓
┌─────────────────────────────────────────┐
│          GENERAL PRACTIONER              │
│           FAMILY DOCTOR                   │
└─────────────────────────────────────────┘
                    ↓
┌─────────────────────────────────────────┐
│    RESPIRATORY CHEST PHYSICIAN           │
│                OR                         │
│         THORACIC SURGEON                  │
│  For Investigation:                       │
└─────────────────────────────────────────┘
                    ↓
┌─────────────────────────────────────────┐
│              TREATMENT                    │
│               Surgery                     │
│             Radiotherapy                  │
│            Cytotoxic drugs                │
└─────────────────────────────────────────┘
                    ↓
```

Fig. (1). The pathway from Symptoms to treatment for lung cancer patients. Circa 1950s–1960s.

1. Visit to family General Practitioner

2. GP referral to specialist Physician or Thoracic Surgeon for investigations.

3. Treatment, which was essentially surgery; unresectable cases (inoperable patients) were referred to what was known as Deep X-ray Therapy (DXT-Radiotherapy).

In most countries, the pathway for lung cancer patients from investigation to treatment, with some variation, was similar to that of the UK. However, in the UK because of the NHS, there was a more uniform and standardised arrangement. In essence, the initial pattern of referral to the specialist depended on the GP's choice and preference. At this time, Surgeons, together with Respiratory Physicians, carried out the investigation and decided on surgical treatment. Radiotherapy had a subsidiary role and Chemotherapy was in its infancy, to be considered in some inoperable cases. Chemotherapy arose from the deadly experiences of mustard gas in the First World War. However, up until the 1950s, there were few cytotoxic drugs available and the role of Chemotherapy was established towards the end of the 20th Century with the availability of a number of agents; with it arose a new medical specialty - Oncology.

By the beginning of the 21st Century, there had been an eruption of new technologies with further developments and evolution in a number of domains such as genetics and immunology, which resulted in better understanding and management of lung cancer. The concept of screening, the progress in imaging, the advent of minimal access surgery and expansion of chemo- radiation, as well as alternative methods of treatment either general or local, such as Photodynamic therapy (PDT), inevitably brought a diverse referral pattern. In developed countries, there remained a basic pathway for suspected lung cancer cases to follow from presentation through investigation and treatment, though this pathway was longer, with more steps for investigation and diagnosis. There were, nevertheless, more precise and targeted therapies which, additionally, needed to take account of health economics, evidence-based treatment and the patient's rights, whilst efforts were made to incorporate the translatable products of the various developments in early diagnosis, rapid referral and multidisciplinary expertise.

These comprised of:

• The TNM stage classification and stage-related outcome [5].

• Inclusion of sophisticated imaging equipment in diagnosis.

• The attempt at introducing screening programmes for the population at risk of lung cancer development.

• Introduction of a Multi-Disciplinary Team (MDT) approach to the planning of treatment, once preliminary investigations were completed.

• Taking account of health economics and, in some cases 'health rationing'.

• Applying evidence-based principles before selecting a treatment option.

• Introduction of Regulatory Science in medicine.

• Application of day or short-stay surgery and minimal access operations.

• Respecting the right of patients to accept, reject or choose a treatment option.

At the beginning of the 21C, the pathway of referral management in the UK, with some local variations, is shown in Fig. (**2**).

The major benefit of the system, which is currently in progress, is the team approach to diagnosis and management of lung cancer and the patient's right to participation in decision making.

In this scheme, the pathway (Fig. **2**) consists of:

1. Referral to a Physician in a respiratory unit.

2. Diagnostic investigation including imaging and bronchoscopy by or through the Respiratory Physician (RP).

Some of the increasingly sophisticated investigations need to be undertaken in separate institutions, in diverse locations which can be far from the residence of the patient, in a different region.

3. Referral to MDT for discussion and to decide on treatment.

4. Referral for treatment to an appropriate department.

Such a department may be in the same locality or at a distance.

5. Patient participation in decision making and informed consent to the suggested treatment.

Neither the aims and objective of this book nor the space in this chapter allow expansion of discussion on historical background or efforts which have been put in to solve the issues of lack of progress in improving lung cancer survival despite the progress in diagnostic imaging and attempts at screening the population at risk.

1. **PRESENTATION**

   - SCREENING
   - SELF-REFERRAL
   - GP (FAMILY PRACTITIONER) FINDING
   - INCIDENTAL DISCOVERY

2: **REFERRAL TO RESPIRATORY MEDICINE DEPARTMENT OF GENERAL/CITY HOSPITAL FOR:**

   - COMPLETE WORK UP
   - DIAGNOSIS
   - STAGING
   - DECISION MAKING (THROUGH MDT) FOR TREATMENT

3: **STANDARD TREATMENT: AT CITY HOSPITAL OR THE REGIONAL CENTRE:**

   - SURGERY (INCLUDING VATS)
   - RADIOTHERAPY
   - CHEMOTHERAPY

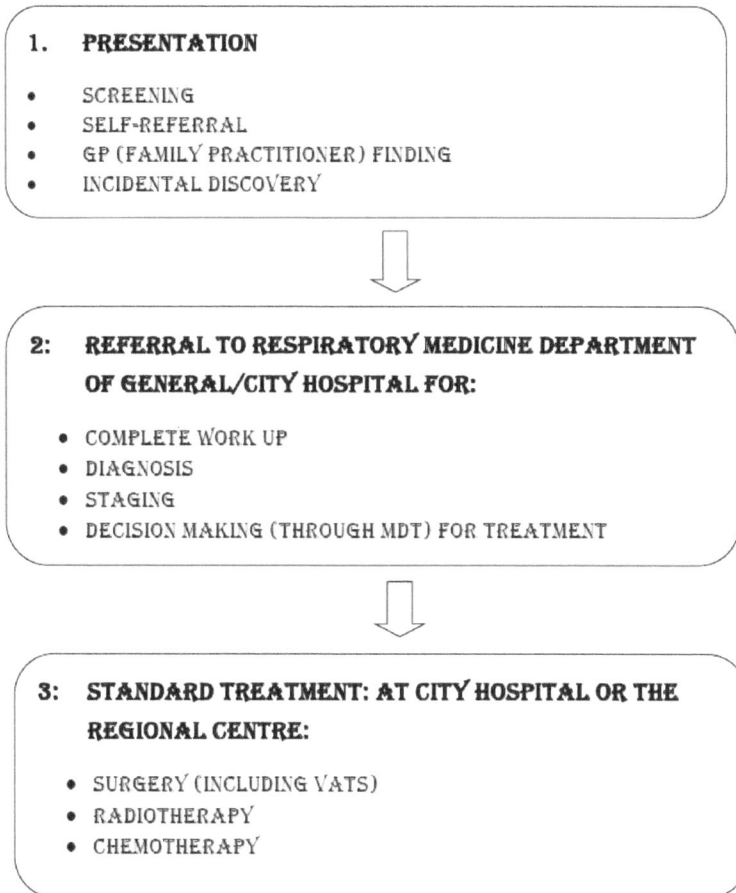

Fig. (2). Current pathway for patients with suspected lung cancer from presentation to diagnosis and treatment.

Nevertheless, this seemingly rational scheme has practical advantages over the previous pathway in a number of ways, but its practical application presents with deficiencies that have become apparent in the past few years.

Some advantages are:

• The patient is investigated fully

• The case is exposed to the comprehensive and diverse opinions of MDT.

• The lung cancer subject is likely to receive appropriate treatment

• Patient's participation and informed consent to therapy.

Disadvantages of the system are that:

• In practice, patients have little choice other than the pathway offered by the general practitioner

• The GP cannot select the respiratory physician/unit they feel to be most suitable for their patient.

• Investigations may involve travel for the patient, to a number of venues; this takes time, expense and personal effort – with additional stress – as well as delay in commencement of treatment

• A patient may not be offered treatment options other than the so-called, 'standard' treatment. In the UK, the NHS provides only treatment – and funding for – 'recommended' treatments; in some other countries, this is also the case when insurances limit payment, based on what they accept as 'standard'.

• Expensive treatment can be bought by more affluent patients but not by the less well off who may benefit equally from them.

• More importantly, 'Research and Development' and 'Clinical Trials' are either divorced from a centre of activity or are not included at all.

Disappointingly, despite all efforts and notwithstanding the inclusion of costly technical equipment and devices in healthcare, the overall outcome of lung cancer patients in terms of cancer-free survival has not changed significantly over the past 10-20 years.

Surgical treatment of lung cancer remains the first-line treatment and the therapy which provides the best chance of long cancer-free survival. In early - stage 1 - cancer. It is the general agreement, backed by experience and statistics, that early diagnosis and submission to treatment should be the goal. There is universal agreement, with ample evidence, to show that treatment of early-stage lung cancer is a recipe for long cancer-free survival amounting to the cure of the disease. Therefore, the above Fig. (**2**) scheme, with the involvement of too many tiers with the time between every step, is giving time during which, cancer continues to grow and spread. Various plans are mooted to accelerate the pathway of patients from the initial referral to diagnosis and treatment.

One option under consideration is to establish an optimal lung cancer pathway, allowing for comprehensive and timely investigations and delivery of treatment for patients. To that end, a number of models are being tried around the world.

In the USA, there is a National Cancer Institute Cancer Centre Programme, with around 70 designated blocks in 36 states; this is an important base, not only for national cancer research but also allows for improved cancer investigations and treatments [6]. Overall, this seems to lead to better cancer survival rates. Similar programmes are under investigation in other countries. These models are all looking at centralisation of manpower and devices or equipment to offer lung cancer patients a truly Mega Establishment.

However, in the real world, one has to reconcile with the fact that the lung cancer population is scattered over villages and towns, many are amongst financially disadvantaged people and the infirm, who will not have the possibility of benefitting from a few super-regional centres.

Any mega-establishment which basically uses finances from the population at large must aim to benefit that population and not a selected cohort that happens to be able to access that establishment.

The available publications seem to indicate - as expected - that the outcome in terms of survival of suspected and diagnosed lung cancer patients are statistically better in lager academic centres compared with those treated in a smaller centre. This is supported by publication from the National Comprehensive Care Network, that patients treated in designated centres have better outcomes and survival [7]. A review of the National Cancer database of 193,279 patients with stage IV lung cancer found that those treated in designated Academic Centres had an improved 2-year survival of 17.4% compared to that of 13.1% for those undergoing treatment in community-based centres [8]. In addition, between 1998 and 2010, the improvement in the 2-year survival was higher in academic centres compared to those that were community-based. The survival improvement was particularly noted in patients with stage IV adenocarcinoma due to better advances in treatment in those patients compared to squamous cell cancer during that period. These findings, therefore, raise a question of potential disparity in outcomes between academic and community-based centres. Similarly, a recent report from the UK using the National Lung Cancer Audit showed that units with high organisational scores had better patient outcomes, including higher 1-year survival, probably related to the fact that in these units the patients had a higher likelihood of receiving the treatment within 62 days and higher curative-intent treatment rate [9].

Alternatively, a better outcome results in large academic centres which could simply be due to the fact that such large centres are better equipped and have more availability of diverse non-surgical methods of therapy than the smaller units.

The issue is not about the creation of a multitude of centres of excellence, even if health care had unlimited funds, to afford such developments. The argument should be based on whether such centres are going to serve a "few instead of the many and/or all". In short, how such a centre can be of benefit across the population spectrum, particularly those in lower-income groups, handicapped and disabled living in remote areas and at a distance from a centre.

The idea that one would bring a patient for a day or a few days attendance at a centre and then discharge them to the isolation of an urban area is unworkable.

There are some observational studies to suggest that the creation of comprehensive regional centres might be the answer to solving the long-standing poor outcome of lung cancer patients - which has hardly changed for the past several decades. However, there are a number of issues that need to be addressed before diverting manpower and financial resources to a few centres of excellence for a few, at the expense of alternative schemes of less grandiose units for the majority.

The questions are:

• How to deliver the best lung cancer care that is not affected by the patients' geographical or socio-economic factors

• How to incorporate evolving and rapidly changing new technologies and therapies at the point of delivery to patients

• How to carry out translational clinical studies within a

Wide lung cancer population.

One track may be:

1) Family practitioners' units: these units would be visited by a 'Family Practice Lung Cancer Specialist' (Oncologist/Respiratory Physician), who is attached to a unit.

2) Local / City/ Regional Lung Cancer Centres. These centres would accommodate dedicated lung cancer expertise and devices for rapid investigation and diagnostic, as well as provision of standard treatment

3) Comprehensive Supra Regional Lung Cancer Centre. These centres would possess a comprehensive range of imaging and investigational tools and expertise, as well as surgical and other therapeutic facilities, staffed by dedicated specialists. Relevant science laboratories and technology and a 'hybrid' operating theatre should be within the provision of such a Regional Comprehensive Lung Cancer

Centre (Fig. **3**).

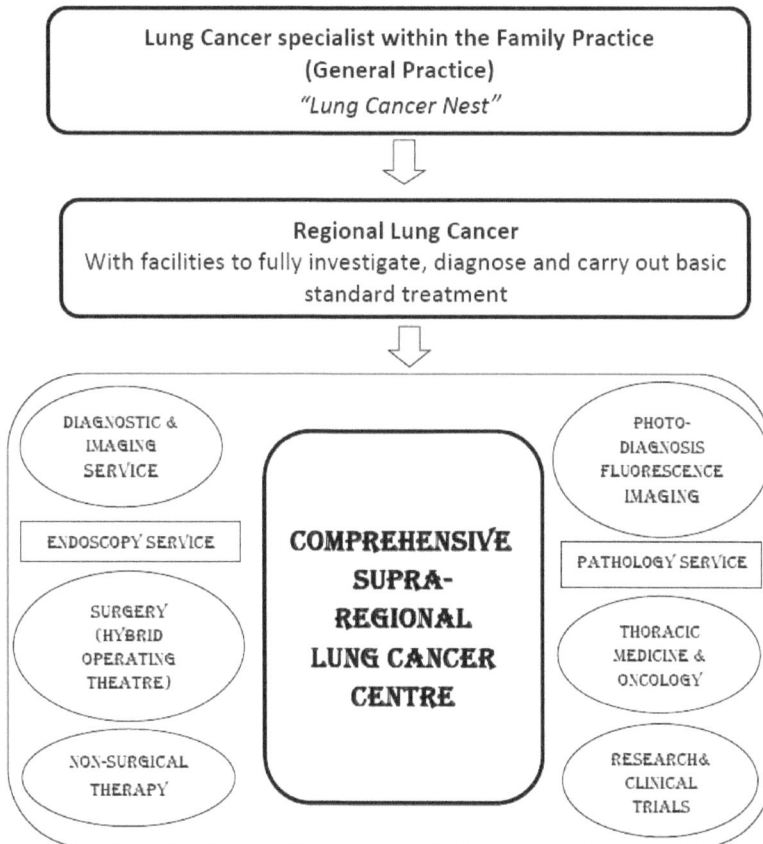

Fig. (3). Comprehensive supra-regional centre & pathway for lung cancer.

Building this kind of model for lung cancer takes time, effort and a considerable infrastructure. Therefore, there remain questions whether they would be justifiable, affordable and achievable in our ever perturbed, and repeated "current financial climate".

CONCLUSION

Based on joint experience of over 80 years on lung cancer the authors of this chapter propose a futuristic scheme of lung cancer organisation. Basically there propose a system in which there should be a dedicated team for Lung Cancer. Patients will be seen by a visiting specialist, chest physician at family practitioners or group practice. From that initial entry to the system, the patient continues not as a referred subject to a Multidisciplinary Dedicated Team, but follows the path specific for suspected or diagnosed lung Cancer Patients, through; District, Regional and Supra Regional Lung Cancer Centres. Easy access to Specialist Lung Cancer Group, Centres and Multidisciplinary Team for Diagnosis and Treatment are the key elements in such a scheme.

CONSENT FOR PUBLICATION

Not applicable.

CONFLICT OF INTEREST

The author declares that there is no conflict of interest in this chapter.

ACKNOWLEDGEMENTS

Declared none.

REFERENCES

[1]   Graham EA, Singer TJ. Successful removal of the entire lung for carcinoma of the bronchus. JAMA J Am Med Assoc 1993; 101: 13-7.

[2]   History of Radiation Therapy. http://wikipedia.org/wiki/history/history

[3]   Baguley BC. A brief history of cancer chemotherapy.Anticancer Drug Development. Academic Press 2002; pp. 1-11.
[http://dx.doi.org/10.1016/B978-012072651-6/50002-4]

[4]   K Moghissi personal observation and presentation on lung cancer. Abstract PDT @ RSM November 2018.

[5]   American Joint Committee for Cancer (AJCC), Staging and End Results Reporting 1stedn. 1977.http://cancerstaging.org

[6]   Balata H, Fong KM, Hendriks LE, *et al.* Prevention and early detection for non-small cell lung cancer: Advances in thoracic oncology 2018. J Thorac Oncol 2019 Jun 19. pii: S1556-0864(19)30476-9.

[7]   National Cancer Institute. Comprehensive Cancer Information https://www.cancer.gov

[8]   Ramalingam S, Dinan MA, Crawford J. Survival comparison in patients with stage iv lung cancer in academic versus community centers in the united states. J Thorac Oncol 2018; 13(12): 1842-50.
[http://dx.doi.org/10.1016/j.jtho.2018.09.007] [PMID: 30312680]

[9]   Adizie JB, Khakwani A, Beckett P, *et al.* Impact of organisation and specialist service delivery on lung cancer outcomes. Thorax 2019; 74(6): 546-50.
[http://dx.doi.org/10.1136/thoraxjnl-2018-212588] [PMID: 30661021]

SUBJECT INDEX

A

Activity 23, 24, 32, 70, 71, 72, 73, 99, 104, 254, 267, 317
  abnormal 70
  constitutive 24
  cytokines 99
  demonstrated 254
  innate metabolic 70
  intense metabolic 71
  mediastinal blood pool 70
  physical 267
  reduced 72
  thymidine kinase 73
Acute myeloid leukaemia 24
Additional tips on pulmonary resection 175
Adenocarcinomas 24, 27, 28, 33, 46, 71, 99, 243, 244, 250, 253, 255
  lower grade 71
Adjuvant 98, 228, 246, 247, 248, 249
  chemotherapy 98, 228, 242, 246, 247, 248, 249
  systemic anti-cancer therapy 242
Agents 29, 73, 80, 103, 245, 251, 253, 304, 306, 314
  chemotherapeutic 29
  cytotoxic 283
  fluorescent chemical 80, 306
  frequent imaging 73
  platinum 251
  sclerosing 103
ALK mutant 242, 244, 254, 255
  adenocarcinoma 242
  cancers 255
  disease 254
  lung cancers 242, 244
Alveolar 191, 121
  capillary transfer 91
  proteinosis 121
American college of chest physicians (ACCP) 93, 119
American thoracic society (ATS) 88, 118
Amino 73, 291

acid transport 73
  levulinic acid 291
Amplicon 24
Anaesthesia 180, 182, 185
Anaplastic lymphoma kinase (ALK) 25, 119, 243, 254, 255
Anastomosis 176, 177, 178, 180, 181, 182, 183, 186, 188
Anterior wall anastomosis 182
Anticipatory medicines 271
Antifibrinolytic agents 269
Antigen-presenting cells (APCs) 31, 32, 123, 245
Anti-tumour immunity 32
Anxiolytic medication 269
Apoptosis 32, 33, 127
  accelerated 127
  increased 32
Atelectasis 69, 93, 121, 285
Atypical adenomatous hyperplasia (AAH) 27
Auto fluorescence bronchoscopy (AFB) 78, 79, 114, 116, 129, 130, 176, 180, 305, 306, 307
Auto fluorescence endoscopy 184

B

Beam's eye view (BEV) 222
Benzodiazepines 267
Bevacizumab carboplatin, paclitaxel (BCP) 251
Body mass index (BMI) 53, 91
Bone marrow 37, 244
  aspirates 37
  suppression 244
Brachytherapy and photodynamic therapy 126
Brain magnetic resonance imaging 230
Brain metastases 72, 88, 230, 231, 254
Breathing cycles 219
  respiratory 219
British thoracic society (BTS) 68, 93, 98, 132, 266, 298
Bronchial carcinoma 291

F

Fibrosarcoma cell line 36
Fibrosis 73, 76, 103, 122, 233
  cystic 122
  induced pulmonary 233
  pleural 103
  post radiation 73
Fine needle aspiration (FNA) 72, 74, 116
Flexible fibreoptic bronchoscope (FFB) 11,
     115, 116, 118, 119, 120, 121, 123, 125,
     130, 131, 180, 286
Fluorescence 36, 45, 47, 48, 63, 77, 78, 80,
     116, 117, 120, 132, 301, 304, 308, 309
  abnormal 117
  acquired 36
  bronchoscopy 45, 47, 48, 57, 116, 120, 132
  emission, molecular system 77
  guided surgery (FGS) 80
  imaging 77, 80, 116, 132, 308
Fluorescent chemical agent (FCA) 80, 306
Forced vital capacity (FVC) 91
Function-based methods 23

G

Generation ALK inhibitor 255
Genes 23, 24, 25, 26, 28, 31, 34, 46, 47
  cancer-causing 26
  candidate 47
  driver 24
  epidermal growth factor receptor 24
  growth-promoting 23
  plausible 25
  -probe assays 47
   suppressor 46
  tissue-restricted 31
Genetic 23, 32, 46
  abnormalities 46
  cascade 46
  deletion 32

  instability 23
Genomic 24, 29, 33
  amplification events 24
  event 29
  instability 33
Glomeruloid microvascular proliferations
     (GMPs) 34
Graft 174, 178, 186
  pedicle intercostal 174, 178
  pedicle omental 174
Granulomatous 56
Gross tumour volume (GTV) 219, 220, 221
Growth 47, 68, 75, 244, 245
  asymmetrical 68
  disrupt cell 244
  invasive cell 47
Guided 89, 90, 96, 100, 105, 106
  biopsy 89, 90, 96, 100, 105, 106
  drainage regimens 105

H

Haematological 76, 86
  abnormalities 86
  malignancies 76
Haematopoietic stem cells (HSCs) 37
Haematoporphyrin derivatives 291
Haemodynamic instability 268
Haemoglobin 78, 80, 99
Haemoptysis 86, 114, 122, 123, 127, 231, 262,
     264, 268, 269, 286
  fatal 268
  life-threatening 268
Haemorrhage 90, 101, 123, 126, 130, 163,
     283, 297
  major vascular accidental 163
  pulmonary 90
Haemostasis 155, 283, 290
HIF alpha subunit 34
Histoplasmosis 71
Horner's syndrome 86, 188
Hypermethylation 46, 47

www.ingramcontent.com/pod-product-compliance
Lightning Source LLC
Chambersburg PA
CBHW050806220326
41598CB00006B/129